Handbook of Cancer Bioinformatics

Handbook of Cancer Bioinformatics

Editor: Page Pollard

AMERICAN
MEDICAL PUBLISHERS
www.americanmedicalpublishers.com

AMERICAN
MEDICAL PUBLISHERS
www.americanmedicalpublishers.com

Cataloging-in-Publication Data

Handbook of cancer bioinformatics / edited by Page Pollard.
p. cm.
Includes bibliographical references and index.
ISBN 978-1-63927-613-4
1. Cancer--Treatment--Data processing. 2. Bioinformatics. 3. Computational biology. I. Pollard, Page.
RC270.8 .H36 2023
616.994 06--dc23

American Medical Publishers,
41 Flatbush Avenue,
1st Floor, New York,
NY 11217, USA

ISBN 978-1-63927-613-4 (Hardback)

Contents

Preface

Cancer is a broad term for a variety of diseases characterized by the formation of aberrant cells that divide uncontrollably. It has the capacity for infiltrating and destroying normal body tissues. Cancer bioinformatics is an evolving field which amalgamates omics science, clinical informatics, mathematics, bioinformatics, information technology and medical informatics for addressing challenges in diagnosis, therapies and prognosis in cancer patients. It is also a primary instrument and method for conducting cancer research in systems medicine. Cancer bioinformatics is one of the strategies to focus on bioinformatics methods in cancer based on the specificity of communication, metabolisms, proliferations and signaling of disease. It plays a larger role in the identification and validation of biomarkers specific to clinical phenotypes associated with early diagnoses. Furthermore, cancer bioinformatics is also expected to measure disease progression and therapy response, as well as indicators for improving patients' quality of life. This book covers in detail some innovative concepts revolving around cancer bioinformatics. The readers would gain knowledge that would broaden their perspective in this area of study.

All of the data presented henceforth, was collaborated in the wake of recent advancements in the field. The aim of this book is to present the diversified developments from across the globe in a comprehensible manner. The opinions expressed in each chapter belong solely to the contributing authors. Their interpretations of the topics are the integral part of this book, which I have carefully compiled for a better understanding of the readers.

At the end, I would like to thank all those who dedicated their time and efforts for the successful completion of this book. I also wish to convey my gratitude towards my friends and family who supported me at every step.

Editor

1

Application of Artificial Intelligence Technology in Oncology: Towards the Establishment of Precision Medicine

Ryuji Hamamoto [1,2,3,*], Kruthi Suvarna [4], Masayoshi Yamada [1,5], Kazuma Kobayashi [1,2,3], Norio Shinkai [1,2,3], Mototaka Miyake [6], Masamichi Takahashi [1,7], Shunichi Jinnai [8], Ryo Shimoyama [1], Akira Sakai [1,3], Ken Takasawa [1,2], Amina Bolatkan [1,2], Kanto Shozu [1], Ai Dozen [1], Hidenori Machino [1,2], Satoshi Takahashi [1,2], Ken Asada [1,2], Masaaki Komatsu [1,2], Jun Sese [1,9] and Syuzo Kaneko [1,2]

1 Division of Molecular Modification and Cancer Biology, National Cancer Center Research Institute, 5-1-1 Tsukiji, Chuo-ku, Tokyo 104-0045, Japan; masyamad@ncc.go.jp (M.Y.); kazumkob@ncc.go.jp (K.K.); norio.shinkai@riken.jp (N.S.); masataka@ncc.go.jp (M.T.); rshimoya@ncc.go.jp (R.S.); dr200004@tmd.ac.jp (A.S.); ktakazaw@ncc.go.jp (K.T.); abolatka@ncc.go.jp (A.B.); kshozu@ncc.go.jp (K.S.); ai.okky61@gmail.com (A.D.); hmachino@ncc.go.jp (H.M.); sing.monotonyflower@gmail.com (S.T.); ken.asada@riken.jp (K.A.); maskomat@ncc.go.jp (M.K.); sesejun@humanome.jp (J.S.); sykaneko@ncc.go.jp (S.K.)

2 Cancer Translational Research Team, RIKEN Center for Advanced Intelligence Project, 1-4-1 Nihonbashi, Chuo-ku, Tokyo 103-0027, Japan

3 Department of NCC Cancer Science, Graduate School of Medical and Dental Sciences, Tokyo Medical and Dental University, 1-5-45 Yushima, Bunkyo-ku, Tokyo 113-8510, Japan

4 Indian Institute of Technology Bombay, Powai, Mumbai 400 076, India; kruthisuvarna5@gmail.com

5 Department of Endoscopy, National Cancer Center Hospital, 5-1-1 Tsukiji, Chuo-ku Tokyo 104-0045, Japan

6 Department of Diagnostic Radiology, National Cancer Center Hospital, 5-1-1 Tsukiji, Chuo-ku, Tokyo 104-0045, Japan; mmiyake@ncc.go.jp

7 Department of Neurosurgery and Neuro-Oncology, National Cancer Center Hospital, 5-1-1 Tsukiji, Chuo-ku, Tokyo 104-0045, Japan

8 Department of Dermatologic Oncology, National Cancer Center Hospital, 5-1-1 Tsukiji, Chuo-ku, Tokyo 104-0045, Japan; sjinnai@ncc.go.jp

9 Humanome Lab, 2-4-10 Tsukiji, Chuo-ku, Tokyo 104-0045, Japan

* Correspondence: rhamamot@ncc.go.jp;

Simple Summary: Artificial intelligence (AI) technology has been advancing rapidly in recent years and is being implemented in society. The medical field is no exception, and the clinical implementation of AI-equipped medical devices is steadily progressing. In particular, AI is expected to play an important role in realizing the current global trend of precision medicine. In this review, we introduce the history of AI as well as the state of the art of medical AI, focusing on the field of oncology. We also describe the current status of the use of AI for drug discovery in the oncology field. Furthermore, while AI has great potential, there are still many issues that need to be resolved; therefore, we would provide details on current medical AI problems and potential solutions.

Abstract: In recent years, advances in artificial intelligence (AI) technology have led to the rapid clinical implementation of devices with AI technology in the medical field. More than 60 AI-equipped medical devices have already been approved by the Food and Drug Administration (FDA) in the United States, and the active introduction of AI technology is considered to be an inevitable trend in the future of medicine. In the field of oncology, clinical applications of medical devices using AI technology are already underway, mainly in radiology, and AI technology is expected to be positioned as an important core technology. In particular, "precision medicine," a medical treatment that selects the most appropriate treatment for each patient based on a vast amount of medical data such as genome information, has become a worldwide trend; AI technology is expected to be utilized in the process of extracting truly useful information from a large amount of medical data and applying it to diagnosis and treatment. In this review, we would like to introduce the history of AI technology and the current state of medical AI, especially in the oncology field, as well as discuss the possibilities and challenges of AI technology in the medical field.

Keywords: machine learning; deep learning; artificial intelligence; precision medicine; radiology; pathology; omics

---

1. Introduction

The rapid progress in machine learning technologies, especially deep learning, along with the development of information infrastructure technologies such as the graphics processing unit (GPU), and the development of public databases, have made it possible to make use of large scale data called big data and have aroused a great deal of interest in artificial intelligence (AI) technology worldwide [1]. Historically, AI research has been conducted for a relatively long time, and the term "artificial intelligence" was already being used as an academic term by the 1950s [2]. However, AI research has not been a smooth road, and it has gone through a difficult period known as the AI winter period. The current boom is being dubbed the third AI boom [3], but this one differs from the previous booms in which many AI technologies in that it is being implemented in society. Face recognition technology based on AI technology is actively being used in airports and other areas, and AI is currently being used in various fields of society, including voice recognition, automatic translation, and automated driving. In fact, more than 60 medical devices with AI have been approved by the FDA in the United States, and the aggressive introduction of AI technology into the medical field in the future is inevitable. The field of oncology is no exception to this trend, and several AI-equipped medical devices are already being used for clinical applications, especially in radiology.

Current AI uses machine learning technology as the core technology [1]. Machine learning techniques are methods that learn from sample data, find patterns in these, and apply them to new data for analysis and prediction [4]. Whereas traditional statistics is often used primarily for explanatory purposes, machine learning uses it primarily for predictive purposes. There is a variety of machine learning techniques, which can be divided into two main types: supervised and unsupervised learning [5]. Supervised learning is a method of extracting features from given information to make predictions, which can be divided into classification and regression problems. The classification problem is used to predict discrete data, for example, distinguishing between benign and malignant tumors [4]. The regression problem is used to predict continuous data, for example, contrast effects. Unsupervised learning is a method of summarizing similarities for a given set of data on a problem for which no answer has been given. Because the classification problem of supervised learning is close to diagnosis, it is also considered to be the most familiar problem for clinicians, such as radiologists [4]. Deep learning technology is a part of machine learning technology; it currently holds great promise in the medical field. Deep learning techniques are used for medical image classification, image quality improvement, and segmentation because they are particularly good for image analysis. There are various types of deep learning techniques, and depending on the type of data to be handled, it is necessary to select the structure of the neural network that best suits the data [4]. Typical deep learning techniques used in medical imaging include convolutional neural networks for image classification [6], recurrent neural networks for reporting tasks [7], and a U-net for image segmentation [8].

In the field of oncology, the promotion of "precision medicine," which refers to the medical care optimized for each patient by extracting important information from medical big data, especially genomic information, has become a global trend. "Precision oncology" and "precision cancer medicine" are also increasingly being used as academic terms [9–13]. However, the selection of treatment options based on a targeted-gene panel (TGP) coupled with next-generation sequencing, which is the core method of precision medicine, has become a major issue in promoting precision medicine because there is only a limited number of patients for whom the most appropriate treatment is suggested [14–16]. In order to increase the number of patients who may benefit from precision medicine, it is considered essential to extract pertinent information from additional medical data, including whole genome and epigenome information, in addition to limited genetic mutation information. However, the amount of information that needs processing has increased significantly; for example, whole genome analysis can yield up to 3 billion base pairs of information. To analyze these very large data efficiently and accurately, the use of cutting-edge AI and information and communications technology (ICT) technologies is required.

In this review, we introduced the history of AI technology and discussed how AI technology is currently being applied in the medical field and implemented in society, with a focus on the field of oncology. In addition, while AI technology has great potential, it is still associated with many issues that need to be resolved. We discussed the current issues in the field of medical AI and what kind of efforts are needed to continue to resolve these issues.

2. History of Artificial Intelligence and Its Application in Medicine

2.1. From the 18th Century to the 19th Century: Bayes' Theorem and Pierre-Simon Laplace

In 1763, "An Essay towards solving a Problem in the Doctrine of Chances," including theorems of conditional probability which form the basis of Bayes' Theorem, was published [17]. This work is based on the mathematical theory of probability by the Reverend Thomas Bayes, with multiple revisions and additions by his friend Richard Price, and was not published until 2 years after Thomas Bayes' death. Meanwhile, the theory itself did not receive attention for a while after publication. In 1814, Pierre-Simon Laplace, a French scholar and polymath, set out a mathematical system of inductive reasoning based on probability as follows: where event $A_j \in \{A_1, A_2, \ldots, A_n\}$ exhausts the list of possible causes for event B, $\Pr(B) = \Pr(A_1, A_2, \ldots, A_n)$. Then:

$$\Pr(A_i \mid B) = \Pr(A_i) \frac{\Pr(B \mid A_i)}{\sum_j \Pr(A_j) \Pr(B \mid A_j)} \tag{1}$$

This formula is now widely known as Bayes' Theorem. Pierre-Simon Laplace used what would now be considered Bayesian methods to solve many statistical problems, and a number of Bayesian methods have been developed by later authors. On the other hand, as the frequentist statisticians, represented by Karl Pearson, Ronald Fisher and Jerzy Neyman, came to be at the core of statistics, Bayesianism was considered unfavorable by many statisticians based on philosophical and practical considerations. As a result, the term "Bayesian method" was not commonly used to describe such a method until the 1950s. However, with the advent of powerful computers and new algorithms (especially the significant contribution of the Markov chain Monte Carlo method), Bayesian methods are still being used in statistics in the 21st century [18,19].

2.2. The Birth of AI, First AI Boom, and First Phase of the AI Winter

When computers became accessible in the mid-1950s, several scientists intuitively realized that two machines that could manipulate numbers could also manipulate symbols, and that the manipulation of symbols could represent the essence of human thought. This became a new way of approaching "thinking machines." In 1956, Dr. John McCarthy proposed the name "Artificial Intelligence (AI)" at the Dartmouth Workshop, and the study of AI as an academic field was launched [2,20]. The years after the Dartmouth Conference were an era of discovery, and the momentum was such that computer scientists were galloping through new horizons. Programs developed in this era relied on reasoning and exploration, and even the best computers of the time, which were developed at great expense, could only solve problems in a very limited domain because the amount of computation they could handle was very small; however, they were still "astounding" to people at the time. The computers showed people how to solve algebra problems, prove geometry theorems, and learn to speak English [21]. However, in the 1970s, AI was subjected to criticism and shrinking funding. One reason was that the AI researchers failed to properly assess the difficulty of the problem they were facing. Expectations of the results were too optimistic and high; however, the results failed to meet these expectations, and funding for AI research largely disappeared.

2.3. *The Second AI Boom and Second Phase of the AI Winter*

In the 1980s, knowledge representation became a focus of AI research as "expert systems," a form of AI program, were adopted by companies around the world [21–23]. An expert system is a program that answers questions and solves problems in a specific domain of knowledge and uses logical rules extracted from expert knowledge. Early examples include the Dendral (1965), which identifies compounds from spectrometer measurements and was developed by Dr. Edward Feigenbaum and colleagues [24], and MYCIN (1972), which diagnoses contagious blood diseases and was developed by Dr. Edward Shortliffe and colleagues [25]. MYCIN used a fairly simple reasoning engine and had a knowledge base consisting of about 500 rules [26]. This expert system asked the physician a number of questions that could be answered with a simple "yes/no" answer or some kind of written answer and finally gave a list of the names of bacteria that could be responsible (in order of probability), the confidence level of each, reasons why they were considered in the list, and the recommended course of drug therapy [27]. Despite its success, MYCIN is now sometimes regarded as an example of the risks of creating ad hoc probabilistic frameworks, such as in artificial intelligence lectures. One of the reasons for this is that MYCIN's depth of inference was limited because of the noise introduced by the confidence coefficient system. This problem can be prevented by adopting a rigorous probabilistic framework, such as the Bayesian estimation [28].

The growing interest in AI in the 1980s was temporary and followed the classic pattern of the bubble economy. In the end, expert systems were only effective in very limited circumstances, and in the 1980s and early 1990s, AI research again ran into a funding crisis.

2.4. *The Third AI Boom and Era of Deep Learning*

In 2006, deep learning using auto-encoders was invented by the Dr. Jeffrey Hinton group [29]. This invention was a major breakthrough in AI because it could extract features without human intervention, eliminating the need for human knowledge representation. In addition, this invention also solved the problem of symbolic grounding, which was caused by human knowledge representation. In 2010, the term "big data" was proposed in response to the increasing amount of data transfer through the Internet. The 2012 ImageNet Large Scale Visual Recognition Competition (ILSVRC) competition for object recognition rates, which featured a major breakthrough in large-scale GPU-based deep learning (led by Dr. Jeffrey Hinton's research team on Alex-net) [30], and Google's announcement in the same year of its success in recognizing a cat from YouTube images using deep learning, led to a renewed interest in artificial intelligence research around the world [31]. AI technology is actively used in the medical field as well, and its effectiveness has been demonstrated in various results such as medical image analysis and omics analysis [1,32–39]. In the field of oncology, the introduction of AI is also being actively studied in tumor screening, including lung and breast cancer [40,41]. Practically, as of 2020, more than 60 AI-powered medical devices have been approved by the US FDA (Table 1). One important thing that sets the third AI boom apart from the previous AI booms is that it is actually being implemented in society. Dr. Demis Hassabis, the CEO and co-founder of DeepMind, mentioned that throughout the history of AI, we have repeatedly climbed up and down the wrong ladder, but it is important that we have finally arrived at the "right ladder." Additionally, Bayesian statistics is also currently receiving a lot of attention due to the advances in AI technology. The reason for this is that in Bayesian statistics, the probability is set at the beginning, and subsequently the probability at that point of time can be changed as more information becomes available. This phenomenon itself resembles the "learning ability" of humans. It is this feature of Bayesian statistics that is the basis of deep learning and machine learning, which is an important feature of AI.

Table 1. List of AI-equipped medical devices approved by the US FDA.

No.	FDA Approval Number	Product Name (Company)	Description	Regulation Medical Specialty	Decision Date	Regulatory Class (Submission Type)
1	K140933	AliveCor Heart Monitor (AliveCor)	An ECG recording device using machine learning techniques to detect abnormal heart rhythms.	Cardiovascular	08/15/2014	Class II (510(k))
2	K143468	QbCheck (Qbtech)	A non-invasive test using AI for diagnosis and treatment of ADHD in children.	Neurology	03/22/2016	Unclassified (510(k))
3	K160016	Steth IO (StratoScientific)	An acoustic device using AI to aid in the identification of abnormal heart and lung sounds.	Cardiovascular	07/15/2016	Class II (510(k))
4	K163253	Arterys Cardio DL (Arterys)	A software using deep learning to visualize and quantify cardiovascular MR images.	Radiology	01/05/2017	Class II (510(k))
5	K161328	CANTAB Mobile (Cambridge Cognition)	An iPad-based memory-assessment tool for older adults.	Neurology	01/13/2017	Class II (510(k))
6	K162627	EnsoSleep (EnsoData)	An AI sleep scoring and analysis solution that automates event detection during sleep.	Neurology	03/31/2017	Class II (510(k))
7 *	K162574	AmCAD-US (AmCad BioMed Corporation)	A software to visualize and quantify ultrasound image data with backscattered signals.	Radiology	05/30/2017	Class II (510(k))
8 *	DEN170022	QuantX (Quantitative Insights)	An AI-equipped diagnosis system to aid in accurate diagnosis of breast cancer.	Radiology	07/19/2017	Class II (De Novo)
9	K172311	BioFlux Device (Biotricity)	A remote patient monitoring platform with AI.	Cardiovascular	12/15/2017	Class II (510(k))
10	K171056	WAVE Clinical Platform (Excel Medical Electronics)	A patient surveillance and predictive algorithm platform using AI.	Cardiovascular	01/04/2018	Class II (510(k))

Table 1. *Cont.*

No.	FDA Approval Number	Product Name (Company)	Description	Regulation Medical Specialty	Decision Date	Regulatory Class (Submission Type)
11 *	K173542	Arterys Oncology DL (Arterys)	An AI-based, cloud-based medical imaging software that automatically measures and tracks lesions and nodules in MRI and CT scans.	Radiology	01/25/2018	Class II (510(k))
12	DEN170073	ContaCT (Viz.AI)	An AI algorithm to analyze CT scans and detect signs of stroke.	Radiology	02/13/2018	Class II (De Novo)
13	K170540	DM-Density (Densitas)	A machine learning application that provides on demand automated breast density assessments at point-of-care.	Radiology	02/23/2018	Class II (510(k))
14	P160007	Guardian Connect System (Medtronic MiniMed)	A continuous glucose monitor with AI assistance.	Clinical Chemistry	03/08/2018	PMA
15	DEN180001	IDx-DR (IDx)	A software program that uses an AI algorithm to analyze retinal images.	Ophthalmic	04/11/2018	Class II (De Novo)
16	K173931	MindMotion GO (MindMaze)	A gamified neurorehabilitation therapy platform using AI.	Physical Medicine	05/17/2018	Class II (510(k))
17	K180455	NeuralBot (Neural Analytics)	A lucid robotic ultrasound system for brain blood flow assessment.	Radiology	05/22/2018	Class II (510(k))
18	DEN180005	OsteoDetect (Imagen Technologies)	A computer-aided detection and diagnostic software that uses an AI algorithm to analyze two-dimensional X-ray images for signs of distal radius fracture.	Radiology	05/24/2018	Class II (De Novo)
19	K173821	LungQ (Thirona Corporation)	A lung quantification software to analyze chest CT scans.	Radiology	06/05/2018	Class II (510(k))
20	DEN170043	DreaMed Advisor Pro (DreaMed Diabetes)	An AI-powered technology to seamlessly treat patients remotely with its virtual diabetes management service.	Clinical Chemistry	06/12/2018	Class II (De Novo)

Table 1. *Cont.*

No.	FDA Approval Number	Product Name (Company)	Description	Regulation Medical Specialty	Decision Date	Regulatory Class (Submission Type)
21	K172983	HealthCCS (Zebra Medical Vision)	An AI-powered software that can be used to evaluate calcified plaques in the coronary arteries.	Radiology	06/13/2018	Class II (510(k))
22	K173780	EchoMD Automated Ejection Fraction Software (Bay Labs)	A system that enables fully automated AI echocardiogram analysis.	Radiology	06/14/2018	Class II (510(k))
23	K180647	BriefCase (Aidoc Medical)	An AI algorithm to detect and triage abnormal findings in non-enhanced head CT images.	Radiology	08/01/2018	Class II (510(k))
24	DEN180042	Irregular Rhythm Notification Feature (Apple)	An application to detect irregular heart rhythms in pulse rate data collected by the Apple Watch photoplethysmograph sensors.	Cardiovascular	09/11/2018	Class II (De Novo)
25	DEN180044	ECG App (Apple)	Applications to detect atrial fibrillations and sinus rhythms in ECG data from an Apple Watch and display the results on an iPhone.	Cardiovascular	09/11/2018	Class II (De Novo)
26	K173872	FibriCheck (Qompium)	A smartphone application for the detection of heart rhythm disorders such as atrial fibrillation.	Cardiovascular	09/28/2018	Class II (510(k))
27	K181771	RightEye Vision System (RightEye)	A cloud-based system that uses objective eye movement measurements to aid in the evaluation of Parkinson's disease.	Neurology	09/28/2018	Class II (510(k))
28 *	K182034	Arterys MICA (Arterys)	An AI-based platform for analyzing medical images such as MRI and CT.	Radiology	10/17/2018	Class II (510(k))

Table 1. *Cont.*

No.	FDA Approval Number	Product Name (Company)	Description	Regulation Medical Specialty	Decision Date	Regulatory Class (Submission Type)
29	K182177	Accipio Ix (MaxQ-AI)	An AI-enabled software workflow tool that aids in identifying acute intracranial hemorrhage and prioritizing the treatment of strokes or head trauma.	Radiology	10/26/2018	Class II (510(k))
30	K181939	icobrain (icometrix)	A software that extracts clinically meaningful information from brain CT or MRI scans of patients with multiple sclerosis, dementia or brain injury.	Radiology	11/06/2018	Class II (510(k))
31	K180432	AI-ECG Platform (Shenzhen Carewell Electronics)	A software package which is a distributed ECG auto analysis system designed to assist in measuring and interpreting 12-lead resting ECG with an AI algorithm.	Cardiovascular	11/19/2018	Class II (510(k))
32	K182218	FerriSmart Analysis System (Resonance Health Analysis Service)	An automated system for measuring liver iron concentration.	Radiology	11/30/2018	Class II (510(k))
33 *	K182336	SubtlePET (Subtle Medical)	An AI-powered technology that enables centers to deliver a faster and safer patient scanning experience, while enhancing exam throughput and provider profitability.	Radiology	11/30/2018	Class II (510(k))
34	K173681	reSET-O (Pear Therapeutics)	A Prescription Digital Therapeutic (PDT) platform for the treatment of Opioid Use Disorder.	Neurology	12/10/2018	Class II (510(k))
35	K181861	Embrace (Empatica)	An epilepsy smartband that detects patterns in motion and physiological signals that may be associated with generalized tonic-clonic seizures, and immediately alerts caregivers.	Neurology	12/20/2018	Class II (510(k))

Table 1. *Cont.*

No.	FDA Approval Number	Product Name (Company)	Description	Regulation Medical Specialty	Decision Date	Regulatory Class (Submission Type)
36	K182130	iSchemaView RAPID (iSchemaView)	An AI-enhanced advanced medical imaging for stroke.	Radiology	12/27/2018	Class II (510(k))
37	K182564	Quantib ND (Quantib)	An AI solution that helps radiologists read MRI brain scans.	Radiology	12/27/2018	Class II (510(k))
38	K182456	Study Watch (Verily Life Sciences)	A wearable device to record, store, transfer, and display ECG rhythms.	Cardiovascular	01/17/2019	Class II (510(k))
39	K182344	RhythmAnalytics (Biofourmis Singapore)	An AI-powered software to detect irregular heart rhythms when ECG data are uploaded.	Cardiovascular	03/07/2019	Class II (510(k))
40 *	K183285	cmTriage (CureMetrix)	An AI-based triage software for mammography.	Radiology	03/08/2019	Class II (510(k))
41	K181823	KardiaAI (AliveCor)	An AI-based software analysis library to assess ambulatory ECG rhythms from adult subjects.	Cardiovascular	03/11/2019	Class II (510(k))
42	K181352	Loop System (Spry Health)	A tool to collect and transfer physiological data of patients in the home environment.	Cardiovascular	03/29/2019	Class II (510(k))
43 *	K183202	Deep Learning Image Reconstruction (GE Medical Systems)	A deep learning-based CT image reconstruction technology.	Radiology	04/12/2019	Class II (510(k))
44	K181988	eMurmur ID (CSD Labs)	A software screening device that uses a smartphone, electronic stethoscope and machine learning to automate the detection of heart murmurs.	Cardiovascular	04/17/2019	Class II (510(k))
45	K190362	HealthPNX (Zebra Medical Vision)	A radiological computer-assisted triage and notification software system.	Radiology	05/06/2019	Class II (510(k))

Table 1. *Cont.*

No.	FDA Approval Number	Product Name (Company)	Description	Regulation Medical Specialty	Decision Date	Regulatory Class (Submission Type)
46 *	K183046	Aquilion ONE (TSX-305A/6) V8.9 with AiCE (Canon Medical Systems Corporation)	A device to acquire and display cross-sectional volumes of the whole body, including the head, with the capability of imaging whole organs in a single rotation.	Radiology	06/12/2019	Class II (510(k))
47 *	K191384	RayCare 2.3 (RaySearch Laboratories)	An oncology information system used to support workflows, scheduling and clinical information management for oncology care and follow-up.	Radiology	07/08/2019	Class II (510(k))
48	K183322	physIQ Heart Rhythm and Respiratory Module (physIQ)	A device for the calculation of heart rate and heart rate variability, the detection of atrial fibrillation and the determination of respiration rate using ambulatory ECG and triaxial accelerometer data.	Cardiovascular	07/10/2019	Class II (510(k))
49	K191272	Current Wearable Health Monitoring System (Current Health)	A device for reusable bedside, mobile and central multi-parameter, physiologic patient monitoring of adult patients in professional healthcare facilities.	Cardiovascular	07/12/2019	Class II (510(k))
50	K182384	ACR | LAB Urine Analysis Test System (Healthy.io)	A device for the semi-quantitative detection of albumin and creatinine in urine, using a smartphone application, a proprietary Color-Board, and ACR Reagent Strips.	Clinical Chemistry	07/26/2019	Class II (510(k))

Table 1. *Cont.*

No.	FDA Approval Number	Product Name (Company)	Description	Regulation Medical Specialty	Decision Date	Regulatory Class (Submission Type)
51	K183271	AI-Rad Companion (Pulmonary) (Siemens Medical Solutions USA)	An image processing software that provides a quantitative and qualitative analysis from previously acquired CT DICOM images to support radiologists and physicians in the evaluation and assessment of lung disease.	Radiology	07/26/2019	Class II (510(k))
52	K183282	Biovitals Analytics Engine (Biofourmis Singapore)	An AI-based software engine used with continuous biometric data from already cleared sensors measuring heart rate, respiratory rate, and activity in ambulatory patients being monitored in a healthcare facility or at home, during periods of minimal activity.	Cardiovascular	08/15/2019	Class II (510(k))
53	K183268	AI-Rad Companion (Cardiovascular) (Siemens Medical Solutions USA)	An image processing software that provides quantitative and qualitative analysis from previously acquired CT DICOM images to support radiologists and physicians in the evaluation and assessment of cardiovascular diseases.	Radiology	09/10/2019	Class II (510(k))
54	K190815	BrainScope TBI (BrainScope Company)	A portable, non-invasive, non-radiation emitting, point of care device intended to provide results and measures to support clinical assessments and aid in the diagnosis of concussion/mild traumatic brain injury (mTBI).	Neurology	09/11/2019	Class II (510(k))
55	K191688	SubtleMR (Subtle Medical)	An image processing software that can be used for image enhancement in MRI images.	Radiology	09/16/2019	Class II (510(k))

Table 1. *Cont.*

No.	FDA Approval Number	Product Name (Company)	Description	Regulation Medical Specialty	Decision Date	Regulatory Class (Submission Type)
56 *	K191994	ProFound AI Software V2.1 (iCAD)	A CAD software device intended to be used concurrently by interpreting physicians while reading digital breast tomosynthesis (DBT) exams from compatible DBT systems.	Radiology	10/04/2019	Class II (510(k))
57	K191713	CS-series-FP Radiographic/Fluoroscopic Systems with Optional CA-100S/FluoroShield (Omega Medical Imaging)	A modification device to provide an automated region of interest that reduces exposure to the patient and operator.	Radiology	10/04/2019	Class II (510(k))
58	K191171	EchoGo Core (Ultromics)	A software for use in quantification and reporting of results of cardiovascular function to support physician diagnosis.	Radiology	11/13/2019	Class II (510(k))
59 *	K192287	Transpara (ScreenPoint Medical)	A device for use as a concurrent reading aid for physicians interpreting screening mammograms from compatible FFDM systems to identify regions suspicious for breast cancer and assess their likelihood of malignancy.	Radiology	12/10/2019	Class II (510(k))
60	K192004	Eko Analysis Software (Eko Devices)	A software to provide support to the physician in the evaluation of patients' heart sounds and ECG's.	Cardiovascular	01/15/2020	Class II (510(k))
61	DEN190040	Caption Guidance (Caption Health)	A software to assist in the acquisition of cardiac ultrasound images.	Radiology	02/07/2020	Class II (De Novo)

*: The product involved in the field of oncology. Abbreviations: AI, artificial intelligence; US FDA, United States Food and Drug Administration; CT, computed tomography; MRI, magnetic resonance imaging; DICOM, Digital Imaging and Communications in Medicine; ECG, electrocardiogram; FFDM, full-field digital mammography; ADHD, attention deficit hyperactivity disorder.

3. Introducing AI Technology in Oncology

3.1. Radiology

In terms of the medical applications of AI, radiology is one of the areas where AI technology has been maximally adopted [42]. In fact, most of the medical devices with AI approved by the FDA that are related to oncology are in the field of radiology (Table 1). The reason for this is that deep learning technology is prominent in image analysis, and radiation image analysis is one of the historically advanced ICT fields such as computer-assisted detection/diagnosis (CAD), which has a strong affinity for AI [43]. Figure 1 shows a typical CADx workflow for detecting prostate cancer [44]. In cancer diagnosis, CAD has been expected to improve productivity in image reading by improving the diagnostic accuracy and reproducibility of image reading, as well as reducing the reading time [45,46].

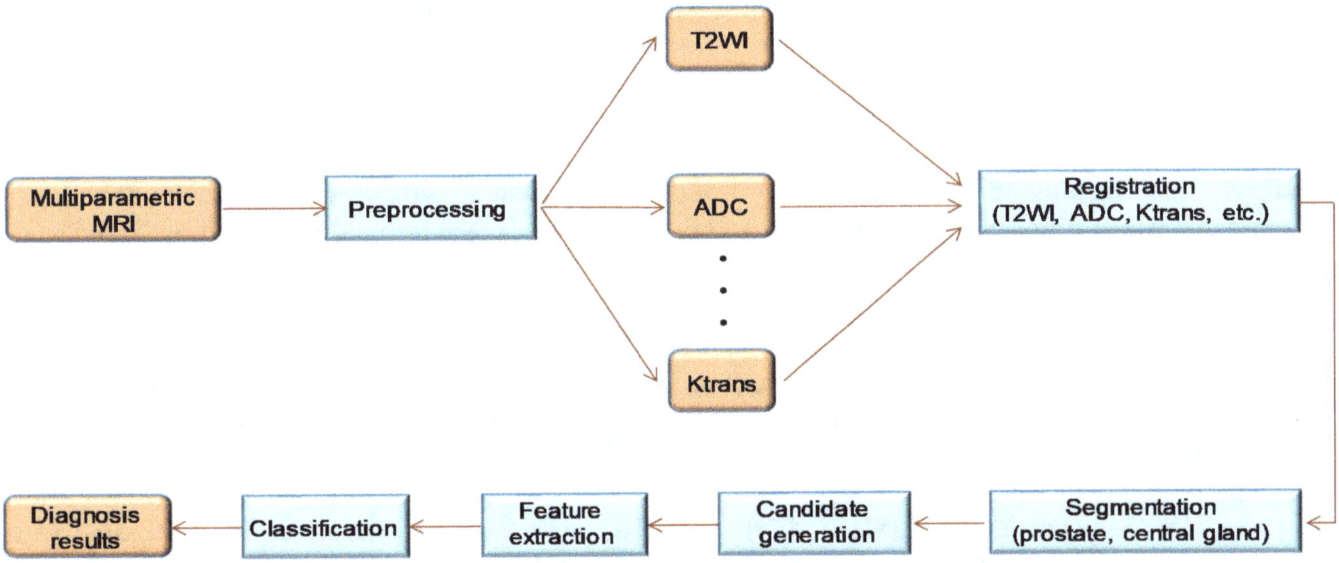

Figure 1. Workflow diagram of a typical prostate CADx system in Reference 44 (Wang et al., 2014); this is a modified figure from the reference. The orange squares indicate the data (original scan and pre-processed image), and the light blue squares indicate the data and processing applied to the image.

Approved by the FDA in May 2017, AmCAD-US (AmCad BioMed Corporation) is a software device that visualizes and quantifies the statistical distribution of backscattered signals echoed by tissue compositions in the body from ultrasound systems [47]. AmCad BioMed Corporation has also developed and received FDA approval for AmCAD-UT, primarily for the detection of thyroid cancer [48]. In July 2017, the Second Reader type CADx (QuantX) by Quantitative Insights received its first FDA approval [49]. This device is designed to target breast magnetic resonance imaging (MRI) and assist physicians in the differential diagnosis of breast cancer. In January 2018, Arterys Oncology DL (Arterys), which can help clinicians to rapidly measure and track lesions and nodules on MRI and computed tomography (CT) scans, received FDA approval [50]. This device was developed to support the diagnosis of solid tumors in general, and is in the first stage of clinical application for liver and lung cancer. In November 2018, SubtlePET (Subtle Medical), an AI-based high-speed positron emission tomography (PET) imaging technology, was approved by the FDA [51]. SubtlePet is an AI technology that enables four times faster imaging, especially during PET imaging, which plays an important role in cancer diagnosis. In March 2019, cmTriage (CureMetrix) was approved by the FDA for the triage of mammography images [52]. cmTriage is a workflow optimization tool that allows radiologists to customize, sort, and prioritize mammography worklists, allowing them to prioritize cases that require immediate attention. In addition, cmTriage can be used to optimize clinical workflows by sending suspicious cases to experienced radiologists or by immediately notifying them of suspicious cases even just before a patient is discharged. In April 2019, Deep Learning Image Reconstruction (DLIR: GE

Medical Systems) was approved by the FDA for use as a specialized deep neural network (DNN) to generate TrueFidelity CT images [53]. TrueFidelity CT imaging has the potential to improve reading reliability in patients of all ages in a wide range of clinical applications, including head, systemic, and cardiovascular applications. In June 2019, the Advanced Intelligent Clear-IQ Engine (AiCE: Canon Medical Systems Corporation) was approved by the FDA [51]. AiCE is a state-of-the-art image reconstruction technique for CT designed using deep learning, which uses a process that discriminates between noise and signal components to selectively remove noise while maintaining spatial resolution. By using AiCE, a high noise reduction effect can be obtained while maximizing the spatial resolution of the CT scanner. In addition, a high noise reduction effect is achieved in low-contrast regions while maintaining the granularity, and stable image quality improvement is achieved even in low-dose regions. ProFound™ AI Software V2.1 (iCAD), approved by the FDA in October 2019, is a CAD software that assists physicians during digital breast tomosynthesis (DBT) [54]. The system is capable of detecting soft tissue density (masses, architectural distortions, and asymmetries) and calcifications within 3D DBT slices, with the aim of improving breast cancer detection rates and making a more accurate diagnosis. Approved by the FDA in December 2019, Transpara (ScreenPoint Medical) is an AI system that specializes in image interpretation in mammography [54]. Studies on the Transpara system showed that using this system to assist in image interpretation can significantly improve the area under the receiver operating characteristic curve (AUC) and diagnostic sensitivity without increasing the interpretation time. Additionally, the AUC of the Transpara system alone was comparable to the average AUC of radiologists.

3.2. *Endoscopy*

Endoscopic images are also an important target of AI analysis. In particular, given that Japanese medical equipment manufacturers hold a 99.1% share of the global market for endoscopes, endoscopic AI development is being actively conducted in Japan [55]. At present, there is an example of clinical implementation of endoscopic AI in Japan after receiving regulatory approval from the Pharmaceuticals and Medical Devices Agency (PMDA) [56]. We also developed a real-time endoscopic diagnostic support system for the detection of colorectal cancer (CRC) and precancerous lesions using AI technology in order to improve the lesion detection rate by colonoscopy, eliminate technology gaps among physicians, and prevent missed lesions [36]. When developing endoscopic AI, we planned to first target CRC; one of the reasons was its high frequency. The latest data show that CRC affects about 130,000 people in Japan annually, and the number of deaths exceeds 50,000 per year [57]. Additionally, the number continues to rise. Meanwhile, CRC and other cancers of the gastrointestinal tract can be controlled if they are detected early with endoscopic intervention. In fact, in the United States, the results of the National Polyp Study reported in 1993 and its cohort study reported in 2012 demonstrated that the endoscopic removal of adenomatous polyps, a precursor lesion to CRC, reduced the morbidity of CRC by 76–90% and mortality by 53% [58,59]. Therefore, endoscopy is actively used for physical examination as well as gastric and colorectal cancer screening, and when adenomatous polyps are found in the colon, they are removed endoscopically. In other words, two things are important for the prevention of CRC: (1) undergoing a colonoscopy; and (2) not missing a lesion during the examination. Interventions to increase the uptake of countermeasure screening are necessary to promote colonoscopy. However, the process from colonoscopy to polypectomy consists of five major stages: 1. lesion detection, 2. qualitative and quantitative diagnosis, 3. treatment, 4. pathological diagnosis, and 5. surveillance. This means that the first thing to do is not to miss any lesions during the examination. The endoscopist can easily detect the so-called "polyps" if they are protruding in shape; however, flat-shaped lesions or lesions that are the same color tone as the surrounding mucosa are less visible and require a certain amount of experience for detection. In addition, the colon has many anatomical blind spots and requires techniques to observe the lumen in every corner of the colon, including between the mucosal folds in the wall. For these reasons, a colonoscopy is a test in which there is a technical gap on the part of the physician, which can be a major source of concern for the patient. Using the latest technology of deep learning, the Department of Endoscopy at the National Cancer Center's Central Hospital trained AI on a large number of endoscopic images of early-stage colorectal cancer and precancerous lesions accumulated to date. In order to study a large number of unbiased cases, we first collected at least one still image of each consecutive early-stage colorectal cancer and precancerous lesion over a period of time. The location of the lesions in the images was then checked, and a line was drawn at the boundary between the surrounding mucosa and each lesion with a marker for all lesions, thus surrounding the lesions. Although it might seem to be a simple and steady task, it was important that there were no mistakes during this work because these data were used as training data for deep learning. We used our own convolutional neural network as a deep learning technique [36]. In conventional machine learning, the extraction of the lesion features in images is done manually by humans, but in deep learning, AI automatically generates a variety of lesion features. The input images are extracted as features in the convolution and pooling layers and their classification is presented in the output layer. Moreover, the AI automatically learns from the training data using the back-propagation method. A performance evaluation test on the developed AI system was performed on 705 images with lesions and 4135 images without lesions obtained at our hospital over a period of time that were not used for training. For the evaluation study, the researchers involved in the analysis of the AI were completely blind to lesion and clinical information. The overall sensitivity and specificity of the AI for colorectal lesions were 98.8 and 99%, respectively, and a correct answer was considered to be correct if the AI correctly detected the location of the lesion. Furthermore, we succeeded in analyzing a single frame of video (lesion detection and result display) within 33 milliseconds (30 frames per second). Therefore, we believe that the system has reached a stage where it can be developed for clinical implementation as an endoscopic diagnostic support system [36].

3.3. *Pathological Images*

Pathological diagnosis is the final diagnosis of a lesion and therefore plays an important role in determining the subsequent treatment strategy and the effectiveness of treatment. However, there is currently a shortage of pathologists in the United States, United Kingdom, Japan, Canada, and other countries around the world, and this has become a problem for maintaining the quality of medical care in each country [60,61]. Under these circumstances, research and development in pathological diagnosis using AI technology is of paramount importance. However, there are some problems that need to be solved, such as how to standardize the pathological images, because the methods for preparing pathological specimens and staining methods vary from institution to institution. Therefore, pathological diagnosis using AI technology has not yet been actively introduced into clinical practice. However, there is no doubt that the utilization of AI for pathological diagnosis is one way to compensate for the shortage of pathologists, and it is likely that pathological diagnosis using AI technology will gradually advance in clinical practice in the future. An important finding on pathological diagnosis using AI technology was recently published by New York University, USA [62]. In this study, Coudray et al. trained a large number of high-definition digitally imaged pathology glass slide specimen images (also known as Virtual Slides) using a deep learning algorithm called InceptionV3 for histopathological classification (lung cancer (adenocarcinoma and squamous cell carcinoma) and normal lung). The results revealed a very high accuracy with 0.97 AUC for tissue classification [62]. Both frozen and formalin-fixed paraffin-embedded sections were available for analysis as specimens. Furthermore, using the developed AI analysis system, six gene mutations, STK11, EGFR, FAT1, SETBP1, KRAS, and TP53, could be accurately predicted from the pathological images (AUC: 0.733–0.856). These results suggest that the analysis of pathological virtual slide images using AI technology may enable the accurate classification of lung cancer tissues and prediction of genetic mutations. As a next step, it is important to conduct prospective studies to ensure the robustness of results across institutions; however, this is not limited to pathological image analysis, and we believe that this should apply to all medical image analysis systems that utilize AI technology.

3.4. Skin Images

Skin cancer is the most common malignancy in Western countries, with melanoma in particular accounting for the majority of skin cancer-related deaths worldwide [63]. Melanoma is a highly malignant skin cancer of melanocyte origin that is similar in shape to a mole; therefore, it is very important to distinguish between moles (benign) and melanomas (malignant). The early detection of skin cancer, including melanoma, is particularly crucial because the early detection of skin cancer makes it easier to treat and significantly improves prognosis [64]. However, melanoma is sometimes difficult to diagnose clinically because of its similarity to other brown to black pigmented lesions such as pigmented nevi, seborrheic keratosis, and basal cell carcinoma. Consequently, we developed a skin tumor determination system for brown to black pigmented lesions [33]. In this study, out of the data of 120,000 images of patients seen at our hospital from 2001 to 2017, we extracted images of brown to black pigmented skin lesions (malignant melanoma and basal cell carcinoma for malignant tumors, nevus pigmentosus, senile pigmentation, seborrheic keratosis, hematoma, and hemangioma for benign tumors), which were the diseases to be analyzed. After the extraction, each image was annotated by a dermatologist with a bounding-box to indicate the location in the image where the lesion was located. We then applied general object detection techniques to train a neural network to predict the location and type of lesion in the image. At the end of the training, the AI predicted the type of lesion for validation data (images not used for training), while clinicians (10 dermatologists and 10 non-specialists) were also tested using the same images. The results showed that the discrimination accuracy of the AI was comparable to that of dermatologists as well as non-specialists. Our goal is to make our skin tumor determination system available to the public so that users can become more aware of their own symptoms and skin tumors in general. Additionally, we hope to establish a framework that encourages them to seek medical attention when necessary. This can help reduce the proportion of patients with advanced stages of the disease and reduce the rising cost of healthcare.

Esteva et al. also attempted to classify skin diseases using AI by analyzing a database of about 130,000 images and their corresponding 2000 diseases, using one of the deep learning algorithms, convolutional neural network [65]. In this study, 127,463 images were trained and validated, and 1942 images were used to compare the diagnoses by AI and dermatologists. The results showed that the AUC values of 135 skin cancer cases and of 130 melanoma cases diagnosed by AI were 0.96 and 0.94, which were almost the same as that of the diagnosed by dermatologists [65].

4. Application of Machine Learning and Deep Learning Techniques to Omics Analysis

With the completion of the International Human Genome Project in 2003 [66], we entered an era known as the post-genome era, and the momentum for the application of genomic information in medicine has increased. As a result, the term "genomic medicine" has emerged, proposing a new type of medical treatment that provides patients with optimal treatment options based on the genome information [67]. In 2015, the Precision Medicine Initiative was announced by US President Barack Obama for cancer and rare diseases, dividing patients/potential sufferers into subgroups of disease morbidity and developing appropriate treatments and prevention methods for each group [68]. This initiative had a great impact on the global medical policy, and since then, the establishment of precision medicine has become one of the major goals of research in the field of oncology. However, the current state of precision medicine has many problems that need to be addressed. One of the main problems is that although the provision of optimal anticancer drugs based on TGP is the current mainstay of precision medicine, the number of patients who receive the most appropriate treatment is low [14–16]. Increasing the number of patients who benefit from precision medicine is considered an important issue; however, it is believed that treatment selection based on the current TGPs alone is insufficient to address this issue [15]. It is essential to integrate whole genome sequencing (WGS) data as well as other omics data, such as epigenomic, proteomic, and metabolomic data, for multimodal analysis. In particular, recent rapid advances in epigenomic analysis techniques have revealed that cancer cells accumulate a variety of epigenomic abnormalities in addition to genetic abnormalities [69–82]. Epigenomic aberrations have a significant impact on the characteristics of cancer from the early stages of development to developmental progression [83–99]. In addition, owing to development and progress in medical epigenetics, which targets epigenome abnormalities, it is important to analyze the pathogenesis of cancer with an appropriate consideration of epigenetic information [100–104].

As mentioned above, in order to promote precision medicine, it is necessary to take into account omics information such as epigenomic information and WGS information in addition to genomic information obtained by panel inspection, and this is a huge amount of data. In order to efficiently and accurately analyze this vast amount of medical big data, that is, in a sense, beyond human capabilities, it is essential to utilize the most advanced AI and ICT technologies. In particular, as we have previously mentioned, machine learning and deep learning technologies have the following four features, and are expected to play an important role in the multimodal analysis of medical big data [1]:

a. Multimodal learning: different types of medical data (e.g., genomic, epigenomic, and proteomic data) can be integrated and treated as inputs;
b. Multitasking learning: multiple different tasks can be learned simultaneously by sharing parts of the model;
c. Representational and semi-supervised learning: acquire a way to represent data from large amounts of unlabeled data, making it possible to learn from small amounts of labeled data;
d. It is possible to capture higher order correlations of inputs.

The above properties have led to the introduction of machine learning and deep learning techniques in medical large data analysis. In particular, machine learning and deep learning techniques are being widely used for dimensionality reduction and feature extraction in the stage of extracting important information from vast amounts of data, as well as for the stratification of patients based on the extracted features (Figure 2). For example, a method for dimensionality reduction using an autoencoder has been proposed for large amounts of multi-omics data [105], and we have also used this method to stratify lung cancer patients [32]. In this study, we combined RNA-seq and miRNA expression data from The Cancer Genome Atlas (TCGA), while focusing on lung adenocarcinoma (LUAD) with clinical information and performed a multi-omics analysis using an autoencoder. Consequently, we successfully subclassified patients according to survival (categorizing good and poor lung cancer prognosis groups). The classifier was developed using estimated labels derived from patient subtypes, the support vector machine (SVM) gave the best classification results, with an accuracy of 0.82 for the test data set. These subtypes were used to rank genes based on their RNA expression levels. The top 25 genes were investigated to identify the mechanisms that influence patient prognosis. Bioinformatics analysis showed that the expression levels of six of the 25 genes (*ERO1B*, *DPY19L1*, *NCAM1*, *RET*, *MARCH1*, and *SLC7A8*) were associated with survival in LUAD patients, and pathway analysis indicated that major cancer signaling pathways were altered in the subtypes. Expanding on this method, we identified survival-related subtypes of non-small cell lung cancer from six categories of TCGA multi-omics datasets (miRNA, mRNA, DNA methylation, somatic mutation, copy number variation, and reverse phase protein array) [106]. As a result, the subtype named the Integrated Survival Subtype, which combined the six types of data, successfully separated the poor and good prognosis groups of lung cancer patients with a statistically significant difference. We also confirmed that this was independent of the histopathological classification. In addition, the predicted subtypes were able to distinguish between high- and low-risk patients. Through the above studies, we presented a new potential multi-omics analysis to accurately predict the prognosis of lung cancer patients.

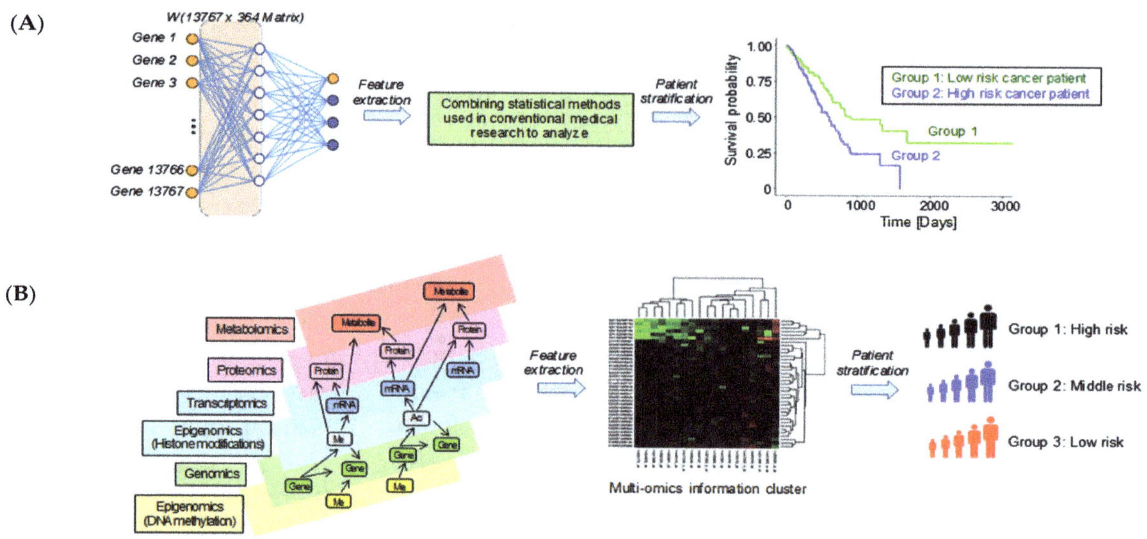

Figure 2. Examples of how machine learning and deep learning techniques are being used to reduce the dimensionality of massive omics data to extract features and then stratify the patients. (**A**) An example of analysis using Kaplan–Meier curves after dimensionality reduction and feature concentration using machine learning and deep learning techniques applied to genetic mutation information. (**B**) An example information. (**B**) An example of patient stratification using machine learning techniques to extract

There are also several challenges in the application of deep learning for medical omics data, such as genomic data. First, the dimensions of the input are in orders of magnitude larger than the number of samples (Large p, Small n Problems) [107], and the model tends to overfit the training dataset. Second, the contribution of each input variable to the prediction is usually difficult to interpret because of the multiple nonlinear operations. Third, genetic data may not be characterized by an innate structure. To mitigate these problems, we proposed a genomic analysis method using a modified diet network by adding per-element input scaling [34]. The original concept of Diet Networks, with transposed data matrices as inputs to the auxiliary network, can significantly reduce the number of parameters in a fully connected layer [108]. The effectiveness of our proposed method was assessed in a binary classification task based on the somatic mutation profile of lung cancer histopathology, i.e., adenocarcinoma and squamous cell carcinoma [34]. The dataset consisted of 950 cases and was subjected to 5-fold cross-validation to assess the performance of the model. The results showed that the prediction accuracy was about 80%, and the addition of per-element input scaling contributed significantly to the stability of the learning process [34]. The latent representation obtained inside the model allowed us to interpret and predict relationships between somatic mutation sites.

For the realization of precision medicine, predicting the effects of anticancer drugs is a vital issue, and attempts have been made to predict the effects of large-scale omics data using machine learning and deep learning techniques [109–114]. Shukla et al. analyzed the chromosome arm aneuploidy (CAA) profiles of 23,427 tumors to identify the aspects of tumor evolution, including the order in which CAAs can occur and the CAAs that can predict tissue-specific metastases [115]. In this study, the authors used machine learning techniques (deep neural network models) to identify 31 CAAs that powerfully altered the response to 56 chemotherapy drugs in cell lines representing 17 cancer types. The authors also found 1024 potentially lethal drug interactions. Notably, CAAs significantly outperformed mutations and local deletions/amplifications combined in predicting the drug response [115]. Thus, CAAs have the potential to predict cancer prognosis, shape tumor evolution, metastasis, and drug response and thus advance precision oncology.

The Bruton tyrosine kinase inhibitor ibrutinib is an effective treatment for patients with chronic lymphocytic leukemia (CLL); however, there is extensive heterogeneity in this disease. Rendeiro et al. attempted to predict the response to ibrutinib treatment by analyzing multi-layered omics data (immunophenotyping, single-cell RNA-seq, and ATAC-seq) together with clinical information using machine learning techniques [116]. Non-malignant B cell changes reflected changes in the CLL cells, with CD4+ T cells, CD8+ T cells, natural killer (NK) cells, and myeloid cells responding in a cell type-specific manner [116]. They also identified a gene expression signature that captures the ibrutinib-induced widespread downregulation of immune cell function and the acquisition of a quiescent state in response to ibrutinib therapy. There was patient-specific variability in the speed of execution of the program, and this variability could be used to predict patient-specific dynamics of the response to ibrutinib based on the pre-treatment patient sample [116]. This study revealed time-dependent cellular, molecular, and regulatory effects on the therapeutic inhibition of B-cell receptor signaling in CLL using machine learning multi-omics analysis and established a widely applicable method for epigenomic/transcriptomic-based therapeutic monitoring.

Recently, the establishment of precision oncology based on large-scale omics analysis using machine learning and deep learning techniques has been actively studied; however, the research is still in its infancy. One of the current problems is that the biological properties of a gene mutation vary depending on the function of the gene and the location of the mutation, but we have not been able to take such detailed information into account, and all the mutations are lumped together for analysis. In the future, we need to consider methods to effectively introduce this kind of domain knowledge into the analysis. In addition, omics information, such as genomic and epigenomic information, has a large number of parameters compared to the number of samples, which is always a problem (Large p, Small n Problems) [107]. This makes it difficult to analyze the raw data as it is, and dimensionality reduction is necessary. An important point is the need to select a model that allows the compression of parameters without compromising the expressive power of the model; therefore, further study is needed. The explanatory and interpretive nature of the results also requires further exploration and is discussed in detail in Section 6.2. Furthermore, recent studies have identified important molecular mechanisms/signaling pathways in cancer development and progression [71,117–138], and several pathway analysis methods have been reported to elucidate the true nature of cancer and identify drug targets by using features extracted from large-scale data. The methodology is correct, and several results have been published that have contributed greatly to the development of the field of oncology [139–150]. However, it should be adequately recognized that there are limitations to the results obtained by a dry lab approach, and it is important to validate the results obtained by the dry lab approach using appropriate wet lab experiments (cell-level studies or animal-level studies using mice). By feeding back the results of the wet lab experiments to the dry lab approach, it is expected that the accuracy of the results of the dry lab approach itself can be improved. This can be said of AI in general, and no matter how much progress AI makes in the future, it is very risky for humans to rely on AI's judgment for everything. We believe that there should always be a human verification step. Ideally, we should have an accurate understanding of the strengths and weaknesses of humans and AI, making it possible to learn together and complement each other.

5. Drug Development Using Machine Learning and Bayesian Statistics in Oncology

Drug development is a costly and time-consuming process that can last up to 15 years. The development pipeline starts with the initial phase 0, comprising basic research or drug discovery. The next three stages (phase I, phase II, and phase III) are clinical trials, while phase IV includes a pharmacovigilance study. Phase I involves the study of dose-toxicity and short-term side effects; the determination of drug performance occurs in phase II and phase III and involves comparing the drug to standard therapies for the disease being studied. Phase IV is to monitor the long-lasting side effects of the drug. The major challenge in the drug development process is the high failure rate and consequent financial loss in the final stages of development [151]. With the recent advances in AI platforms and machine learning techniques, it is now possible to fasten the pace of development as well as reduce the likelihood of failure. The machine learning models such as support vector machine, random forest, Bayes' theorem, and many others find application in all the stages of drug development leading to accurate prediction and insights (Figure 3) [152]. The Bayesian approach is an emerging technique used by medical researchers in the field of oncology drug development. The issues of case fatality, survival analysis, dropouts from clinical observations, and complex computational problems can be effortlessly handled using Bayesian techniques. In the era of big data, the Bayesian statistical approach is better suited for combining the current data with prior knowledge and for creating posterior probabilities for both drug effectiveness and its safety [153].

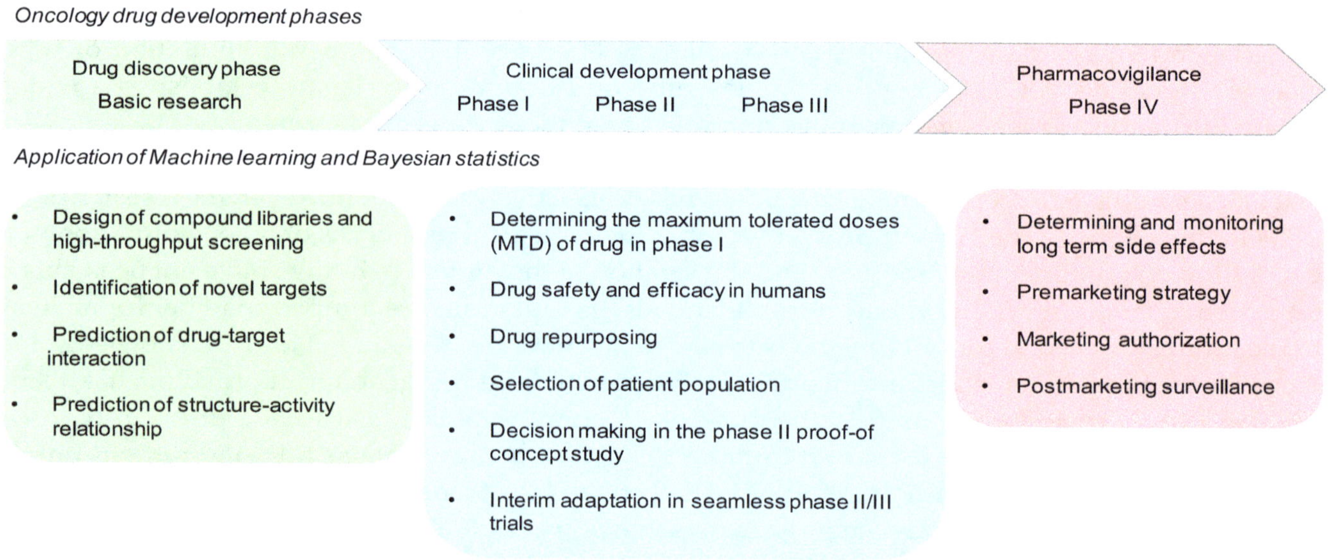

Figure 3. Application of machine learning and Bayesian statistics in different phases of drug development.

The mathematical method using Bayesian statistics can be implemented at the design stage, during the conduct of the trial, at the analysis stage, for post-marketing surveillance purposes, and in meta-analysis. Recently, Bayesian Analysis to determine Drug Interaction Targets (BANDIT), an integrative big data approach, was developed for drug target prediction, validation for clinical development, and drug repurposing. This machine learning algorithm identified a novel microtubule inhibitor with activity against breast cancer cells that were resistant to all other clinically approved anti-microtubule drugs [154]. The Bayesian adaptive design can also be applied in phase I oncology trials, which are conducted in a small number of patients to determine the maximum tolerated dose (MTD) of the drug molecule [155]. A multicentered and non-randomized Bayesian adaptive design study on the γ-secretase inhibitor MK-0752 in combination with gemcitabine was conducted in patients with pancreatic ductal adenocarcinoma and successfully determined the safety of the combination treatment as well as identified the recommended dose for the phase II trial [156]. Yan et al. proposed an intuitive Bayesian keyboard decision method, which relies on the posterior distribution of the toxicity probability and can identify the true MTD with high accuracy [157]. The development of the oncology drugs usually involves a proof-of-concept study (PoC) at the end of the phase I or phase II trial. The PoC study is carried out to obtain an early evidence of the clinical efficacy using a small number of patients. Using a Bayesian framework, the decision making in PoC can be more effective since the direct estimation of evidence is possible for the effect of interest [158]. The Bayesian design can also shorten the duration of a cancer clinical trial by integrating the phase II/III trials into a single confirmatory study. Recently, ComPAS, a novel adaptive shrinkage method was developed using Bayesian model selection and hierarchical methods. This model allows for the dropping of ineffective drugs and the addition of new combinations to ongoing clinical pipelines based on accumulating trial data in an adaptive and seamless fashion [159].

The flexibility of the Bayesian statistics also makes it suitable for the network meta-analysis of pooled data that allows for the simultaneous comparison of multiple treatments. The characteristics of such pooled data are random from trial to trial, differing in the size of the trial, study design, and methodology. The random effects are best handled using Bayesian statistics, which can help to address unanswered questions from controversial clinical trials. The Bayesian network meta-analysis has been applied to assess the role of immunotherapies and targeted therapies in advanced melanoma. This model compared the therapies using the hazard ratio for the overall survival and progression-free survival and the odds ratio for the response rate and probabilities of the drug outperforming others. This meta-analysis suggested that combined BRAF-MEK targeted therapy is optimal for BRAF-mutant patients and can enhance the favorable outcomes in advanced melanoma [160].

Although the Bayesian method has been applied effectively in all phases of drug development in oncology, it is associated with several challenges. The application of the Bayesian method requires decision making regarding prior information, information obtained from the trial and the mathematical model to be used, at the initial design stage itself. A change in the prior information and the quality of the data at a later stage might affect the scientific validity of the trial results. It has been suggested that the type of statistical analysis used in cancer clinical trials should be determined at an earlier stage. The Bayesian adaptive design may suffer from operational biases; thus, the confidentiality of the data needs to be maintained [161]. The recent advances in machine learning algorithms and computational speed have made it possible to carry out calculations for complex Bayesian models. Furthermore, the integration of machine learning methods and statistical tools in drug development pipelines might decrease the cost and time of drug development and also enhance the development of precision medicine for cancer treatment.

6. Issues to Be Overcome in the Application of AI to Oncology

The importance of AI technology has been recognized worldwide, and several countries are promoting AI research as a national policy. Considering its great potential, there are high expectations from AI technology, and it is likely that AI technology will be increasingly introduced in the oncology field in the future. Despite the great potential of AI technology, there is still a number of challenges that need to be overcome. Therefore, we described the key challenges that need to be overcome on an ongoing basis.

6.1. Overfitting

In machine learning and deep learning techniques, overfitting refers to a situation where the training error is small, but the generalization error (the error in determining unknown data) is not small. Particularly in the medical field, where the amount of training data is limited, it is always necessary to carefully judge the generalization performance of the constructed model. We feel that validation is especially important when aiming for the clinical implementation of medical devices with AI; we need to confirm the general performance of these devices through clinical trials more carefully than we have done with conventional medical devices.

6.2. Black Box Problem

Since the analysis process of the machine learning and deep learning techniques is very complex, a black box problem arises in that humans cannot understand the analysis process of the results obtained. The presence of a black box in the system makes it difficult for the designer or user to predict the behavior of the system at the time of design or use and hinders the safety of the system. In Europe, the General Data Protection Regulation (GDPR), which came into force in May 2018, included an article (Article 22) requiring the transparency of AI; consequently, it is necessary to address the black box issue in terms of GDPR regulation compliance [162]. The following three approaches are mainly implemented to improve the interpretability of machine learning and deep learning.

Deep explanation: deep learning state analysis to generate attention heat maps and natural language explanations [163–165].

Interpretable models: machine learning using originally interpretable models (to improve the accuracy of white-box machine learning) [166,167].

Model induction: Create an interpretive model externally that approximates the behavior of black-box machine learning [168–170].

6.3. Discrepancies among Facilities, especially in Medical Imaging (Domain Shift and Domain Adaptation)

Medical imaging analysis is prone to facility characteristics (e.g., different manufacturers of devices, different model numbers of devices, differences in protocols, and differences in operators), and, we along with others, have observed in various studies that the accuracy of predicting data from other facilities is significantly reduced when a trainer built by training on data from one facility is used to predict data from another facility. In general, this problem is called the domain shift problem, and it is an important issue that needs to be resolved for the promotion of medical AI [171–174]. As an important study, we present the results of the analysis and validation of a large number of chest X-ray images using deep learning techniques, published by Pooch et al. [175]. They attempted to evaluate models trained independently on each of A, B, and C, using three large datasets from the U.S. National Institutes of Health (A: 112,120 images), Stanford University Hospital (B: 224,316 images), and the Massachusetts Institute of Technology (C: 379,920 images), with all of the A, B, and C data. When the data were evaluated by splitting the data into 80% training (10% of which were validated) and 20% testing, it was found that the models trained with the data from the same facility as the test data were more accurate, whereas the models trained with data from a different facility were found to be less accurate [175]. The results of this study show that even with such a large set of data, the generalization performance may not be properly evaluated owing to overfitting for each of the datasets. This can be attributed to the fact that the learning sets are independent of each other due to domain shifts. In other words, it was suggested that the model trained with data from each facility was overestimated when tested only with data from the same facility.

Domain adaptation has been proposed as one of the methods to solve the domain shift problem and is being actively studied [172,176–187]. Domain adaptation is a type of transfer learning in which knowledge obtained from a domain with sufficient labeled training data (source domain) is applied to a target domain that lacks sufficient information (target domain) to learn things such as discriminators that work with high accuracy in the target domain (here, a domain is a collection of data). There are several contexts of domain adaptation, and it is necessary to select an appropriate method for the target task.

Unsupervised domain adaptation: the training sample includes a set of labeled source examples, a set of unlabeled source examples, and a set of unlabeled target examples.

Semi-supervised domain adaptation: we also consider a "small" set of labeled target examples.

Supervised domain adaptation: all examples considered are assumed to be labeled.

As an example of the application of domain adaptation to medical image analysis, Qin et al. recently published an interesting study on the multi-center computer-assisted diagnosis of lymph nodes using unsupervised domain adaptation networks based on cross-domain confounding representation (Figure 4) [188]. In general, in order to achieve a robust, high performance computer-aided diagnostic system for lymph nodes, CT images may be collected from multicenter data, which can lead to model isolation based on different data source centers (the domain shift problem described above). However, the lymph node data variation adaptation problem related to the domain adaptation problem in deep learning is different from the general domain adaptation problem because the size of CT images is typically larger and the data distribution is more complex. Therefore, domain adaptation for this problem needs to take into account the shared feature representation of each region, as well as the conditioning information, so that the adaptive network can capture a significant discriminative representation in the domain invariant space. In this study, the authors extracted domain-invariant features based on cross-domain confounding representations, and proposed a cycle-consistency learning framework that encourages the network to retain class conditioning information through cross-domain image translations [188]. Figure 4A shows a conceptual diagram of the method adopted in this study. This method provided a better and more stable performance than did the conventional domain adaptation methods such as gradient reversal layer [189], maximum mean discrepancy [190], and Generate To Adapt [191] for high-resolution medical images with complex feature distribution. Figure 4B shows the process of extracting the cross-region confounding representation of the entire network and the classification cycle consistency after image reconstruction through the source image phase. Compared with the performance of different domain adaptation methods, this method achieved at least 4.4 percentage points higher accuracy for multicenter lymph node data. This method enables the stable domain adaptation of high-resolution images in complex medical fields. Experimental results on simple data distributions also show the generality of the proposed method. Furthermore, the stability of the learning process makes it possible to easily obtain the optimal model under the target domain, which may further realize the integration of multidisciplinary medical data.

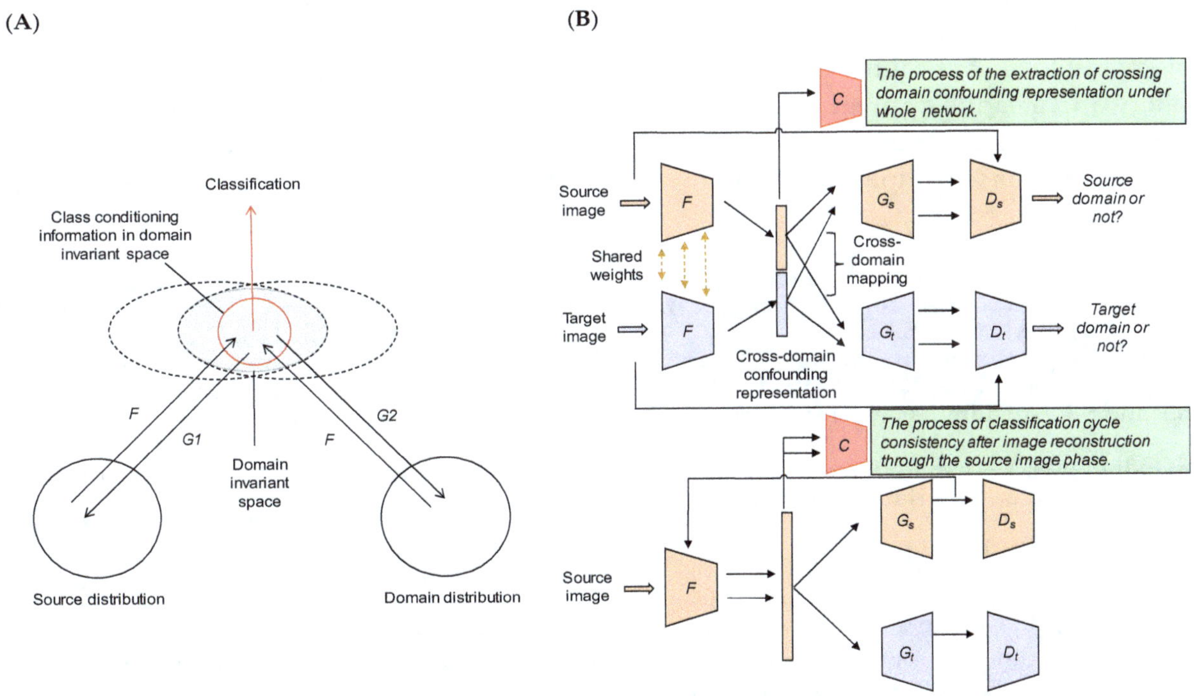

Figure 4. Illustration of the proposed network in Reference 188 (Qin et al., 2020); this is a modified figure from the reference. (**A**) Illustration of the proposed method: a cross-domain confounding representation is generated by constraining the cross-domain mapping reconstruction. (**B**) Domain confounding representation through cross-domain mapping and classification cycle consistency. Encoder F and decoder G constitute the variational automatic encoder (VAE) architecture for unsupervised representation learning. The D module constitutes the GAN discriminator and the C module constitutes the classifier.

Judging from the concept of Bayesian statistics, which is to make predictions based on the prior distribution of probabilities, it can be concluded that having a single algorithm with generalized performance for events with different prior distributions of probabilities from one facility to another is in itself a difficult task. Since AI technology is different from other technologies in that it has the ability to learn on its own, we believe that it is necessary to re-learn and optimize the training data, including the characteristics of each facility, in order to increase the potential of AI as much as possible. In this case, because medical devices themselves continue to evolve, which is a characteristic that conventional medical devices do not have, a multifaceted study that includes not only research and development but also the formulation of guidelines and legislation is necessary.

7. Concluding Remarks and Future Perspectives

In this review article, we described the application of AI technologies in the field of oncology, focusing on machine learning and deep learning technologies. Given that more than 60 types of AI-equipped medical devices have already been approved by the FDA, we believe that AI technology will be used as a core technology in the field of oncology and that the clinical implementation of this technology will steadily increase. Compared with medical image analysis, the introduction of machine learning and deep learning technologies for omics analysis, such as genomics and epigenomics, has lagged behind. However, with the realization of precision medicine as a goal all over the world, the utilization of AI technologies for omics analysis is expected to progressively rise in the future. Furthermore, as we have mentioned in this review, the introduction of AI in drug discovery is an important direction. Nevertheless, as mentioned previously, AI technology still has many problems that need to be addressed. Accordingly, it is important not to have excessive expectations of AI technology but to always calmly and objectively understand the advantages and disadvantages of the technology and steadily apply it to medicine. If humans become dependent on AI as a result of the development of AI, it will not lead to the establishment of an ideal human society. We believe that the ideal situation is for humans and AI to work together to improve the quality of cancer treatment and research.

Author Contributions: Conceptualization: R.H., K.S. (Kruthi Suvarna), M.Y., K.K., N.S., M.M., M.T., S.J., R.S., A.S., K.T., A.B., K.S. (Kanto Shozu), A.D., H.M., S.T., K.A., M.K., J.S. and S.K.; investigation: R.H., K.S. (Kruthi Suvarna), M.Y., K.K., N.S., M.M., M.T., S.J., R.S., A.S., K.T., A.B., K.S. (Kanto Shozu), A.D., H.M., S.T., K.A., M.K., J.S. and S.K.; writing—original draft preparation: R.H. and K.S.(Kruthi Suvarna); writing—review and editing: R.H., K.S. (Kruthi Suvarna), M.Y., K.K., N.S., M.M., M.T., S.J., R.S., A.S., K.T., A.B., K.S. (Kanto Shozu), A.D., H.M., S.T., K.A., M.K., J.S. and S.K. All authors have read and agreed to the published version of the manuscript.

Acknowledgments: We would like to thank all members of the Hamamoto Laboratory. All members provided valuable advice and a comfortable research environment to us.

References

1. Hamamoto, R.; Komatsu, M.; Takasawa, K.; Asada, K.; Kaneko, S. Epigenetics Analysis and Integrated Analysis of Multiomics Data, Including Epigenetic Data, Using Artificial Intelligence in the Era of Precision Medicine. *Biomolecules* **2020**, *10*, 62. [CrossRef] [PubMed]
2. Moor, J. The Dartmouth College Artificial Intelligence Conference: The Next Fifty years. *AI Mag.* **2006**, *27*, 87–89.
3. Fujita, H. AI-based computer-aided diagnosis (AI-CAD): The latest review to read first. *Radiol. Phys. Technol.* **2020**, *13*, 6–19. [CrossRef] [PubMed]
4. Nakaura, T.; Higaki, T.; Awai, K.; Ikeda, O.; Yamashita, Y. A primer for understanding radiology articles about machine learning and deep learning. *Diagn. Interv. Imaging* **2020**. [CrossRef] [PubMed]
5. Chen, X.W.; Gao, J.X. Big Data Bioinformatics. *Methods* **2016**, *111*, 1–2. [CrossRef]
6. Kumar, A.; Kim, J.; Lyndon, D.; Fulham, M.; Feng, D. An Ensemble of Fine-Tuned Convolutional Neural Networks for Medical Image Classification. *IEEE J. Biomed. Health Inform.* **2017**, *21*, 31–40. [CrossRef] [PubMed]
7. Monshi, M.M.A.; Poon, J.; Chung, V. Deep learning in generating radiology reports: A survey. *Artif. Intell. Med.* **2020**, *106*, 101878. [CrossRef]
8. Falk, T.; Mai, D.; Bensch, R.; Cicek, O.; Abdulkadir, A.; Marrakchi, Y.; Bohm, A.; Deubner, J.; Jackel, Z.; Seiwald, K.; et al. U-Net: Deep learning for cell counting, detection, and morphometry. *Nat. Methods* **2019**, *16*, 67–70. [CrossRef]
9. Prasad, V.; Fojo, T.; Brada, M. Precision oncology: Origins, optimism, and potential. *Lancet Oncol.* **2016**, *17*, e81–e86. [CrossRef]
10. Senft, D.; Leiserson, M.D.M.; Ruppin, E.; Ronai, Z.A. Precision Oncology: The Road Ahead. *Trends Mol. Med.* **2017**, *23*, 874–898. [CrossRef]
11. Ku, S.Y.; Gleave, M.E.; Beltran, H. Towards precision oncology in advanced prostate cancer. *Nat. Rev. Urol.* **2019**, *16*, 645–654. [CrossRef] [PubMed]
12. Markman, M. Precision Cancer Medicine. *MD Advis.* **2018**, *11*, 4–6. [PubMed]

13. Rodon, J.; Soria, J.C.; Berger, R.; Miller, W.H.; Rubin, E.; Kugel, A.; Tsimberidou, A.; Saintigny, P.; Ackerstein, A.; Brana, I.; et al. Genomic and transcriptomic profiling expands precision cancer medicine: The WINTHER trial. *Nat. Med.* **2019**, *25*, 751–758. [CrossRef] [PubMed]
14. Zhang, X.; Yang, H.; Zhang, R. Challenges and future of precision medicine strategies for breast cancer based on a database on drug reactions. *Biosci. Rep.* **2019**, *39*. [CrossRef]
15. Prasad, V. Perspective: The precision-oncology illusion. *Nature* **2016**, *537*, S63. [CrossRef]
16. Meric-Bernstam, F.; Brusco, L.; Shaw, K.; Horombe, C.; Kopetz, S.; Davies, M.A.; Routbort, M.; Piha-Paul, S.A.; Janku, F.; Ueno, N.; et al. Feasibility of Large-Scale Genomic Testing to Facilitate Enrollment Onto Genomically Matched Clinical Trials. *J. Clin. Oncol.* **2015**, *33*, 2753–2762. [CrossRef]
17. Bayes, T. An Essay towards solving a Problem in the Doctrine of Chance. *Philos. Trans. R. Soc. Lond.* **1763**, *53*, 370–418. [CrossRef]
18. Gelman, A.; Stern, H.S.; Carlin, J.B.; Dunson, D.B.; Vehtari, A.; Rubin, D.B. *Bayesian Data Analysis*; Chapman and Hall/CRC: Boca Raton, FL, USA, 2013.
19. Fienberg, S.E. When did Bayesian inference become "Bayesian"? *Bayesian Anal.* **2006**, *1*, 1–40. [CrossRef]
20. Solomonoff, R.J. The Time Scale of Artificial Intelligence; Reflections on Social Effects. *Hum. Syst. Manag.* **1985**, *5*, 149–153. [CrossRef]
21. Russell, S.; Norvig, P. *Artificial Intelligence: A Modern Approach*; Prentice Hall: Upper Saddle River, NJ, USA, 1995.
22. Luger, G.; Stubblefield, W. *Artificial Intelligence: Structures and Strategies for Complex Problem Solving*; Benjamin/Cummings: San Francisco, CA, USA, 2004.
23. Nillson, M. *Artificial Intelligence: A New Synthesis*; Morgan Kaufmann: Burlington, MA, USA, 1998.
24. Lindsay, R.; Buchanan, B.; Feigenbaum, E.; Lederberg, J. *Applications of Artificial Intelligence for Organic Chemistry: The DENDRAL Project*; McGraw-Hill: New York, NY, USA, 1980.
25. Shortliffe, E.H. *Computer-Based Medical Consultations: MYCIN*; Elsevier: North Holland, NY, USA, 1976.
26. Feigenbaum, E.A. Knowledge Engineering: The Applied Side of Artificial Intelligence. *Ann. N. Y. Acad. Sci.* **1984**, *1*, 91–107. [CrossRef]
27. Karimi, A.M.; Çelebi, F.V.; Mohammed, A.S. Software Development for Blood Disease Expert System. *Lect. Notes Softw. Eng.* **2016**, *4*, 179–183.
28. Heckerman, D.; Shortliffe, E. From Certainty Factors to Belief Networks. *Artif. Intell. Med.* **1992**, *4*, 35–52. [CrossRef]
29. Hinton, G.E.; Salakhutdinov, R.R. Reducing the Dimensionality of Data with Neural Networks. *Science* **2006**, *313*, 504–507. [CrossRef] [PubMed]
30. Krizhevsky, A.; Sutskever, I.; Hinton, G.E. ImageNet classification with deep convolutional neural networks. *Adv. Neural Inf. Process. Syst.* **2012**, 1097–1105. [CrossRef]
31. Markoff, J. How Many Computers to Identify a Cat? 16,000. *The New York Times*, 25 June 2012.
32. Asada, K.; Kobayashi, K.; Joutard, S.; Tubaki, M.; Takahashi, S.; Takasawa, K.; Komatsu, M.; Kaneko, S.; Sese, J.; Hamamoto, R. Uncovering Prognosis-Related Genes and Pathways by Multi-Omics Analysis in Lung Cancer. *Biomolecules* **2020**, *10*, 524. [CrossRef]
33. Jinnai, S.; Yamazaki, N.; Hirano, Y.; Sugawara, Y.; Ohe, Y.; Hamamoto, R. The Development of a Skin Cancer Classification System for Pigmented Skin Lesions Using Deep Learning. *Biomolecules* **2020**, *10*, 1123. [CrossRef]
34. Kobayashi, K.; Bolatkan, A.; Shiina, S.; Hamamoto, R. Fully-Connected Neural Networks with Reduced Parameterization for Predicting Histological Types of Lung Cancer from Somatic Mutations. *Biomolecules* **2020**, *10*, 1249. [CrossRef]
35. Kobayashi, K.; Hataya, R.; Kurose, Y.; Bolatkan, A.; Miyake, M.; Watanabe, H.; Takahashi, M.; Mihara, N.; Itami, J.; Harada, T.; et al. Unsupervised Brain Abnormality Detection Using High Fidelity Image Reconstruction Networks. *arXiv* **2020**, arXiv:2005.12573.
36. Yamada, M.; Saito, Y.; Imaoka, H.; Saiko, M.; Yamada, S.; Kondo, H.; Takamaru, H.; Sakamoto, T.; Sese, J.; Kuchiba, A.; et al. Development of a real-time endoscopic image diagnosis support system using deep learning technology in colonoscopy. *Sci. Rep.* **2019**, *9*, 14465. [CrossRef]
37. Yasutomi, S.; Arakaki, T.; Hamamoto, R. Shadow Detection for Ultrasound Images Using Unlabeled Data and Synthetic Shadows. *arXiv* **2019**, arXiv:1908.01439.

38. Weisberg, E.M.; Chu, L.C.; Park, S.; Yuille, A.L.; Kinzler, K.W.; Vogelstein, B.; Fishman, E.K. Deep lessons learned: Radiology, oncology, pathology, and computer science experts unite around artificial intelligence to strive for earlier pancreatic cancer diagnosis. *Diagn. Interv. Imaging* **2020**, *101*, 111–115. [CrossRef] [PubMed]
39. Dong, J.; Geng, Y.; Lu, D.; Li, B.; Tian, L.; Lin, D.; Zhang, Y. Clinical Trials for Artificial Intelligence in Cancer Diagnosis: A Cross-Sectional Study of Registered Trials in ClinicalTrials.gov. *Front. Oncol.* **2020**, *10*, 1629. [CrossRef] [PubMed]
40. Blanc, D.; Racine, V.; Khalil, A.; Deloche, M.; Broyelle, J.A.; Hammouamri, I.; Sinitambirivoutin, E.; Fiammante, M.; Verdier, E.; Besson, T.; et al. Artificial intelligence solution to classify pulmonary nodules on CT. *Diagn. Interv. Imaging* **2020**. [CrossRef] [PubMed]
41. Jiang, Y.; Edwards, A.V.; Newstead, G.M. Artificial Intelligence Applied to Breast MRI for Improved Diagnosis. *Radiology* **2020**, 200292. [CrossRef]
42. European Society of Radiology. What the radiologist should know about artificial intelligence—An ESR white paper. *Insights Imaging* **2019**, *10*, 44. [CrossRef]
43. Qin, C.; Yao, D.; Shi, Y.; Song, Z. Computer-aided detection in chest radiography based on artificial intelligence: A survey. *Biomed. Eng. Online* **2018**, *17*, 113. [CrossRef]
44. Wang, S.; Burtt, K.; Turkbey, B.; Choyke, P.; Summers, R.M. Computer aided-diagnosis of prostate cancer on multiparametric MRI: A technical review of current research. *Biomed. Res. Int.* **2014**, *2014*, 789561. [CrossRef]
45. Transin, S.; Souchon, R.; Gonindard-Melodelima, C.; de Rozario, R.; Walker, P.; de la Vega, M.F.; Loffroy, R.; Cormier, L.; Rouviere, O. Computer-aided diagnosis system for characterizing ISUP grade>/=2 prostate cancers at multiparametric MRI: A cross-vendor evaluation. *Diagn. Interv. Imaging* **2019**, *100*, 801–811. [CrossRef]
46. Hizukuri, A.; Nakayama, R.; Nara, M.; Suzuki, M.; Namba, K. Computer-Aided Diagnosis Scheme for Distinguishing Between Benign and Malignant Masses on Breast DCE-MRI Images Using Deep Convolutional Neural Network with Bayesian Optimization. *J. Digit. Imaging* **2020**. [CrossRef]
47. Huang, F.; Zhang, Z.; Wang, N.; Li, N.; Du, M.; Hao, T.; Zhan, J. A new direction to promote the implementation of artificial intelligence in natural clinical settings. *arXiv* **2019**, arXiv:1905.02940.
48. Ha, E.J.; Baek, J.H. Application of machine learning and deep learning to thyroid imaging: Where do we stand? *Ultrasonography* **2020**. [CrossRef] [PubMed]
49. Dlamini, Z.; Francies, F.Z.; Hull, R.; Marima, R. Artificial intelligence (AI) and big data in cancer and precision oncology. *Comput. Struct. Biotechnol. J.* **2020**, *18*, 2300–2311. [CrossRef] [PubMed]
50. Hwang, T.J.; Kesselheim, A.S.; Vokinger, K.N. Lifecycle Regulation of Artificial Intelligence- and Machine Learning-Based Software Devices in Medicine. *JAMA* **2019**. [CrossRef] [PubMed]
51. Tanenbaum, L.N. Artificial Intelligence and Medical Imaging: Image Acquisition and Reconstruction. *Appl. Radiol.* **2020**, *49*, 34–35.
52. Bryant, M. The Potential and Reality of AI in Clinical Application. *Appl. Radiol.* **2020**, *49*, 10–11.
53. Hsieh, J.; Liu, E.; Nett, B.; Tang, J.; Thibault, J.B.; Sahney, S. *A New Era of Image Reconstruction: TrueFidelity™. Technical White Paper on Deep Learning Image Reconstruction*; GE Healthcare: Chicago, IL, USA, 2019.
54. Bryant, M.; Massat, M.B. The Ubiquity of AI at RSNA 2019. *Appl. Radiol.* **2020**, *49*, 32–38.
55. Ministry of Economy, Trade and Industry. The Medical Device Industry in Japan. Report from the Medical and Assistive Device Industries Office, 2018. Available online: https://www.meti.go.jp/committee/kenkyukai/iryou_innovation/pdf/002_05_00.pdf (accessed on 8 February 2018).
56. Kudo, S.E.; Misawa, M.; Mori, Y.; Hotta, K.; Ohtsuka, K.; Ikematsu, H.; Saito, Y.; Takeda, K.; Nakamura, H.; Ichimasa, K.; et al. Artificial Intelligence-assisted System Improves Endoscopic Identification of Colorectal Neoplasms. *Clin. Gastroenterol. Hepatol.* **2020**, *18*, 1874–1881.e2. [CrossRef]
57. Hori, M.; Matsuda, T.; Shibata, A.; Katanoda, K.; Sobue, T.; Nishimoto, H.; Japan Cancer Surveillance Research Group. Cancer incidence and incidence rates in Japan in 2009: A study of 32 population-based cancer registries for the Monitoring of Cancer Incidence in Japan (MCIJ) project. *Jpn. J. Clin. Oncol.* **2015**, *45*, 884–891. [CrossRef]
58. Winawer, S.J.; Zauber, A.G.; Ho, M.N.; O'Brien, M.J.; Gottlieb, L.S.; Sternberg, S.S.; Waye, J.D.; Schapiro, M.; Bond, J.H.; Panish, J.F.; et al. Prevention of colorectal cancer by colonoscopic polypectomy. The National Polyp Study Workgroup. *N. Engl. J. Med.* **1993**, *329*, 1977–1981. [CrossRef]
59. Zauber, A.G.; Winawer, S.J.; O'Brien, M.J.; Lansdorp-Vogelaar, I.; van Ballegooijen, M.; Hankey, B.F.; Shi, W.; Bond, J.H.; Schapiro, M.; Panish, J.F.; et al. Colonoscopic polypectomy and long-term prevention of colorectal-cancer deaths. *N. Engl. J. Med.* **2012**, *366*, 687–696. [CrossRef]

60. Metter, D.M.; Colgan, T.J.; Leung, S.T.; Timmons, C.F.; Park, J.Y. Trends in the US and Canadian Pathologist Workforces From 2007 to 2017. *JAMA Netw. Open* **2019**, *2*, e194337. [CrossRef] [PubMed]
61. Yoshizawa, A. A trial of integrated telepathology (iTP) in Nagano prefecture. *Rinsho. Byori.* **2013**, *61*, 65–73. [PubMed]
62. Coudray, N.; Ocampo, P.S.; Sakellaropoulos, T.; Narula, N.; Snuderl, M.; Fenyo, D.; Moreira, A.L.; Razavian, N.; Tsirigos, A. Classification and mutation prediction from non-small cell lung cancer histopathology images using deep learning. *Nat. Med.* **2018**, *24*, 1559–1567. [CrossRef] [PubMed]
63. Schadendorf, D.; van Akkooi, A.C.J.; Berking, C.; Griewank, K.G.; Gutzmer, R.; Hauschild, A.; Stang, A.; Roesch, A.; Ugurel, S. Melanoma. *Lancet* **2018**, *392*, 971–984. [CrossRef]
64. Melanoma of the Skin 2019 . In *Cancer Stat Facts*; National Cancer Institute: Bethesda, MD, USA, 2019.
65. Esteva, A.; Kuprel, B.; Novoa, R.A.; Ko, J.; Swetter, S.M.; Blau, H.M.; Thrun, S. Dermatologist-level classification of skin cancer with deep neural networks. *Nature* **2017**, *542*, 115–118. [CrossRef]
66. Collins, F.S.; Morgan, M.; Patrinos, A. The Human Genome Project: Lessons from large-scale biology. *Science* **2003**, *300*, 286–290. [CrossRef]
67. Auffray, C.; Caulfield, T.; Khoury, M.J.; Lupski, J.R.; Schwab, M.; Veenstra, T. Genome Medicine: Past, present and future. *Genome Med.* **2011**, *3*, 6. [CrossRef]
68. Ashley, E.A. The precision medicine initiative: A new national effort. *JAMA* **2015**, *313*, 2119–2120. [CrossRef]
69. Oki, S.; Sone, K.; Oda, K.; Hamamoto, R.; Ikemura, M.; Maeda, D.; Takeuchi, M.; Tanikawa, M.; Mori-Uchino, M.; Nagasaka, K.; et al. Oncogenic histone methyltransferase EZH2: A novel prognostic marker with therapeutic potential in endometrial cancer. *Oncotarget* **2017**, *8*, 40402–40411. [CrossRef]
70. Saloura, V.; Vougiouklakis, T.; Zewde, M.; Deng, X.; Kiyotani, K.; Park, J.H.; Matsuo, Y.; Lingen, M.; Suzuki, T.; Dohmae, N.; et al. WHSC1L1-mediated EGFR mono-methylation enhances the cytoplasmic and nuclear oncogenic activity of EGFR in head and neck cancer. *Sci. Rep.* **2017**, *7*, 40664. [CrossRef]
71. Yoshioka, Y.; Suzuki, T.; Matsuo, Y.; Nakakido, M.; Tsurita, G.; Simone, C.; Watanabe, T.; Dohmae, N.; Nakamura, Y.; Hamamoto, R. SMYD3-mediated lysine methylation in the PH domain is critical for activation of AKT1. *Oncotarget* **2016**, *7*, 75023–75037. [CrossRef] [PubMed]
72. Saloura, V.; Vougiouklakis, T.; Zewde, M.; Kiyotani, K.; Park, J.H.; Gao, G.; Karrison, T.; Lingen, M.; Nakamura, Y.; Hamamoto, R. WHSC1L1 drives cell cycle progression through transcriptional regulation of CDC6 and CDK2 in squamous cell carcinoma of the head and neck. *Oncotarget* **2016**, *7*, 42527–42538. [CrossRef] [PubMed]
73. Shigekawa, Y.; Hayami, S.; Ueno, M.; Miyamoto, A.; Suzaki, N.; Kawai, M.; Hirono, S.; Okada, K.I.; Hamamoto, R.; Yamaue, H. Overexpression of KDM5B/JARID1B is associated with poor prognosis in hepatocellular carcinoma. *Oncotarget* **2018**, *9*, 34320–34335. [CrossRef] [PubMed]
74. Kim, S.K.; Kim, K.; Ryu, J.W.; Ryu, T.Y.; Lim, J.H.; Oh, J.H.; Min, J.K.; Jung, C.R.; Hamamoto, R.; Son, M.Y.; et al. The novel prognostic marker, EHMT2, is involved in cell proliferation via HSPD1 regulation in breast cancer. *Int. J. Oncol.* **2019**, *54*, 65–76. [CrossRef]
75. Toyokawa, G.; Takada, K.; Tagawa, T.; Hamamoto, R.; Yamada, Y.; Shimokawa, M.; Oda, Y.; Maehara, Y. A Positive Correlation Between the EZH2 and PD-L1 Expression in Resected Lung Adenocarcinomas. *Ann. Thorac. Surg.* **2019**, *107*, 393–400. [CrossRef]
76. Toyokawa, G.; Takada, K.; Tagawa, T.; Kinoshita, F.; Kozuma, Y.; Matsubara, T.; Haratake, N.; Takamori, S.; Akamine, T.; Hirai, F.; et al. Prevalence of Enhancer of Zeste Homolog 2 in Patients with Resected Small Cell Lung Cancer. *Anticancer Res.* **2018**, *38*, 3707–3711. [CrossRef]
77. Ryu, J.W.; Kim, S.K.; Son, M.Y.; Jeon, S.J.; Oh, J.H.; Lim, J.H.; Cho, S.; Jung, C.R.; Hamamoto, R.; Kim, D.S.; et al. Novel prognostic marker PRMT1 regulates cell growth via downregulation of CDKN1A in HCC. *Oncotarget* **2017**, *8*, 115444–115455. [CrossRef]
78. Kim, S.; Bolatkan, A.; Kaneko, S.; Ikawa, N.; Asada, K.; Komatsu, M.; Hayami, S.; Ojima, H.; Abe, N.; Yamaue, H.; et al. Deregulation of the Histone Lysine-Specific Demethylase 1 Is Involved in Human Hepatocellular Carcinoma. *Biomolecules* **2019**, *9*, 810. [CrossRef]
79. Saloura, V.; Vougiouklakis, T.; Bao, R.; Kim, S.; Baek, S.; Zewde, M.; Bernard, B.; Burkitt, K.; Nigam, N.; Izumchenko, E.; et al. WHSC1 monomethylates histone H1 and induces stem-cell like features in squamous cell carcinoma of the head and neck. *Neoplasia* **2020**, *22*, 283–293. [CrossRef]
80. Asada, K.; Bolatkan, A.; Takasawa, K.; Komatsu, M.; Kaneko, S.; Hamamoto, R. Critical Roles of N(6)-Methyladenosine (m(6)A) in Cancer and Virus Infection. *Biomolecules* **2020**, *10*, 1071. [CrossRef]

81. Kojima, M.; Sone, K.; Oda, K.; Hamamoto, R.; Kaneko, S.; Oki, S.; Kukita, A.; Kawata, A.; Honjoh, H.; Kawata, Y.; et al. The histone methyltransferase SMYD2 is a novel therapeutic target for the induction of apoptosis in ovarian clear cell carcinoma cells. *Oncol. Lett.* **2020**, *20*, 153. [CrossRef] [PubMed]
82. Sone, K.; Piao, L.; Nakakido, M.; Ueda, K.; Jenuwein, T.; Nakamura, Y.; Hamamoto, R. Critical role of lysine 134 methylation on histone H2AX for gamma-H2AX production and DNA repair. *Nat. Commun.* **2014**, *5*, 5691. [CrossRef] [PubMed]
83. Cho, H.S.; Kelly, J.D.; Hayami, S.; Toyokawa, G.; Takawa, M.; Yoshimatsu, M.; Tsunoda, T.; Field, H.I.; Neal, D.E.; Ponder, B.A.; et al. Enhanced expression of EHMT2 is involved in the proliferation of cancer cells through negative regulation of SIAH1. *Neoplasia* **2011**, *13*, 676–684. [CrossRef] [PubMed]
84. Cho, H.S.; Toyokawa, G.; Daigo, Y.; Hayami, S.; Masuda, K.; Ikawa, N.; Yamane, Y.; Maejima, K.; Tsunoda, T.; Field, H.I.; et al. The JmjC domain-containing histone demethylase KDM3A is a positive regulator of the G1/S transition in cancer cells via transcriptional regulation of the HOXA1 gene. *Int. J. Cancer* **2012**, *131*, E179–E189. [CrossRef] [PubMed]
85. Hamamoto, R.; Furukawa, Y.; Morita, M.; Iimura, Y.; Silva, F.P.; Li, M.; Yagyu, R.; Nakamura, Y. SMYD3 encodes a histone methyltransferase involved in the proliferation of cancer cells. *Nat. Cell Biol.* **2004**, *6*, 731–740. [CrossRef]
86. Hamamoto, R.; Silva, F.P.; Tsuge, M.; Nishidate, T.; Katagiri, T.; Nakamura, Y.; Furukawa, Y. Enhanced SMYD3 expression is essential for the growth of breast cancer cells. *Cancer Sci.* **2006**, *97*, 113–118. [CrossRef]
87. Hayami, S.; Kelly, J.D.; Cho, H.S.; Yoshimatsu, M.; Unoki, M.; Tsunoda, T.; Field, H.I.; Neal, D.E.; Yamaue, H.; Ponder, B.A.; et al. Overexpression of LSD1 contributes to human carcinogenesis through chromatin regulation in various cancers. *Int. J. Cancer* **2011**, *128*, 574–586. [CrossRef]
88. Hayami, S.; Yoshimatsu, M.; Veerakumarasivam, A.; Unoki, M.; Iwai, Y.; Tsunoda, T.; Field, H.I.; Kelly, J.D.; Neal, D.E.; Yamaue, H.; et al. Overexpression of the JmjC histone demethylase KDM5B in human carcinogenesis: Involvement in the proliferation of cancer cells through the E2F/RB pathway. *Mol. Cancer* **2010**, *9*, 59. [CrossRef]
89. Kang, D.; Cho, H.S.; Toyokawa, G.; Kogure, M.; Yamane, Y.; Iwai, Y.; Hayami, S.; Tsunoda, T.; Field, H.I.; Matsuda, K.; et al. The histone methyltransferase Wolf-Hirschhorn syndrome candidate 1-like 1 (WHSC1L1) is involved in human carcinogenesis. *Genes Chromosomes Cancer* **2013**, *52*, 126–139. [CrossRef]
90. Mutonga, M.; Tamura, K.; Malnassy, G.; Fulton, N.; de Albuquerque, A.; Hamamoto, R.; Stock, W.; Nakamura, Y.; Alachkar, H. Targeting Suppressor of Variegation 3-9 Homologue 2 (SUV39H2) in Acute Lymphoblastic Leukemia (ALL). *Transl. Oncol.* **2015**, *8*, 368–375. [CrossRef]
91. Saloura, V.; Cho, H.S.; Kyiotani, K.; Alachkar, H.; Zuo, Z.; Nakakido, M.; Tsunoda, T.; Seiwert, T.; Lingen, M.; Licht, J.; et al. WHSC1 Promotes Oncogenesis through Regulation of NIMA-related-kinase-7 in Squamous Cell Carcinoma of the Head and Neck. *Mol. Cancer Res.* **2015**, *13*, 293–304. [CrossRef] [PubMed]
92. Silva, F.P.; Hamamoto, R.; Kunizaki, M.; Tsuge, M.; Nakamura, Y.; Furukawa, Y. Enhanced methyltransferase activity of SMYD3 by the cleavage of its N-terminal region in human cancer cells. *Oncogene* **2008**, *27*, 2686–2692. [CrossRef] [PubMed]
93. Toyokawa, G.; Cho, H.S.; Iwai, Y.; Yoshimatsu, M.; Takawa, M.; Hayami, S.; Maejima, K.; Shimizu, N.; Tanaka, H.; Tsunoda, T.; et al. The histone demethylase JMJD2B plays an essential role in human carcinogenesis through positive regulation of cyclin-dependent kinase 6. *Cancer Prev. Res.* **2011**, *4*, 2051–2061. [CrossRef] [PubMed]
94. Toyokawa, G.; Cho, H.S.; Masuda, K.; Yamane, Y.; Yoshimatsu, M.; Hayami, S.; Takawa, M.; Iwai, Y.; Daigo, Y.; Tsuchiya, E.; et al. Histone Lysine Methyltransferase Wolf-Hirschhorn Syndrome Candidate 1 Is Involved in Human Carcinogenesis through Regulation of the Wnt Pathway. *Neoplasia* **2011**, *13*, 887–898. [CrossRef]
95. Takawa, M.; Masuda, K.; Kunizaki, M.; Daigo, Y.; Takagi, K.; Iwai, Y.; Cho, H.S.; Toyokawa, G.; Yamane, Y.; Maejima, K.; et al. Validation of the histone methyltransferase EZH2 as a therapeutic target for various types of human cancer and as a prognostic marker. *Cancer Sci.* **2011**, *102*, 1298–1305. [CrossRef] [PubMed]
96. Tsuge, M.; Hamamoto, R.; Silva, F.P.; Ohnishi, Y.; Chayama, K.; Kamatani, N.; Furukawa, Y.; Nakamura, Y. A variable number of tandem repeats polymorphism in an E2F-1 binding element in the 5′ flanking region of SMYD3 is a risk factor for human cancers. *Nat. Genet.* **2005**, *37*, 1104–1107. [CrossRef]
97. Miles, W.O.; Lepesant, J.M.; Bourdeaux, J.; Texier, M.; Kerenyi, M.A.; Nakakido, M.; Hamamoto, R.; Orkin, S.H.; Dyson, N.J.; Di Stefano, L. The LSD1 Family of Histone Demethylases and the Pumilio Posttranscriptional Repressor Function in a Complex Regulatory Feedback Loop. *Mol. Cell. Biol.* **2015**, *35*, 4199–4211. [CrossRef]

98. Yoshimatsu, M.; Toyokawa, G.; Hayami, S.; Unoki, M.; Tsunoda, T.; Field, H.I.; Kelly, J.D.; Neal, D.E.; Maehara, Y.; Ponder, B.A.; et al. Dysregulation of PRMT1 and PRMT6, Type I arginine methyltransferases, is involved in various types of human cancers. *Int. J. Cancer* **2011**, *128*, 562–573. [CrossRef]
99. Toyokawa, G.; Taguchi, K.; Edagawa, M.; Shimamatsu, S.; Toyozawa, R.; Nosaki, K.; Hirai, F.; Yamaguchi, M.; Shimokawa, M.; Seto, T.; et al. The Prognostic Impact of Jumonji Domain-containing 2B in Patients with Resected Lung Adenocarcinoma. *Anticancer Res.* **2016**, *36*, 4841–4846. [CrossRef]
100. Hamamoto, R.; Saloura, V.; Nakamura, Y. Critical roles of non-histone protein lysine methylation in human tumorigenesis. *Nat. Rev. Cancer* **2015**, *15*, 110–124. [CrossRef]
101. Hamamoto, R.; Nakamura, Y. Dysregulation of protein methyltransferases in human cancer: An emerging target class for anticancer therapy. *Cancer Sci.* **2016**, *107*, 377–384. [CrossRef] [PubMed]
102. Vougiouklakis, T.; Hamamoto, R.; Nakamura, Y.; Saloura, V. The NSD family of protein methyltransferases in human cancer. *Epigenomics* **2015**, *7*, 863–874. [CrossRef] [PubMed]
103. Berdasco, M.; Esteller, M. Clinical epigenetics: Seizing opportunities for translation. *Nat. Rev. Genet.* **2019**, *20*, 109–127. [CrossRef] [PubMed]
104. Kukita, A.; Sone, K.; Oda, K.; Hamamoto, R.; Kaneko, S.; Komatsu, M.; Wada, M.; Honjoh, H.; Kawata, Y.; Kojima, M.; et al. Histone methyltransferase SMYD2 selective inhibitor LLY-507 in combination with poly ADP ribose polymerase inhibitor has therapeutic potential against high-grade serous ovarian carcinomas. *Biochem. Biophys. Res. Commun.* **2019**, *513*, 340–346. [CrossRef]
105. Chaudhary, K.; Poirion, O.B.; Lu, L.; Garmire, L.X. Deep Learning-Based Multi-Omics Integration Robustly Predicts Survival in Liver Cancer. *Clin. Cancer Res.* **2018**, *24*, 1248–1259. [CrossRef]
106. Takahashi, S.; Asada, K.; Takasawa, K.; Shimoyama, R.; Sakai, A.; Bolatkan, A.; Shinkai, N.; Kobayashi, K.; Komatsu, M.; Kaneko, S.; et al. Predicting Deep Learning Based Multi-Omics Parallel Integration Survival Subtypes in Lung Cancer Using Reverse Phase Protein Array Data. *Biomolecules* **2020**, *10*, 1460. [CrossRef]
107. Diao, G.; Vidyashankar, A.N. Assessing genome-wide statistical significance for large p small n problems. *Genetics* **2013**, *194*, 781–783. [CrossRef]
108. Romero, A.; Carrier, P.L.; Erraqabi, A.; Sylvain, T.; Auvolat, A.; Dejoie, E.; Legault, M.A.; Dubé, M.P.; Hussin, J.G.; Bengio, Y. Diet Networks: Thin Parameters for Fat Genomics. *arXiv* **2016**, arXiv:1611.09340.
109. Clayton, E.A.; Pujol, T.A.; McDonald, J.F.; Qiu, P. Leveraging TCGA gene expression data to build predictive models for cancer drug response. *BMC Bioinform.* **2020**, *21*, 364. [CrossRef]
110. Naulaerts, S.; Menden, M.P.; Ballester, P.J. Concise Polygenic Models for Cancer-Specific Identification of Drug-Sensitive Tumors from Their Multi-Omics Profiles. *Biomolecules* **2020**, *10*, 963. [CrossRef]
111. Tolios, A.; De Las Rivas, J.; Hovig, E.; Trouillas, P.; Scorilas, A.; Mohr, T. Computational approaches in cancer multidrug resistance research: Identification of potential biomarkers, drug targets and drug-target interactions. *Drug Resist. Updat.* **2020**, *48*, 100662. [CrossRef] [PubMed]
112. Liu, Q.; Muglia, L.J.; Huang, L.F. Network as a Biomarker: A Novel Network-Based Sparse Bayesian Machine for Pathway-Driven Drug Response Prediction. *Genes* **2019**, *10*, 602. [CrossRef] [PubMed]
113. Song, P.; Cui, X.; Bai, L.; Zhou, X.; Zhu, X.; Zhang, J.; Jin, F.; Zhao, J.; Zhou, C.; Zhou, Y.; et al. Molecular characterization of clinical responses to PD-1/PD-L1 inhibitors in non-small cell lung cancer: Predictive value of multidimensional immunomarker detection for the efficacy of PD-1 inhibitors in Chinese patients. *Thorac. Cancer* **2019**, *10*, 1303–1309. [CrossRef] [PubMed]
114. Ali, M.; Aittokallio, T. Machine learning and feature selection for drug response prediction in precision oncology applications. *Biophys. Rev.* **2019**, *11*, 31–39. [CrossRef]
115. Shukla, A.; Nguyen, T.H.M.; Moka, S.B.; Ellis, J.J.; Grady, J.P.; Oey, H.; Cristino, A.S.; Khanna, K.K.; Kroese, D.P.; Krause, L.; et al. Chromosome arm aneuploidies shape tumour evolution and drug response. *Nat. Commun.* **2020**, *11*, 449. [CrossRef]
116. Rendeiro, A.F.; Krausgruber, T.; Fortelny, N.; Zhao, F.; Penz, T.; Farlik, M.; Schuster, L.C.; Nemc, A.; Tasnady, S.; Reti, M.; et al. Chromatin mapping and single-cell immune profiling define the temporal dynamics of ibrutinib response in CLL. *Nat. Commun.* **2020**, *11*, 577. [CrossRef]
117. Sever, R.; Brugge, J.S. Signal transduction in cancer. *Cold Spring Harb. Perspect. Med.* **2015**, *5*, a006098. [CrossRef]

118. Chiyoda, T.; Hart, P.C.; Eckert, M.A.; McGregor, S.M.; Lastra, R.R.; Hamamoto, R.; Nakamura, Y.; Yamada, S.D.; Olopade, O.I.; Lengyel, E.; et al. Loss of BRCA1 in the Cells of Origin of Ovarian Cancer Induces Glycolysis: A Window of Opportunity for Ovarian Cancer Chemoprevention. *Cancer Prev. Res.* **2017**, *10*, 255–266. [CrossRef]
119. Cho, H.S.; Hayami, S.; Toyokawa, G.; Maejima, K.; Yamane, Y.; Suzuki, T.; Dohmae, N.; Kogure, M.; Kang, D.; Neal, D.E.; et al. RB1 methylation by SMYD2 enhances cell cycle progression through an increase of RB1 phosphorylation. *Neoplasia* **2012**, *14*, 476–486. [CrossRef]
120. Cho, H.S.; Shimazu, T.; Toyokawa, G.; Daigo, Y.; Maehara, Y.; Hayami, S.; Ito, A.; Masuda, K.; Ikawa, N.; Field, H.I.; et al. Enhanced HSP70 lysine methylation promotes proliferation of cancer cells through activation of Aurora kinase B. *Nat. Commun.* **2012**, *3*, 1072. [CrossRef]
121. Cho, H.S.; Suzuki, T.; Dohmae, N.; Hayami, S.; Unoki, M.; Yoshimatsu, M.; Toyokawa, G.; Takawa, M.; Chen, T.; Kurash, J.K.; et al. Demethylation of RB regulator MYPT1 by histone demethylase LSD1 promotes cell cycle progression in cancer cells. *Cancer Res.* **2011**, *71*, 655–660. [CrossRef] [PubMed]
122. Deng, X.; Hamamoto, R.; Vougiouklakis, T.; Wang, R.; Yoshioka, Y.; Suzuki, T.; Dohmae, N.; Matsuo, Y.; Park, J.H.; Nakamura, Y. Critical roles of SMYD2-mediated beta-catenin methylation for nuclear translocation and activation of Wnt signaling. *Oncotarget* **2017**, *8*, 55837–55847. [CrossRef] [PubMed]
123. Deng, X.; Von Keudell, G.; Suzuki, T.; Dohmae, N.; Nakakido, M.; Piao, L.; Yoshioka, Y.; Nakamura, Y.; Hamamoto, R. PRMT1 promotes mitosis of cancer cells through arginine methylation of INCENP. *Oncotarget* **2015**. [CrossRef] [PubMed]
124. Deng, Z.; Matsuda, K.; Tanikawa, C.; Lin, J.; Furukawa, Y.; Hamamoto, R.; Nakamura, Y. Late Cornified Envelope Group I, a novel target of p53, regulates PRMT5 activity. *Neoplasia* **2014**, *16*, 656–664. [CrossRef]
125. Hamamoto, R.; Toyokawa, G.; Nakakido, M.; Ueda, K.; Nakamura, Y. SMYD2-dependent HSP90 methylation promotes cancer cell proliferation by regulating the chaperone complex formation. *Cancer Lett.* **2014**, *351*, 126–133. [CrossRef]
126. Kunizaki, M.; Hamamoto, R.; Silva, F.P.; Yamaguchi, K.; Nagayasu, T.; Shibuya, M.; Nakamura, Y.; Furukawa, Y. The lysine 831 of vascular endothelial growth factor receptor 1 is a novel target of methylation by SMYD3. *Cancer Res.* **2007**, *67*, 10759–10765. [CrossRef]
127. Matsuno, Y.; Atsumi, Y.; Shimizu, A.; Katayama, K.; Fujimori, H.; Hyodo, M.; Minakawa, Y.; Nakatsu, Y.; Kaneko, S.; Hamamoto, R.; et al. Replication stress triggers microsatellite destabilization and hypermutation leading to clonal expansion in vitro. *Nat. Commun.* **2019**, *10*, 3925. [CrossRef]
128. Nakakido, M.; Deng, Z.; Suzuki, T.; Dohmae, N.; Nakamura, Y.; Hamamoto, R. Dysregulation of AKT Pathway by SMYD2-Mediated Lysine Methylation on PTEN. *Neoplasia* **2015**, *17*, 367–373. [CrossRef]
129. Nakakido, M.; Deng, Z.; Suzuki, T.; Dohmae, N.; Nakamura, Y.; Hamamoto, R. PRMT6 increases cytoplasmic localization of p21CDKN1A in cancer cells through arginine methylation and makes more resistant to cytotoxic agents. *Oncotarget* **2015**, *6*, 30957–30967. [CrossRef]
130. Obama, K.; Satoh, S.; Hamamoto, R.; Sakai, Y.; Nakamura, Y.; Furukawa, Y. Enhanced expression of RAD51 associating protein-1 is involved in the growth of intrahepatic cholangiocarcinoma cells. *Clin. Cancer Res.* **2008**, *14*, 1333–1339. [CrossRef]
131. Piao, L.; Fujioka, K.; Nakakido, M.; Hamamoto, R. Regulation of poly(ADP-Ribose) polymerase 1 functions by post-translational modifications. *Front. Biosci.* **2018**, *23*, 13–26.
132. Piao, L.; Kang, D.; Suzuki, T.; Masuda, A.; Dohmae, N.; Nakamura, Y.; Hamamoto, R. The histone methyltransferase SMYD2 methylates PARP1 and promotes poly(ADP-ribosyl)ation activity in cancer cells. *Neoplasia* **2014**, *16*, 257–264. [CrossRef] [PubMed]
133. Piao, L.; Suzuki, T.; Dohmae, N.; Nakamura, Y.; Hamamoto, R. SUV39H2 methylates and stabilizes LSD1 by inhibiting polyubiquitination in human cancer cells. *Oncotarget* **2015**, *6*, 16939–16950. [CrossRef] [PubMed]
134. Takahashi, M.; Fujita, M.; Furukawa, Y.; Hamamoto, R.; Shimokawa, T.; Miwa, N.; Ogawa, M.; Nakamura, Y. Isolation of a novel human gene, APCDD1, as a direct target of the beta-Catenin/T-cell factor 4 complex with probable involvement in colorectal carcinogenesis. *Cancer Res.* **2002**, *62*, 5651–5656. [PubMed]
135. Takawa, M.; Cho, H.S.; Hayami, S.; Toyokawa, G.; Kogure, M.; Yamane, Y.; Iwai, Y.; Maejima, K.; Ueda, K.; Masuda, A.; et al. Histone Lysine Methyltransferase SETD8 Promotes Carcinogenesis by Deregulating PCNA Expression. *Cancer Res.* **2012**, *72*, 3217–3227. [CrossRef] [PubMed]

136. Toyokawa, G.; Masuda, K.; Daigo, Y.; Cho, H.S.; Yoshimatsu, M.; Takawa, M.; Hayami, S.; Maejima, K.; Chino, M.; Field, H.I.; et al. Minichromosome Maintenance Protein 7 is a potential therapeutic target in human cancer and a novel prognostic marker of non-small cell lung cancer. *Mol. Cancer* **2011**, *10*, 65. [CrossRef] [PubMed]
137. Yagyu, R.; Hamamoto, R.; Furukawa, Y.; Okabe, H.; Yamamura, T.; Nakamura, Y.; Osada, H.; Hamamoto, R.; Simizu, S. Isolation and characterization of a novel human gene, VANGL1, as a therapeutic target for hepatocellular carcinoma. *Int. J. Oncol.* **2002**, *20*, 1173–1178. [CrossRef]
138. Yoshioka, Y.; Suzuki, T.; Matsuo, Y.; Tsurita, G.; Watanabe, T.; Dohmae, N.; Nakamura, Y.; Hamamoto, R. Protein lysine methyltransferase SMYD3 is involved in tumorigenesis through regulation of HER2 homodimerization. *Cancer Med.* **2017**, *6*, 1665–1672. [CrossRef]
139. Kim, S.; Bae, W.J.; Ahn, J.M.; Heo, J.H.; Kim, K.M.; Choi, K.W.; Sung, C.O.; Lee, D. MicroRNA signatures associated with lymph node metastasis in intramucosal gastric cancer. *Mod. Pathol.* **2020**. [CrossRef]
140. Kouznetsova, V.L.; Li, J.; Romm, E.; Tsigelny, I.F. Finding distinctions between oral cancer and periodontitis using saliva metabolites and machine learning. *Oral Dis.* **2020**. [CrossRef]
141. Eicher, T.; Kinnebrew, G.; Patt, A.; Spencer, K.; Ying, K.; Ma, Q.; Machiraju, R.; Mathe, A.E.A. Metabolomics and Multi-Omics Integration: A Survey of Computational Methods and Resources. *Metabolites* **2020**, *10*, 202. [CrossRef] [PubMed]
142. Milanez-Almeida, P.; Martins, A.J.; Germain, R.N.; Tsang, J.S. Cancer prognosis with shallow tumor RNA sequencing. *Nat. Med.* **2020**, *26*, 188–192. [CrossRef] [PubMed]
143. Sanchez, R.; Mackenzie, S.A. Integrative Network Analysis of Differentially Methylated and Expressed Genes for Biomarker Identification in Leukemia. *Sci. Rep.* **2020**, *10*, 2123. [CrossRef] [PubMed]
144. Kim, Y.; Bismeijer, T.; Zwart, W.; Wessels, L.F.A.; Vis, D.J. Genomic data integration by WON-PARAFAC identifies interpretable factors for predicting drug-sensitivity in vivo. *Nat. Commun.* **2019**, *10*, 5034. [CrossRef]
145. Keshava, N.; Toh, T.S.; Yuan, H.; Yang, B.; Menden, M.P.; Wang, D. Defining subpopulations of differential drug response to reveal novel target populations. *NPJ Syst. Biol. Appl.* **2019**, *5*, 36. [CrossRef]
146. Norman, T.M.; Horlbeck, M.A.; Replogle, J.M.; Ge, A.Y.; Xu, A.; Jost, M.; Gilbert, L.A.; Weissman, J.S. Exploring genetic interaction manifolds constructed from rich single-cell phenotypes. *Science* **2019**, *365*, 786–793. [CrossRef]
147. Nelson, C.A.; Butte, A.J.; Baranzini, S.E. Integrating biomedical research and electronic health records to create knowledge-based biologically meaningful machine-readable embeddings. *Nat. Commun.* **2019**, *10*, 3045. [CrossRef]
148. Wang, Y.; Wang, Z.; Xu, J.; Li, J.; Li, S.; Zhang, M.; Yang, D. Systematic identification of non-coding pharmacogenomic landscape in cancer. *Nat. Commun.* **2018**, *9*, 3192. [CrossRef]
149. Zhang, W.; Chien, J.; Yong, J.; Kuang, R. Network-based machine learning and graph theory algorithms for precision oncology. *NPJ Precis. Oncol.* **2017**, *1*, 25. [CrossRef]
150. Madubata, C.J.; Roshan-Ghias, A.; Chu, T.; Resnick, S.; Zhao, J.; Arnes, L.; Wang, J.; Rabadan, R. Identification of potentially oncogenic alterations from tumor-only samples reveals Fanconi anemia pathway mutations in bladder carcinomas. *NPJ Genom. Med.* **2017**, *2*, 29. [CrossRef]
151. Réda, C.; Kaufmann, E.; Delahaye-Duriez, A. Machine learning applications in drug development. *Comput. Struct. Biotechnol. J.* **2020**, *18*, 241–252. [CrossRef]
152. Ekins, S.; Puhl, A.C.; Zorn, K.M.; Lane, T.R.; Russo, D.P.; Klein, J.J.; Hickey, A.J.; Clark, A.M. Exploiting machine learning for end-to-end drug discovery and development. *Nat. Mater.* **2019**, *18*, 435–441. [CrossRef] [PubMed]
153. Bhattacharjee, A. Application of Bayesian Approach in Cancer Clinical Trial. *World J. Oncol.* **2014**, *5*, 109–112. [CrossRef] [PubMed]
154. Madhukar, N.S.; Khade, P.K.; Huang, L.; Gayvert, K.; Galletti, G.; Stogniew, M.; Allen, J.E.; Giannakakou, P.; Elemento, O. A Bayesian machine learning approach for drug target identification using diverse data types. *Nat. Commun.* **2019**, *10*, 5221. [CrossRef] [PubMed]
155. Lyu, J.; Curran, E.; Ji, Y. Bayesian Adaptive Design for Finding the Maximum Tolerated Sequence of Doses in Multicycle Dose-Finding Clinical Trials. *JCO Precis. Oncol.* **2018**, *2018*, 1–19. [CrossRef]
156. Cook, N.; Basu, B.; Smith, D.M.; Gopinathan, A.; Evans, J.; Steward, W.P.; Palmer, D.; Propper, D.; Venugopal, B.; Hategan, M.; et al. A phase I trial of the gamma-secretase inhibitor MK-0752 in combination with gemcitabine in patients with pancreatic ductal adenocarcinoma. *Br. J. Cancer* **2018**, *118*, 793–801. [CrossRef]
157. Yan, F.; Mandrekar, S.J.; Yuan, Y. Keyboard: A Novel Bayesian Toxicity Probability Interval Design for Phase I Clinical Trials. *Clin. Cancer Res.* **2017**, *23*, 3994–4003. [CrossRef]

158. Jin, J.; Liu, Q.; Zheng, W.; Shun, Z.; Lin, T.T.; Gao, L.; Dong, Y. A Bayesian Method for the Detection of Proof of Concept in Early Phase Oncology Studies with a Basket Design. *Stat. Biosci. Vol.* **2020**, *12*, 167–179. [CrossRef]
159. Tang, R.; Shen, J.; Yuan, Y. ComPAS: A Bayesian drug combination platform trial design with adaptive shrinkage. *Stat. Med.* **2019**, *38*, 1120–1134. [CrossRef]
160. da Silveira Nogueira Lima, J.P.; Georgieva, M.; Haaland, B.; de Lima Lopes, G. A systematic review and network meta-analysis of immunotherapy and targeted therapy for advanced melanoma. *Cancer Med.* **2017**, *6*, 1143–1153. [CrossRef]
161. Gupta, S.K. Use of Bayesian statistics in drug development: Advantages and challenges. *Int. J. Appl. Basic Med. Res.* **2012**, *2*, 3–6. [CrossRef] [PubMed]
162. Rudin, C. Stop explaining black box machine learning models for high stakes decisions and use interpretable models instead. *Nat. Mach. Intell.* **2019**, *1*, 206–215. [CrossRef]
163. Samek, W.; Montavon, G.; Lapuschkin, S.; Anders, C.J.; Müller, K.R. Toward Interpretable Machine Learning: Transparent Deep Neural Networks and Beyond. *arXiv* **2020**, arXiv:2003.07631.
164. Montavon, G.; Samek, W.; Müller, K.R. Methods for interpreting and understanding deep neural networks. *Digit. Signal Process.* **2018**, *73*, 1–15. [CrossRef]
165. Wang, N.; Chen, M.; Subbalakshmi, K.P. Explainable CNN-attention Networks (C-Attention Network) for Automated Detection of Alzheimer's Disease. *arXiv* **2020**, arXiv:2006.14135.
166. Yang, J.H.; Wright, S.N.; Hamblin, M.; McCloskey, D.; Alcantar, M.A.; Schrubbers, L.; Lopatkin, A.J.; Satish, S.; Nili, A.; Palsson, B.O.; et al. A White-Box Machine Learning Approach for Revealing Antibiotic Mechanisms of Action. *Cell* **2019**, *177*, 1649–1661.e9. [CrossRef]
167. Wu, M.; Zhong, X.; Peng, Q.; Xu, M.; Huang, S.; Yuan, J.; Ma, J.; Tan, T. Prediction of molecular subtypes of breast cancer using BI-RADS features based on a "white box" machine learning approach in a multi-modal imaging setting. *Eur. J. Radiol.* **2019**, *114*, 175–184. [CrossRef]
168. Gunning, D. *Explainable Artificial Intelligence (xAI)*; Technical Report; Defense Advanced Research Projects Agency (DARPA): Arlington County, FL, USA, 2017; Available online: http://www.darpa.mil/program/explainable-artificial-intelligence (accessed on 9 September 2017).
169. Kuhn, D.R.; Kacker, R.N.; Lei, Y.; Simos, D.E. Combinatorial Methods for Explainable AI. In Proceedings of the 2020 IEEE International Conference on Software Testing, Verification and Validation Workshops (ICSTW), Porto, Portugal, 24–28 October 2020.
170. Shakerin, F.; Gupta, G. Induction of Non-Monotonic Logic Programs to Explain Boosted Tree Models Using LIME. *arXiv* **2018**, arXiv:1808.00629. [CrossRef]
171. Stacke, K.; Eilertsen, G.; Unger, J.; Lundstrom, C. Measuring Domain Shift for Deep Learning in Histopathology. *IEEE J. Biomed. Health Inform.* **2020**. [CrossRef]
172. Pandey, P.; Ap, P.; Kyatham, V.; Mishra, D.; Dastidar, T.R. Target-Independent Domain Adaptation for WBC Classification using Generative Latent Search. *IEEE Trans. Med. Imaging* **2020**. [CrossRef]
173. Bian, C.; Yuan, C.; Wang, J.; Li, M.; Yang, X.; Yu, S.; Ma, K.; Yuan, J.; Zheng, Y. Uncertainty-aware domain alignment for anatomical structure segmentation. *Med. Image Anal.* **2020**, *64*, 101732. [CrossRef] [PubMed]
174. Gu, Y.; Ge, Z.; Bonnington, C.P.; Zhou, J. Progressive Transfer Learning and Adversarial Domain Adaptation for Cross-Domain Skin Disease Classification. *IEEE J. Biomed. Health Inform.* **2020**, *24*, 1379–1393. [CrossRef] [PubMed]
175. Pooch, E.H.P.; Ballester, P.L.; Barros, R.C. Can we trust deep learning models diagnosis? The impact of domain shift in chest radiograph classification. *arXiv* **2020**, arXiv:1909.01940.
176. Jiang, J.; Hu, Y.C.; Tyagi, N.; Wang, C.; Lee, N.; Deasy, J.O.; Sean, B.; Veeraraghavan, H. Self-derived organ attention for unpaired CT-MRI deep domain adaptation based MRI segmentation. *Phys. Med. Biol.* **2020**, *65*, 205001. [CrossRef] [PubMed]
177. Choudhary, A.; Tong, L.; Zhu, Y.; Wang, M.D. Advancing Medical Imaging Informatics by Deep Learning-Based Domain Adaptation. *Yearb. Med. Inform.* **2020**, *29*, 129–138. [CrossRef]
178. Li, X.; Gu, Y.; Dvornek, N.; Staib, L.H.; Ventola, P.; Duncan, J.S. Multi-site fMRI analysis using privacy-preserving federated learning and domain adaptation: ABIDE results. *Med. Image Anal.* **2020**, *65*, 101765. [CrossRef]
179. Xia, Y.; Yang, D.; Yu, Z.; Liu, F.; Cai, J.; Yu, L.; Zhu, Z.; Xu, D.; Yuille, A.; Roth, H. Uncertainty-aware multi-view co-training for semi-supervised medical image segmentation and domain adaptation. *Med. Image Anal.* **2020**, *65*, 101766. [CrossRef]

180. Chen, C.; Dou, Q.; Chen, H.; Qin, J.; Heng, P.A. Unsupervised Bidirectional Cross-Modality Adaptation via Deeply Synergistic Image and Feature Alignment for Medical Image Segmentation. *IEEE Trans. Med. Imaging* **2020**, *39*, 2494–2505. [CrossRef]
181. Yan, Z.; Yang, X.; Cheng, K.T. Enabling a Single Deep Learning Model for Accurate Gland Instance Segmentation: A Shape-Aware Adversarial Learning Framework. *IEEE Trans. Med. Imaging* **2020**, *39*, 2176–2189. [CrossRef]
182. Xing, F.; Bennett, T.; Ghosh, D. Adversarial Domain Adaptation and Pseudo-Labeling for Cross-Modality Microscopy Image Quantification. *Med. Image Comput. Comput. Assist. Interv.* **2019**, *11764*, 740–749.
183. Hamed Mozaffari, M.; Lee, W.S. Domain adaptation for ultrasound tongue contour extraction using transfer learning: A deep learning approach. *J. Acoust. Soc. Am.* **2019**, *146*, EL431. [CrossRef] [PubMed]
184. Zhu, Q.; Du, B.; Yan, P. Boundary-Weighted Domain Adaptive Neural Network for Prostate MR Image Segmentation. *IEEE Trans. Med. Imaging* **2020**, *39*, 753–763. [CrossRef] [PubMed]
185. Perone, C.S.; Ballester, P.; Barros, R.C.; Cohen-Adad, J. Unsupervised domain adaptation for medical imaging segmentation with self-ensembling. *Neuroimage* **2019**, *194*, 1–11. [CrossRef] [PubMed]
186. Jiang, J.; Hu, Y.C.; Tyagi, N.; Zhang, P.; Rimner, A.; Mageras, G.S.; Deasy, J.O.; Veeraraghavan, H. Tumor-aware, Adversarial Domain Adaptation from CT to MRI for Lung Cancer Segmentation. *Med. Image Comput. Comput. Assist. Interv.* **2018**, *11071*, 777–785.
187. Mahmood, F.; Chen, R.; Durr, N.J. Unsupervised Reverse Domain Adaptation for Synthetic Medical Images via Adversarial Training. *IEEE Trans. Med. Imaging* **2018**, *37*, 2572–2581. [CrossRef] [PubMed]
188. Qin, R.; Zhang, H.; Jiang, L.; Qiao, K.; Hai, J.; Chen, J.; Xu, J.; Shi, D.; Yan, B. Multicenter Computer-Aided Diagnosis for Lymph Nodes Using Unsupervised Domain-Adaptation Networks Based on Cross-Domain Confounding Representations. *Comput. Math Methods Med.* **2020**, *2020*, 3709873. [CrossRef]
189. Ganin, Y.; Ustinova, E.; Ajakan, H. Domain-adversarial training of neural networks. *J. Mach. Learn. Res.* **2017**, *17*, 2096-2030.
190. Borgwardt, K.M.; Gretton, A.; Rasch, M.J.; Kriegel, H.P.; Scholkopf, B.; Smola, A.J. Integrating structured biological data by Kernel Maximum Mean Discrepancy. *Bioinformatics* **2006**, *22*, e49–e57. [CrossRef]
191. Sankaranarayanan, S.; Balaji, Y.; Castillo, C.D.; Chellappa, R. Generate To Adapt: Aligning Domains using Generative Adversarial Networks. *arXiv* **2017**, arXiv:1704.01705.

2

Predicting 90-Day Mortality in Locoregionally Advanced Head and Neck Squamous Cell Carcinoma after Curative Surgery

Lei Qin [1,†], Tsung-Ming Chen [2,†], Yi-Wei Kao [3], Kuan-Chou Lin [4], Kevin Sheng-Po Yuan [5], Alexander T. H. Wu [6], Ben-Chang Shia [7,*] and Szu-Yuan Wu [8,9,*]

1. School of Statistics, University of International Business and Economics, Beijing 100029, China; qinlei@uibe.edu.cn
2. Department of Otorhinolaryngology, Shuang-Ho Hospital, Taipei Medical University, New Taipei City 23561, Taiwan; 09326@s.tmu.edu.tw
3. Graduate Institute of Business Administration, Fu Jen Catholic University, Taipei 116, Taiwan; kyw498762030@gmail.com
4. Department of Oral and Maxillofacial Surgery, Wanfang Hospital, Taipei Medical University, Taipei 116, Taiwan; kclin0628@hotmail.com
5. Department of Otorhinolaryngology, Wanfang Hospital, Taipei Medical University, Taipei 116, Taiwan; dryuank@gmail.com
6. Ph.D. Program for Translational Medicine, Taipei Medical University, Taipei 116, Taiwan; chaw1211@tmu.edu.tw
7. College of Management, Taipei Medical University, Taipei 106, Taiwan
8. Department of Radiation Oncology, Wanfang Hospital, Taipei Medical University, Taipei 116, Taiwan
9. Department of Internal Medicine, School of Medicine, College of Medicine, Taipei Medical University, Taipei 110, Taiwan

* Correspondence: stat1001@tmu.edu.tw (B.-C.S.); szuyuanwu5399@gmail.com (S.-Y.W.)

† These authors have contributed equally to this study (joint primary authors).

Abstract: *Purpose:* To propose a risk classification scheme for locoregionally advanced (Stages III and IV) head and neck squamous cell carcinoma (LA-HNSCC) by using the Wu comorbidity score (WCS) to quantify the risk of curative surgeries, including tumor resection and radical neck dissection. *Methods:* This study included 55,080 patients with LA-HNSCC receiving curative surgery between 2006 and 2015 who were identified from the Taiwan Cancer Registry database; the patients were classified into two groups, mortality (n = 1287, mortality rate = 2.34%) and survival (n = 53,793, survival rate = 97.66%), according to the event of mortality within 90 days of surgery. Significant risk factors for mortality were identified using a stepwise multivariate Cox proportional hazards model. The WCS was calculated using the relative risk of each risk factor. The accuracy of the WCS was assessed using mortality rates in different risk strata. *Results:* Fifteen comorbidities significantly increased mortality risk after curative surgery. The patients were divided into low-risk (WCS, 0–6; 90-day mortality rate, 0–1.57%), intermediate-risk (7–11; 2.71–9.99%), high-risk (12–16; 17.30–20.00%), and very-high-risk (17–18 and >18; 46.15–50.00%) strata. The 90-day survival rates were 98.97, 95.85, 81.20, and 53.13% in the low-, intermediate-, high-, and very-high-risk patients, respectively (log-rank $p < 0.0001$). The five-year overall survival rates after surgery were 70.86, 48.62, 22.99, and 18.75% in the low-, intermediate-, high-, and very-high-risk patients, respectively (log-rank $p < 0.0001$). *Conclusion:* The WCS is an accurate tool for assessing curative-surgery-related 90-day mortality risk and overall survival in patients with LA-HNSCC.

Keywords: comorbidity score; mortality; locoregionally advanced; HNSCC; curative surgery

---

1. Introduction

The incidence of head and neck squamous cell carcinoma (HNSCC) in Taiwan is different from that in Western countries. Betel nut chewing is endemic to Taiwan and is observed in >90% patients with HNSCC in Taiwan [1–5]. Betel nut chewing results in a high risk of local recurrence and second primary HNSCC in patients with HNSCC in Taiwan [1–5]. Due to betel nut chewing, the proportion of oral cavity and nonoral cavity cancers in patients with HNSCC in Taiwan is approximately 66 and 34%, respectively [1–6]. The proportion of oral cavity cancers in patients with HNSCC is higher in Taiwan than in other countries [1–6]. Treatments for Taiwanese patients with HNSCC might be complicated, and the frequency of reirradiation is higher in Taiwan than in areas where betel nut chewing is not endemic [1–5]. Therefore, comprehensive curative surgery is the main treatment (accounting for 64.09% of all HNSCC treatments) for patients with HNSCC in Taiwan [1–6]. In addition, in Taiwan, at initial diagnosis, >50% of HNSCC cases are locoregionally advanced (Stages III and IV) HNSCC (LA-HNSCC) [6]. Instead of RT or chemotherapy, the initial treatment for LA-HNSCC is surgical resection of the primary tumor and neck dissection, followed by postoperative radiotherapy (RT) or concurrent chemoradiotherapy (CCRT).

Curative head and neck surgery, including radical neck dissection, is associated with a mortality rate of 1.5–8.5% [7–11]; however, the time interval between curative surgery and mortality has not been specified in the literature. Most studies on curative surgery for HNSCC were published in the 1970s to 1980s [7–11]; however, surgical techniques have improved considerably in the past 20 years [12,13]. Definitive data on mortality rates after curative surgery for LA-HNSCC in the past 20 years, particularly in Asia, are not available. In this study, we estimated mortality rates after curative surgery in patients with LA-HNSCC between 2006 and 2015. A new comorbidity score to predict mortality rates in patients with LA-HNSCC receiving curative surgery was also proposed because modern RT techniques, chemotherapy regimens, induction chemotherapy, and immune therapy might be more suitable alternative curative-intent treatments than curative surgery for high-mortality risk patients with LA-HNSCC [2–4,14–21].

The mean age of patients with HNSCC in Taiwan has been reported to be 55 years; consequently, the patients are generally individuals who provide the main economic support to their families [1–6]. We hope to reduce mortality rates after aggressive treatments in LA-HNSCC and propose a new comorbidity score to preoperatively predict 90-day mortality and overall survival in patients with LA-HNSCC who will receive curative surgery. The new comorbidity score can be used to determine whether curative surgery or other curative-intent aggressive treatments are the optimal treatment [2,4,14–21].

2. Patients and Methods

Ethics approval and consent: Our protocols were reviewed and approved by the Institutional Review Board of Taipei Medical University (TMU-JIRB No. 201712019).

2.1. Database

The study population was identified from the Taiwan Cancer Registry database (TCRD). The TCRD is a crucial research resource for epidemiological studies, and the results obtained using the database can be used as a reference when developing medical and health policies. The Cancer Registry database of Collaboration Center of Health Information Application contains detailed cancer-related information on clinical stages, RT doses, habits (smoking, betel nut chewing, and drinking), surgical procedures, techniques, and chemotherapy regimens [2,4,22,23]. The Institutional Review Board of Taipei Medical University approved this study (TMU-No. 201712019). The TCRD is released to the public for research purposes after identification numbers are scrambled and personal information is de-identified.

2.2. Selection of Patients and Controls

This study included 55,080 patients with LA-HNSCC who had received curative surgeries, including tumor resection and ipsilateral radical neck dissection, between 1 January 2006 and 31 December 2015. In the patients with HNSCC, clinical staging was performed according to the American Joint Committee on Cancer (AJCC), Seventh Edition. Squamous cell carcinoma was confirmed in all study patients identified from the TCRD. Patients with the following contraindications for curative surgery were excluded from the study: An Eastern Cooperative Oncology Group performance status of $\geq$2, a fixed neck mass in the deep cervical fascia, skull base involvement, circumferential or near circumferential involvement, and invasion of the carotid vessels if the patient could not tolerate a balloon occlusion test. All head and neck surgeons in Taiwan are head and neck oncology specialists certified by the Taiwan Ministry of Health and Welfare. We only included patients aged >18 years to restrict our study population to adults. Patients with metastatic HNSCC were excluded. The included patients were classified into two groups, namely mortality (n = 1287, mortality rate = 2.34%) and survival (n = 53,793, survival rate = 97.66%) groups, according to the event of mortality within 90 days after curative surgery. For each patient, the index date was designated as the date of curative surgery.

2.3. Statistical Analysis

All statistical analyses were performed using SAS statistical software (SAS for Windows, version 9.2, SAS Institute, Cary, NC, USA). Statistical significance was set at $p \leq 0.05$.

For demographic characteristics, age group (18–29, 30–39, 40–49, 50–59, 60–69, and $\geq$70) and sex were selected as the basic information of the patients. Age was calculated as the time interval between the index date and birth date, and data on sex were extracted from the database. Comorbidities were evaluated using the Charlson comorbidity index (CCI), and before surgery, physical status was determined according to the American Society of Anesthesiologists (ASA) Physical Status Classification System [2,4,24–26]. Patients with recent (within 6 months before the index date) myocardial infarction (MI), cerebral vascular accident (CVA), transient ischemic attack (TIA), or coronal arterial disease (CADs) with stents, ongoing cardiac ischemia or severe valve dysfunction, severe reduction of ejection fraction, sepsis, disseminated intravascular coagulation (DIC), adult respiratory distress syndrome (ARDS), or end-stage renal disease (ESRD) were excluded from the study. Only comorbidities observed 6 months before the index date were included in the analysis; comorbidities were identified and included according to the main International Classification of Diseases, Ninth Revision, Clinical Modification (ICD-9-CM) diagnostic codes for the first admission or 3 or more repeated main diagnosis codes for visits to outpatient departments. The comorbidities of interest were diabetes mellitus (DM), hypertension (HTN), pneumonia, chronic obstructive pulmonary disease (COPD), hepatitis B (HBV) infection, hepatitis C (HCV) infection, implanted pacemaker, MI, CVA, TIA, CADs, angina, heart valve dysfunction, ESRD, sepsis, chronic kidney disease (CKD), heart failure, DIC, ARDS, aortic aneurysm, peripheral vascular disease (PVD), peptic ulcer disease (PUD), dementia, chronic pulmonary disease, connective tissue disease, mild liver disease, hemiplegia, moderate or severe renal disease, any non-HNSCC solid cancer, leukemia, lymphoma, moderate or severe liver disease, metastatic non-HNSCC solid cancer, previous thoracic surgery, smoking, obesity, asthma, and bowel obstruction. The chi-square test was used to compare demographic characteristics and comorbidities between the mortality and survival groups.

In this study, we aimed to identify significant risk factors for mortality within 90 days after curative surgery and proposed the Wu comorbidity score (WCS) to assess mortality risk associated with curative surgery in patients with HNSCC. Univariate and multivariate Cox proportional hazard models were constructed to calculate the hazard ratios (HRs) of the variables and corresponding 95% confidence intervals (CIs). A stepwise selection method was used to select all the variables that exerted significant effects on the survival duration in the patients. Variables with coefficients of >0 or HRs of >1 were selected as risk factors to construct the WCS by adding points according to the HRs. We divided all the patients into different strata according to the WCS and confirmed that the patients with high scores had high mortality risk after curative surgery. The cumulative mortality rate was estimated using the Kaplan–Meier method, and differences among the risk strata were determined using the log-rank test. Two-tailed $p < 0.05$ was considered statistically significant.

3. Results

Table 1 shows a comparison of demographic characteristics and mortality rates within 90 days after curative surgery between the mortality and survival groups. Significant differences were observed between the groups in the age ($p < 0.0001$), sex ($p < 0.0001$), and comorbidities, such as DM, HTN, and pneumonia.

Table 1. Demographic characteristics between death within 90 days and survival groups receiving curative surgery in locoregionally advanced head and neck squamous cell carcinoma patients.

Factor	Death No.	Death Rate	Survival No.	Survival Rate	*p* Value
Number of patients	1287		53,793		
Age (years)					<0.0001
18–29	2	0.16%	696	1.29%	
30–39	40	3.11%	4978	9.25%	
40–49	231	17.95%	14,379	26.73%	
50–59	352	27.35%	16,611	30.88%	
60–69	263	20.44%	10,046	18.68%	
≥70	399	31.00%	7083	13.17%	
Sex					<0.0001
Female	195	7.38%	5697	10.59%	
Male	1192	92.62%	48,096	89.41%	
Comorbidity					
DM	80	6.22%	1804	3.35%	<0.0001
HTN	477	37.06%	16,260	30.23%	<0.0001
Pneumonia	250	19.43%	2665	4.95%	<0.0001
COPD	240	18.65%	4517	8.40%	<0.0001
Hepatitis B	8	0.62%	425	0.79%	0.4989
Hepatitis C	32	2.49%	1003	1.86%	0.1045
Implanted pacemaker	2	0.16%	22	0.04%	0.0518
MI, CVA, TIA, angina, or CAD	280	21.76%	6957	12.93%	<0.0001
Heart valve dysfunction	35	2.72%	659	1.23%	<0.0001
ESRD	0	0.00%	0	0.00%	
Sepsis	172	13.36%	882	1.64%	<0.0001
CKD	165	12.82%	1754	3.26%	<0.0001
Heart failure	92	7.15%	1000	1.86%	<0.0001
DIC	5	0.39%	5	0.01%	<0.0001
ARDS	4	0.31%	18	0.03%	<0.0001
Aortic aneurysm	4	0.31%	58	0.11%	0.0319
PVD	33	2.56%	707	1.31%	0.0001
PUD	268	20.82%	7394	13.75%	<0.0001
Dementia	71	5.52%	1100	2.04%	<0.0001
Chronic pulmonary disease	222	17.25%	4810	8.94%	<0.0001
Connective tissue disease	23	1.79%	614	1.14%	0.0323
Mild liver disease	255	19.81%	7733	14.38%	<0.0001
Hemiplegia	107	8.31%	1970	3.66%	<0.0001
Moderate or severe renal disease	166	12.90%	1757	3.27%	<0.0001
Any non-HNSCC Solid Cancer	659	51.20%	14,591	27.12%	<0.0001
Leukemia	2	0.16%	33	0.06%	0.1858
Lymphoma	22	1.71%	647	1.20%	0.101
Moderate or severe liver disease	89	6.92%	2487	4.62%	0.0001
Metastatic non-HNSCC solid cancer	548	42.58%	13,390	24.89%	<0.0001
Smoking	1158	89.98%	48,413	90.00%	0.8989
Previous thoracic surgery	6	0.47%	268	0.50%	0.6767
Obesity	11	1.24%	699	1.30%	0.7756
Asthma	10	0.78%	429	0.80%	0.9573
Bowel obstruction	3	0.23%	123	0.23%	0.8457

Diabetes mellitus: DM; hypertension: HTN; Chronic Obstructive Pulmonary Disease: COPD; Hepatitis B: HBV; Hepatitis C: HCV; myocardial infarction: MI; cerebral vascular accident: CVA; transient ischemic attack: TIA; coronal arterial disease: CAD; end stage renal disease: ESRD; Chronic kidney disease: CKD; disseminated intravascular coagulation: DIC; adult respiratory distress syndrome: ARDS; peripheral vascular disease: PVD; peptic ulcer disease: PUD.

Tables 2 and 3 present the relative risk for each variable estimated using univariate and multivariate Cox proportional hazard models. Fewer variables were significant in the multivariate model than in the univariate model, indicating strong collinearity between the variables. Therefore, we used a stepwise method in the multivariate model for variable selection (Table 4). Among comorbidities, significant variables were HTN, pneumonia, COPD, sepsis, heart failure, DIC, ARDS, dementia, mild to severe liver disease, hemiplegia, moderate or severe renal disease, any tumor, and metastatic solid tumor.

Table 2. Mortality risk assessment through univariate Cox proportional hazard model in locoregionally advanced head and neck squamous cell carcinoma patients receiving curative surgery.

Factor	HR	95% CI	*p* Value
Age (years)			
18–29	1	(Reference)	
≥30	1.277	2.077, 32.989	0.0027
≥40	1.463	2.546, 4.709	<0.0001
≥50	2.19	1.916, 2.503	<0.0001
≥60	2.245	2.012, 2.504	<0.0001
≥70	2.915	2.59, 3.28	<0.0001
Sex			
Female	1	(Reference)	
Male	1.48	1.201, 1.824	0.0002
Comorbidities			
DM	1.894	1.51, 2.374	<0.0001
HTN	1.356	1.211, 1.518	<0.0001
Pneumonia	4.476	3.898, 5.138	<0.0001
COPD	2.466	2.143, 2.838	<0.0001
Hepatitis B	0.787	0.393, 1.576	0.4986
Hepatitis C	1.342	0.945, 1.905	0.1004
Implanted pacemaker	3.716	0.928, 14.874	0.0636
MI, CVA, TIA, angina, or CAD	1.857	1.627, 2.12	<0.0001
Heart valve dysfunction	2.224	1.589, 3.111	<0.0001
Sepsis	8.647	7.364, 10.153	<0.0001
CKD	4.245	3.605, 4.999	<0.0001
Heart failure	3.965	3.207, 4.902	<0.0001
DIC	32.834	13.643, 79.019	<0.0001
ARDS	9.058	3.395, 24.166	<0.0001
Aortic aneurysm	2.818	1.056, 7.519	0.0385
PAD	1.962	1.389, 2.772	0.0001
PUD	1.64	1.433, 1.876	<0.0001
Dementia	2.735	2.153, 3.475	<0.0001
Chronic pulmonary disease	2.1	1.817, 2.427	<0.0001
Connective tissue disease	1.567	1.037, 2.367	0.0328
Mild liver disease	1.465	1.277, 1.68	<0.0001
Hemiplegia	2.35	1.928, 2.865	<0.0001
Moderate or severe renal disease	4.272	3.629, 5.028	<0.0001
Any non-HNSCC Solid Cancer	2.753	1.917, 3.953	<0.0001
Leukemia	2.506	0.626, 10.032	0.1941
Lymphoma	1.423	0.934, 2.168	0.1008
Moderate or severe liver disease	1.525	1.229, 1.891	0.0001
Metastatic non-HNSCC solid cancer	2.21	1.979, 2.468	<0.0001
Smoking	0.964	0.405, 1.459	0.3571
Previous thoracic surgery	1.168	0.778, 2.589	0.6734
Obesity	1.473	0.746, 1.896	0.8197
Asthma	1.384	0.804, 8.09	0.7592
Bowel obstruction	1.132	0.494, 2.873	0.8112

Diabetes mellitus: DM; hypertension: HTN; Chronic Obstructive Pulmonary Disease: COPD; Hepatitis B: HBV; Hepatitis C: HCV; myocardial infarction: MI; cerebral vascular accident: CVA; transient ischemic attack: TIA; coronal arterial disease: CAD; end stage renal disease: ESRD; Chronic kidney disease: CKD; disseminated intravascular coagulation: DIC; adult respiratory distress syndrome: ARDS; peripheral vascular disease: PVD; peptic ulcer disease: PUD.

Table 3. Mortality risk assessment through multivariate Cox proportional hazard model in locoregionally advanced head and neck squamous cell carcinoma patients receiving curative surgery.

Factor	HR	95% CI	*p* Value
Age (years)			
18–29	1	(Reference)	
≥30	1.012	0.486, 3.336	0.3348
≥40	1.125	1.304, 2.555	0.0004
≥50	1.309	1.107, 1.547	0.0016
≥60	1.218	1.037, 1.432	0.0166
≥70	1.902	1.618, 2.236	<0.0001
Sex			
Female	1	(Reference)	
Male	1.439	1.163, 1.78	0.0008
Comorbidities			
DM	1.188	0.942, 1.5	0.1463
HTN	0.811	0.713, 0.922	0.0014
Pneumonia	2.093	1.79, 2.447	<0.0001
COPD	1.262	1.007, 1.581	0.0431
Hepatitis B	0.864	0.429, 1.741	0.6823
Hepatitis C	0.746	0.488, 1.142	0.1772
Implanted pacemaker	1.453	0.36, 5.873	0.6001
MI, CVA, TIA, angina, or CAD	0.891	0.745, 1.066	0.2072
Heart valve dysfunction	1.215	0.858, 1.721	0.2716
Sepsis	4.079	3.418, 4.869	<0.0001
CKD	1.117	0.658, 1.897	0.6818
Heart failure	2.037	1.617, 2.567	<0.0001
DIC	7.585	3.105, 18.53	<0.0001
ARDS	4.04	1.494, 10.923	0.0059
Aortic aneurysm	1.059	0.394, 2.845	0.9093
PAD	1.107	0.777, 1.578	0.5733
PUD	1.063	0.923, 1.225	0.3953
Dementia	1.583	1.234, 2.029	0.0003
Chronic pulmonary disease	0.97	0.774, 1.216	0.7916
Connective tissue disease	1.173	0.772, 1.781	0.4551
Mild liver disease	1.211	1.043, 1.407	0.0121
Hemiplegia	1.426	1.117, 1.821	0.0044
Moderate or severe renal disease	2.092	1.235, 3.544	0.0061
Any non-HNSCC solid cancer	2.306	1.599, 3.325	<0.0001
Leukemia	1.989	0.496, 7.981	0.332
Lymphoma	1.455	0.952, 2.225	0.0832
Moderate or severe liver disease	1.212	1.104, 1.519	0.0025
Metastatic non-HNSCC solid Cancer	2.144	1.916, 2.399	<0.0001
Smoking	0.846	0.618, 1.126	0.5753
Previous thoracic surgery	0.957	0.901, 1.976	0.8251
Obesity	1.015	0.879, 1.705	0.9088
Asthma	1.203	0.798, 1.511	0.8603
Bowel obstruction	1.047	0.505, 1.984	0.9221

Diabetes mellitus: DM; hypertension: HTN; Chronic Obstructive Pulmonary Disease: COPD; Hepatitis B: HBV; Hepatitis C: HCV; myocardial infarction: MI; cerebral vascular accident: CVA; transient ischemic attack: TIA; coronal arterial disease: CAD; end stage renal disease: ESRD; Chronic kidney disease: CKD; disseminated intravascular coagulation: DIC; adult respiratory distress syndrome: ARDS; peripheral vascular disease: PVD; peptic ulcer disease: PUD.

Table 4. Stepwise selection results and comorbidity score for multivariate Cox proportional hazard model in locoregionally advanced head and neck squamous cell carcinoma patients receiving curative surgery.

Factor	HR	95% CI	*p* Value	Points
Age (years)				
≥40	1.913	1.376, 2.659	0.0001	1
≥50	1.309	1.107, 1.547	0.0016	1
≥60	1.221	1.039, 1.435	0.0154	1
≥70	1.894	1.613, 2.225	<0.0001	1
Sex				
Female	1	(Reference)		
Male	1.425	1.153, 1.76	0.001	1
Comorbidities				
HTN	0.803	0.708, 1.11	0.1006	0
Pneumonia	2.092	1.79, 2.446	<0.0001	2
COPD	1.227	1.052, 1.431	0.0093	1
Sepsis	4.161	3.492, 4.958	<0.0001	4
Heart failure	2.056	1.646, 2.566	<0.0001	2
DIC	7.683	3.152, 18.728	<0.0001	7
ARDS	3.897	1.444, 10.52	0.0073	3
Dementia	1.598	1.247, 2.048	0.0002	1
Mild liver disease	1.251	1.087, 1.439	0.0018	1
Hemiplegia	1.342	1.089, 1.654	0.0059	1
Moderate or severe renal disease	2.361	1.983, 2.81	<0.0001	2
Any non-HNSCC solid cancer	2.289	1.588, 3.3	<0.0001	2
Moderate or severe liver disease	1.284	1.034, 1.473	0.0083	1
Metastatic non-HNSCC solid cancer	2.142	1.915, 2.397	<0.0001	2

Diabetes mellitus: DM; hypertension: HTN; Chronic Obstructive Pulmonary Disease: COPD; Hepatitis B: HBV; Hepatitis C: HCV; myocardial infarction: MI; cerebral vascular accident: CVA; transient ischemic attack: TIA; coronal arterial disease: CAD; end stage renal disease: ESRD; Chronic kidney disease: CKD; disseminated intravascular coagulation: DIC; adult respiratory distress syndrome: ARDS; peripheral vascular disease: PVD; peptic ulcer disease: PUD.

The WCS was calculated using significant variables other than HTN because the HR of HTN was <1. Although HTN increased the risk of outcomes, which can be observed from univariate analysis (Table 2, HR = 1.356, CI: 1.211–1.518), collinearity in multivariate model may have reduced the HR to <1 (Table 4, HR = 0.803, CI: 0.708–0.91), which is a common statistical phenomenon. We calculated the WCS by adding points according to the HR of each risk factor. The points of each risk factor were assigned as the largest integer less than or equal to its HR (last column in Table 4); for example, 2 points for pneumonia with an HR of 2.092 and 3 points for ARDS with an HR of 3.897. In the WSC, a high number of points were assigned to risk factors with high relative mortality risk within 90 days. In our study, the minimum and maximum values of the WCS were 0 and 18+, respectively. We collapsed the range of the WCS into 4 strata, namely the low-risk (WCS, 0–6; 90-day mortality rate, 0–1.57%), intermediate-risk (7–11; 2.71–9.99%), high-risk (12–16, 17.30–20.00%), and very-high-risk (17 to 18+; 46.15–50.00%) strata (Table 4). We used the CCI for scoring to predict 90-day mortality compared with the current scoring system (Figures S1 and S2), the risk groups of CCI were not feasible for predicting 90-day mortality in LA-HNSCC patients receiving curative surgery and could not reach statistical significance. In addition, there were scarcely LA-HNSCC patients with ASA classifications I and IV–V receiving curative surgery in our database. Therefore, we cannot use ASA classifications I–V to predict 90-day mortality in LA-HNSCC patients receiving curative surgery. The 90-day mortality rate tended to increase as the WCS increased, indicating the accuracy of the WCS. The 90-day mortality rate and five-year survival in the patients were estimated using the Kaplan–Meier method to analyze the risk of mortality associated with the 4 risk strata (Figures 1 and 2). The 90-day survival rates were 98.97, 95.85, 81.20, and 53.13% in the low-, intermediate-, high-, and very-high-risk strata, respectively (log-rank test $p < 0.0001$; Figure 1). The five-year overall survival rates were 70.86, 48.62, 22.99, and 18.75% in the low-, intermediate-, high-, and very-high-risk strata, respectively (log-rank $p < 0.0001$; Figure 2).

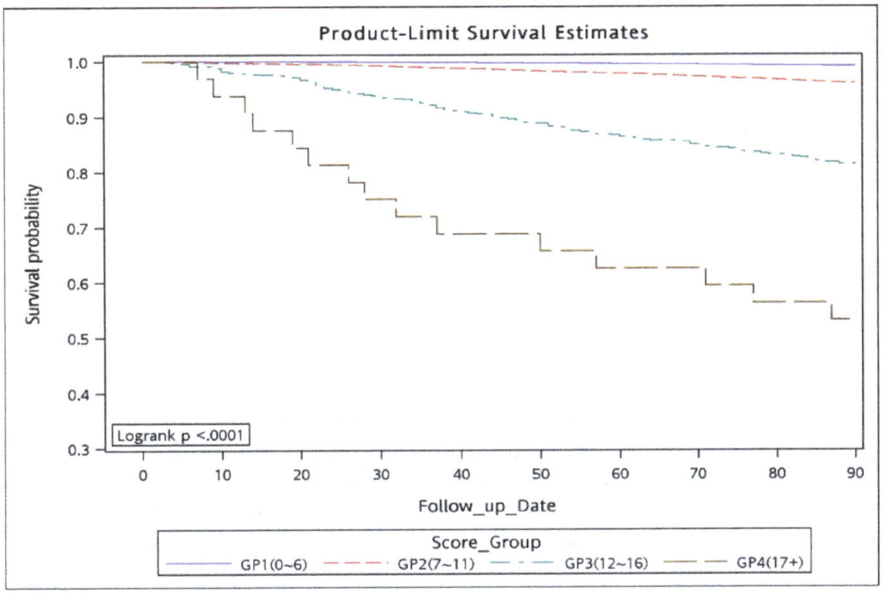

Figure 1. Kaplan–Meier curves for 90-day survival in patients with locoregionally advanced head and neck squamous cell carcinoma receiving curative surgery associated with the four risk groups. Note: *p*-value of Log Rank Test is <0.0001.

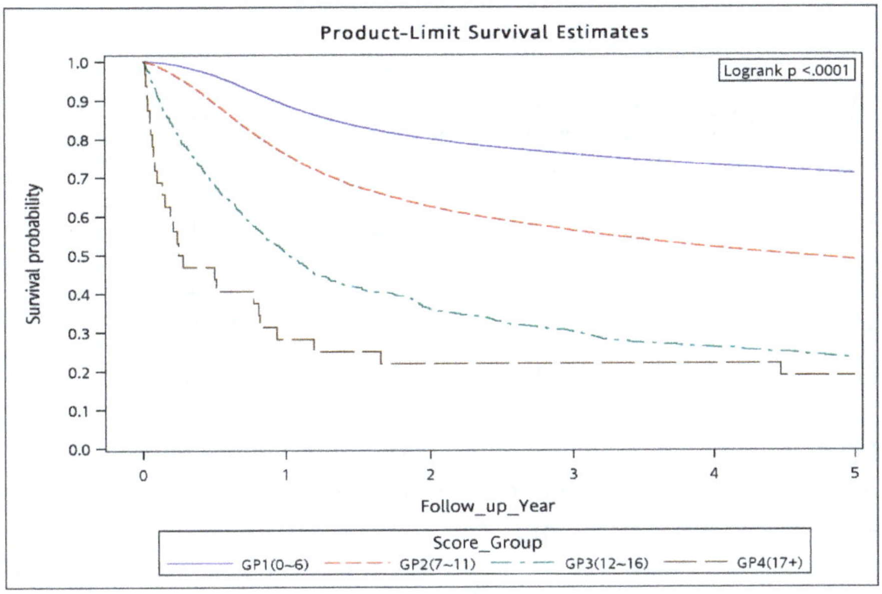

Figure 2. Kaplan–Meier curves for five years overall survival in patients with locoregionally advanced head and neck squamous cell carcinoma receiving curative surgery associated with the four risk groups. Note: *p*-value of Log Rank Test is <0.0001.

4. Discussion

According to the Taiwan Cancer Registry report, 2017 edition [6], >90% of curative surgery procedures for LA-HNSCC are conducted in top-ranking medical centers. The ranking is based on accreditation of hospitals in Taiwan into 4 levels since 1988 (medical center, regional hospitals, local hospital, clinics); the accreditation grade affects the service quality and specific patient volume of the hospital [6]. Most curative surgery procedures were performed in hospitals with sufficient patient volume (>100 newly diagnosed patients with LA-HNSCC per year), thus leading to consistent patient outcomes for LA-HNSCC in Taiwan [6,27–30]. Therefore, in Taiwan, the overall mortality rate within 90 days after curative surgery in the patients with LA-HNSCC was only 2.34% (Table 5) after consultation with a professional head and neck surgeon and anesthesia consultation. In Table 1, <3% of the patients with LA-HNSCC and heart valve dysfunctions and <5% of the patients with LA-HNSCC and moderate or severe liver disease received curative surgery. Surgeons were unwilling to perform curative surgery on the patients with LA-HNSCC and ESRD. However, the 90-day mortality remained 2.34%. Therefore, we wanted to develop a highly accurate predictor score to estimate mortality rates after curative surgery because CCRT or induction chemotherapy, followed by CCRT, might be an alternative treatment for patients with LA-HNSCC [3,4]. The proportion of the patients with LA-HNSCC with smoking habit (approximately 90%) in Table 1 was consistent with that reported in previous studies in Taiwan [1–5]. The 90-day mortality rate was proportional to age, particularly in the patients aged >70 years. This is the first study to show that age is a predictor of 90-day mortality in the patients with LA-HNSCC after curative surgery (Tables 1–3).

Table 5. Mortality (%) by different cumulative comorbidity scores among locoregionally advanced head and neck squamous cell carcinoma patients receiving curative surgery.

Score	No of Patient	No of Death	Death Rate
0	107	0	0.00%
1	277	0	0.00%
2	1104	5	0.45%
3	4289	16	0.37%
4	8948	67	0.75%
5	11,317	124	1.10%
6	10,621	167	1.57%
7	8423	228	2.71%
8	4621	168	3.64%
9	2514	154	6.13%
10	1263	109	8.63%
11	681	68	9.99%
12	393	68	17.30%
13	236	44	18.64%
14	149	32	21.48%
15	70	15	21.43%
16	35	7	20.00%
17	26	12	46.15%
18+	6	3	50.00%
Total	55,080	1287	2.34%

Univariate and multivariate analyses revealed that age is an independent predictor of 90-day mortality after curative surgery in patients (Tables 2 and 3). The male patients had higher 90-day mortality risk than did the female patients after curative surgery. These findings are consistent with those of previous studies, which reported endpoints different from those in our study [31,32]. From Table 3, the patients with LA-HNSCC and pneumonia or COPD exhibited high mortality rates. These findings are consistent with those of previous studies [33,34]. However, this is the first study to demonstrate that preoperative pneumonia increases mortality rates in the patients with LA-HNSCC who received curative surgery. Notably, although heart valve dysfunction, MI, CVA, TIA, angina, or CADs were listed as risk factors in the ASA Physical Status Classification System before surgery [24,26], these factors were not risk factors for 90-day mortality in our study. This discrepancy can be explained by our inclusion of comorbidities observed >6 months before the index date and exclusion of the comorbidities observed within 6 months of the index date. The mortality rates of these acute vascular diseases might decrease considerably after 6 months of having these diseases [35–38]. This is the first study to show the absence of correlations between heart valve dysfunction, MI, CVA,

TIA, angina, or CADs and 90-day mortality rates associated with curative surgery in the patients with LA-HNSCC. These findings are reliable references for head and neck surgeons in the future.

Notably, HF, DIC, and ARDS were independent risk factors for 90-day mortality, even when comorbidities observed 6 months before the index date were included. This is because HF, DIC, and ARDS are chronic diseases [39–42] and not acute vascular diseases. In addition, HF, DIC, and ARDS were also listed in the ASA Physical Status Classification System before surgery [24,26]. Dementia and hemiplegia might affect self-care by patients who receive surgery and might result in an increased mortality rate after surgery [31,43]. Our study is the first to demonstrate that dementia and hemiplegia were independent risk factors for mortality in the patients with LA-HNSCC who had received head and neck curative surgery. Head and neck surgeons should carefully consider curative surgery for patients with LA-HNSCC and dementia or hemiplegia. Furthermore, in our study, liver disease or renal disease were independent risk factors for 90-day mortality. Moreover, Cramer et al. showed that liver disease increases the risk of perioperative mortality in patients with HNSCC, and this risk should be carefully considered during surgical decision-making and postoperative care [44]. ESRD was also an independent 90-day mortality risk factor in our study; this finding is consistent with the results of a previous study, which reported a slightly different endpoint from ours [45]. However, leukemia and lymphoma were not risk factors for 90-day mortality in our study (Table 3). Most patients with leukemia or lymphoma have long survival durations of >1 year [46,47]; this long survival duration might explain why leukemia and lymphoma did not affect 90-day mortality in our study. By contrast, non-HNSCC cancer with or without metastasis was an independent risk factor for 90-day mortality (Table 3). This result may be attributable to the weakening of overall physical health, immunity, and the hematological system owing to previous cancer treatments, such as systemic chemotherapy, major surgical procedures, or RT, which increase 90-day mortality rates because of systemic infection complications, hospitalizations, and uncontrolled coagulation or hematological problems [48–50]. For patients with LA-HNSCC and non-HNSCC cancer with or without metastasis, alternative curative-intent aggressive treatments might be considered [4].

In our analysis, the WCS corresponded with not only the 90-day mortality rates but also with the overall survival rates (Figure 2). Developing a new comorbidity score for predicting 90-day mortality in patients with LA-HNSCC who will receive curative surgery is currently valuable because of the evolution of contemporary chemotherapy, RT techniques, target therapy, or immunotherapy, particularly in the past 10 years [14–21]. An increasing number of alternative curative-intent aggressive treatments are available for patients with LA-HNSCC [14–21].

Because the development of new surgical procedures has minimized surgical morbidity and mortality, the contraindications to curative surgery for LA-HNSCC remain controversial [12,13]. However, patients with LA-HNSCC who have a high surgical risk because of comorbidities and whose condition cannot be optimized preoperatively should not be considered for new surgical procedures. Even after treatment by a professional head and neck surgeon and careful anesthesia consultation, the 90-day mortality in Taiwan remained at 2.34% from 2006 to 2015 (Table 5). The WCS can serve as a valuable tool for preoperative prediction of the risk associated with curative surgery in patients with LA-HNSCC. After predicting the risk, other alternative curative-intent aggressive treatments can be considered in LA-HNSCC patients [4,14–21].

To the best of our knowledge, our study is the first to use a comorbidity score to predict the 90-day mortality in the patients with LA-HNSCC who had received curative surgery. Figures revealed significant differences between low-, intermediate-, high-, and very-high-risk strata. These findings suggest that the WCS is a valid and specific tool for predicting 90-day and overall mortality in patients with LA-HNSCC who will receive curative surgery. Our literature review also revealed that our study also had the largest sample size among the studies that have proposed new comorbidity scores in the past 10 years.

This study has some limitations. First, the morbidity of curative surgery could not be determined because of differences in the levels of experience among surgeons and across hospitals; therefore, head and neck curative-surgery-related mortality estimates may have been biased. However, the Taiwan Cancer Registry report, 2017 edition, revealed that curative surgery for LA-HNSCC in Taiwan are mostly performed in hospitals with high patient volumes and large medical centers [6]. Therefore, the outcomes of head and neck curative surgery would be consistent in Taiwan. Second, because all the patients with LA-HNSCC were enrolled from an Asian population and all the surgical procedures were performed by Taiwanese surgeons, the corresponding ethnic and regional susceptibility to this disease remain unclear; hence, our results should be cautiously extrapolated to non-Asian populations. Third, the diagnoses of all comorbid conditions were based on ICD-9-CM codes. However, the Taiwan Cancer Registry administration randomly reviews charts and interviews patients to verify the accuracy of the diagnoses. Hospitals with outlier chargers or practices may be audited and be subsequently heavily penalized if malpractice or discrepancies are identified. In addition, the quality and precision of ICD-9-CM codes in Taiwan have been verified and proven by previous studies [51,52]. Therefore, to obtain accurate information on population specificity and disease occurrence, large-scale randomized trials that compare carefully selected patients who had received suitable treatments are required. Fourth, we have scarcely very-high WCS patients (32/55,080 = 0.05%) and scarcely high WCS patients (<1000/55,080 = 1.60%). For remaining more than 98 percent of the patients only two risk strata groups are left and this is the same problem what we have with the ASA II and ASA III patients. Nevertheless, the individual 90-day mortality can be predicted upon the findings of this study because a big cancer registry supports this data. Finally, the TCRD does not contain information on dietary habits, socioeconomic status, or body mass index, which may all be risk factors for mortality. However, considering the magnitude and statistical significance of the effects observed in this study, these limitations are unlikely to have affected the conclusions.

5. Conclusions

The WCS is a valid tool for predicting 90-day mortality and overall survival in patients with LA-HNSCC who will receive curative surgery. Other alternative curative-intent aggressive treatments can be considered for patients with LA-HNSCC in the high- to very-high-risk strata instead of curative surgery.

Author Contributions: Study concept and design, S.-Y.W. and L.Q.; financial support, Taipei Medical University. (TMU105-AE1-B26); collection and organization of data, Y.-W.K.; data analysis and interpretation, all authors; administrative Support, S.-Y.W.; manuscript writing, all authors; final approval of manuscript, all authors.

Acknowledgments: We thank National Natural Science Foundation of China (Grant No. 61603092), National Statistical Science Research Key Project (2016LZ35), University of International Business and Economics Huiyuan outstanding young scholars research funding (17YQ15) for the financial support provided to Lei Qin. We also thank Taipei Medical University (TMU105-AE1-B26) and Wanfang Hospital (funding 107-wf-swf-08) for the financial support provided to Szu-Yuan Wu.

Abbreviations

AJCC	American Joint Committee on Cancer
ARDS	Adult Respiratory Distress Syndrome
ASA	American Society of Anesthesiologists
CAD	Coronal Arterial Disease
CCI	Charlson Comorbidity Index
CCRT	Concurrent Chemoradiotherapy
CI	Confidence Interval
CKD	Chronic Kidney Disease
COPD	Chronic Obstructive Pulmonary Disease
CVA	Cerebral Vascular Accident
DIC	Disseminated Intravascular Coagulation
ESRD	End-Stage Renal Disease
HBV	Hepatitis B

HCV	Hepatitis C
HNSCC	Head and Neck Squamous Cell Carcinoma
HR	Hazard Ratio
HTN	Diabetes Mellitus DM Hypertension
ICD-9-CM	International Classification of Diseases Ninth Revision Clinical Modification
LA-HNSCC	Locoregionally Advanced Head and Neck Squamous Cell Carcinoma
MI	Myocardial Infarction
PUD	Peptic Ulcer Disease
PVD	Peripheral Vascular Disease
RT	Radiotherapy
TCRD	Taiwan Cancer Registry Database
TIA	Transient Ischemic Attack

References

1. Chen, J.H.; Yen, Y.C.; Chen, T.M.; Yuan, K.S.; Lee, F.P.; Lin, K.C.; Lai, M.T.; Wu, C.C.; Chang, C.L.; Wu, S.Y. Survival prognostic factors for metachronous second primary head and neck squamous cell carcinoma. *Cancer Med.* **2017**, *6*, 142–153. [CrossRef] [PubMed]
2. Chang, C.L.; Yuan, K.S.; Wu, S.Y. High-dose or low-dose cisplatin concurrent with radiotherapy in locally advanced head and neck squamous cell cancer. *Head Neck* **2017**, *39*, 1364–1370. [CrossRef] [PubMed]
3. Chen, J.H.; Yen, Y.C.; Liu, S.H.; Yuan, S.P.; Wu, L.L.; Lee, F.P.; Lin, K.C.; Lai, M.T.; Wu, C.C.; Chen, T.M.; et al. Outcomes of Induction Chemotherapy for Head and Neck Cancer Patients: A Combined Study of Two National Cohorts in Taiwan. *Medicine (Baltimore)* **2016**, *95*, e2845. [CrossRef] [PubMed]
4. Chen, J.H.; Yen, Y.C.; Yang, H.C.; Liu, S.H.; Yuan, S.P.; Wu, L.L.; Lee, F.P.; Lin, K.C.; Lai, M.T.; Wu, C.C.; et al. Curative-intent aggressive treatment improves survival in elderly patients with locally advanced head and neck squamous cell carcinoma and high comorbidity index. *Medicine (Baltimore)* **2016**, *95*, e3268. [CrossRef] [PubMed]
5. Chang, J.H.; Wu, C.C.; Yuan, K.S.; Wu, A.T.H.; Wu, S.Y. Locoregionally recurrent head and neck squamous cell carcinoma: Incidence, survival, prognostic factors, and treatment outcomes. *Oncotarget* **2017**, *8*, 55600–55612. [CrossRef] [PubMed]
6. Health Promotion Administration, M.o.H.a.W. Taiwan Cancer Registry Report, 2017 Edition. Available online: http://www.hpa.gov.tw/BHPNet/Web/Stat/StatisticsShow.aspx?No=201404160001 (accessed on 28 December 2017).
7. McGuirt, W.F.; Loevy, S.; McCabe, B.F.; Krause, C.J. The risks of major head and neck surgery in the aged population. *Laryngoscope* **1977**, *87*, 1378–1382. [CrossRef] [PubMed]
8. Gueret, G.; Bourgain, J.L.; Luboinski, B. Sudden death after major head and neck surgery. *Curr. Opin. Otolaryngol. Head Neck Surg.* **2006**, *14*, 89–94. [CrossRef] [PubMed]
9. Krause, L.G.; Moreno-Torres, A.; Campos, R. Radical neck dissection. Evaluation of 230 consecutive cases. *Arch. Otolaryngol.* **1971**, *94*, 153–157. [CrossRef] [PubMed]
10. Yarington, C.T., Jr.; Yonkers, A.J.; Beddoe, G.M. Radical neck dissection. Mortality and morbidity. *Arch. Otolaryngol.* **1973**, *97*, 306–308. [CrossRef] [PubMed]
11. MacComb, W.S. Mortality from radical neck dissection. *Am. J. Surg.* **1968**, *115*, 352–354. [CrossRef]
12. Shaha, A.R. Neck dissection: An operation in evolution. *World J. Surg. Oncol.* **2005**, *3*, 22. [CrossRef] [PubMed]
13. Myers, E.N.; Gastman, B.R. Neck dissection: An operation in evolution: Hayes Martin lecture. *Arch. Otolaryngol. Head Neck Surg.* **2003**, *129*, 14–25. [CrossRef] [PubMed]
14. Seiwert, T.Y.; Salama, J.K.; Vokes, E.E. The concurrent chemoradiation paradigm—General principles. *Nat. Clin. Pract. Oncol.* **2007**, *4*, 86–100. [CrossRef] [PubMed]
15. Ang, K.K.; Zhang, Q.; Rosenthal, D.I.; Nguyen-Tan, P.F.; Sherman, E.J.; Weber, R.S.; Galvin, J.M.; Bonner, J.A.; Harris, J.; El-Naggar, A.K.; et al. Randomized phase III trial of concurrent accelerated radiation plus cisplatin with or without cetuximab for stage III to IV head and neck carcinoma: RTOG 0522. *J. Clin. Oncol.* **2014**, *32*, 2940–2950. [CrossRef] [PubMed]

16. Seiwert, T.Y.; Burtness, B.; Mehra, R.; Weiss, J.; Berger, R.; Eder, J.P.; Heath, K.; McClanahan, T.; Lunceford, J.; Gause, C.; et al. Safety and clinical activity of pembrolizumab for treatment of recurrent or metastatic squamous cell carcinoma of the head and neck (KEYNOTE-012): An open-label, multicentre, phase 1b trial. *Lancet Oncol.* **2016**, *17*, 956–965. [CrossRef]
17. Chow, L.Q.M.; Haddad, R.; Gupta, S.; Mahipal, A.; Mehra, R.; Tahara, M.; Berger, R.; Eder, J.P.; Burtness, B.; Lee, S.H.; et al. Antitumor activity of pembrolizumab in biomarker-unselected patients with recurrent and/or metastatic head and neck squamous cell carcinoma: Results from the phase IB KEYNOTE-012 expansion cohort. *J. Clin. Oncol.* **2016**, *34*, 3838–3845. [CrossRef] [PubMed]
18. Bauml, J.; Seiwert, T.Y.; Pfister, D.G.; Worden, F.; Liu, S.V.; Gilbert, J.; Saba, N.F.; Weiss, J.; Wirth, L.; Sukari, A.; et al. Pembrolizumab for Platinum-and Cetuximab-Refractory Head and Neck Cancer: Results from a Single-Arm, Phase II Study. *J. Clin. Oncol.* **2017**, *35*, 1542–1549. [CrossRef] [PubMed]
19. Owen, D.; Iqbal, F.; Pollock, B.E.; Link, M.J.; Stien, K.; Garces, Y.I.; Brown, P.D.; Foote, R.L. Long-term follow-up of stereotactic radiosurgery for head and neck malignancies. *Head Neck* **2015**, *37*, 1557–1562. [CrossRef] [PubMed]
20. Mageras, G.S.; Mechalakos, J. Planning in the IGRT context: Closing the loop. *Semin. Radiat. Oncol.* **2007**, *17*, 268–277. [CrossRef] [PubMed]
21. Lee, N.; Puri, D.R.; Blanco, A.I.; Chao, K.S. Intensity-modulated radiation therapy in head and neck cancers: An update. *Head Neck* **2007**, *29*, 387–400. [CrossRef] [PubMed]
22. Yen, Y.C.; Chang, J.H.; Lin, W.C.; Chiou, J.F.; Chang, Y.C.; Chang, C.L.; Hsu, H.L.; Chow, J.M.; Yuan, K.S.; Wu, A.T.; et al. Effectiveness of esophagectomy in patients with thoracic esophageal squamous cell carcinoma receiving definitive radiotherapy or concurrent chemoradiotherapy through intensity-modulated radiation therapy techniques. *Cancer* **2017**. [CrossRef] [PubMed]
23. Chang, C.L.; Tsai, H.C.; Lin, W.C.; Chang, J.H.; Hsu, H.L.; Chow, J.M.; Yuan, K.S.; Wu, A.T.H.; Wu, S.Y. Dose escalation intensity-modulated radiotherapy-based concurrent chemoradiotherapy is effective for advanced-stage thoracic esophageal squamous cell carcinoma. *Radiother. Oncol.* **2017**. [CrossRef] [PubMed]
24. Wijeysundera, D.N.; Austin, P.C.; Beattie, W.S.; Hux, J.E.; Laupacis, A. A population-based study of anesthesia consultation before major noncardiac surgery. *Arch. Intern. Med.* **2009**, *169*, 595–602. [CrossRef] [PubMed]
25. Lin, W.C.; Ding, Y.F.; Hsu, H.L.; Chang, J.H.; Yuan, K.S.; Wu, A.T.H.; Chow, J.M.; Chang, C.L.; Chen, S.U.; Wu, S.Y. Value and application of trimodality therapy or definitive concurrent chemoradiotherapy in thoracic esophageal squamous cell carcinoma. *Cancer* **2017**, *123*, 3904–3915. [CrossRef] [PubMed]
26. Cohen, M.M.; Duncan, P.G.; Tate, R.B. Does anesthesia contribute to operative mortality? *JAMA* **1988**, *260*, 2859–2863. [CrossRef] [PubMed]
27. Chowdhury, M.M.; Dagash, H.; Pierro, A. A systematic review of the impact of volume of surgery and specialization on patient outcome. *Br. J. Surg.* **2007**, *94*, 145–161. [CrossRef] [PubMed]
28. Lau, R.L.; Perruccio, A.V.; Gandhi, R.; Mahomed, N.N. The role of surgeon volume on patient outcome in total knee arthroplasty: A systematic review of the literature. *BMC Musculoskelet. Disord.* **2012**, *13*, 250. [CrossRef] [PubMed]
29. Wen, H.C.; Tang, C.H.; Lin, H.C.; Tsai, C.S.; Chen, C.S.; Li, C.Y. Association between surgeon and hospital volume in coronary artery bypass graft surgery outcomes: A population-based study. *Ann. Thorac. Surg.* **2006**, *81*, 835–842. [CrossRef] [PubMed]
30. Birkmeyer, J.D.; Siewers, A.E.; Finlayson, E.V.; Stukel, T.A.; Lucas, F.L.; Batista, I.; Welch, H.G.; Wennberg, D.E. Hospital volume and surgical mortality in the United States. *N. Engl. J. Med.* **2002**, *346*, 1128–1137. [CrossRef] [PubMed]
31. Turrentine, F.E.; Wang, H.; Simpson, V.B.; Jones, R.S. Surgical risk factors, morbidity, and mortality in elderly patients. *J. Am. Coll. Surg.* **2006**, *203*, 865–877. [CrossRef] [PubMed]
32. Van Bokhorst-de van der, S.; van Leeuwen, P.A.; Kuik, D.J.; Klop, W.M.; Sauerwein, H.P.; Snow, G.B.; Quak, J.J. The impact of nutritional status on the prognoses of patients with advanced head and neck cancer. *Cancer* **1999**, *86*, 519–527. [CrossRef]
33. Sylvester, M.J.; Marchiano, E.; Park, R.C.; Baredes, S.; Eloy, J.A. Impact of chronic obstructive pulmonary disease on patients undergoing laryngectomy for laryngeal cancer. *Laryngoscope* **2017**, *127*, 417–423. [CrossRef] [PubMed]

34. Patterson, J.T.; Bohl, D.D.; Basques, B.A.; Arzeno, A.H.; Grauer, J.N. Does Preoperative Pneumonia Affect Complications of Geriatric Hip Fracture Surgery? *Am. J. Orthop. (Belle Mead NJ)* **2017**, *46*, E177–E185. [PubMed]
35. Volpi, A.; De Vita, C.; Franzosi, M.G.; Geraci, E.; Maggioni, A.P.; Mauri, F.; Negri, E.; Santoro, E.; Tavazzi, L.; Tognoni, G. Determinants of 6-month mortality in survivors of myocardial infarction after thrombolysis. Results of the GISSI-2 data base. The Ad hoc Working Group of the Gruppo Italiano per lo Studio della Sopravvivenza nell'Infarto Miocardico (GISSI)-2 Data Base. *Circulation* **1993**, *88*, 416–429. [CrossRef] [PubMed]
36. Johansson, S.; Rosengren, A.; Young, K.; Jennings, E. Mortality and morbidity trends after the first year in survivors of acute myocardial infarction: A systematic review. *BMC Cardiovasc. Disord.* **2017**, *17*, 53. [CrossRef] [PubMed]
37. Kwiatkowski, T.G.; Libman, R.B.; Frankel, M.; Tilley, B.C.; Morgenstern, L.B.; Lu, M.; Broderick, J.P.; Lewandowski, C.A.; Marler, J.R.; Levine, S.R.; et al. Effects of tissue plasminogen activator for acute ischemic stroke at one year. National Institute of Neurological Disorders and Stroke Recombinant Tissue Plasminogen Activator Stroke Study Group. *N. Engl. J. Med.* **1999**, *340*, 1781–1787. [CrossRef] [PubMed]
38. Wang, Y.; Zhao, X.; Liu, L.; Wang, D.; Wang, C.; Li, H.; Meng, X.; Cui, L.; Jia, J.; Dong, Q.; et al. Clopidogrel with aspirin in acute minor stroke or transient ischemic attack. *N. Engl. J. Med.* **2013**, *369*, 11–19. [CrossRef] [PubMed]
39. Marwick, T.H. The viable myocardium: Epidemiology, detection, and clinical implications. *Lancet* **1998**, *351*, 815–819. [CrossRef]
40. Allman, K.C.; Shaw, L.J.; Hachamovitch, R.; Udelson, J.E. Myocardial viability testing and impact of revascularization on prognosis in patients with coronary artery disease and left ventricular dysfunction: A meta-analysis. *J. Am. Coll. Cardiol.* **2002**, *39*, 1151–1158. [CrossRef]
41. Sack, G.H., Jr.; Levin, J.; Bell, W.R. Trousseau's syndrome and other manifestations of chronic disseminated coagulopathy in patients with neoplasms: Clinical, pathophysiologic, and therapeutic features. *Medicine (Baltimore)* **1977**, *56*, 1–37. [CrossRef] [PubMed]
42. Katzenstein, A.L.; Myers, J.L.; Mazur, M.T. Acute interstitial pneumonia. A clinicopathologic, ultrastructural, and cell kinetic study. *Am. J. Surg. Pathol.* **1986**, *10*, 256–267. [CrossRef] [PubMed]
43. Kassahun, W.T. The effects of pre-existing dementia on surgical outcomes in emergent and nonemergent general surgical procedures: Assessing differences in surgical risk with dementia. *BMC Geriatr.* **2018**, *18*, 153. [CrossRef] [PubMed]
44. Cramer, J.D.; Patel, U.A.; Samant, S.; Yang, A.; Smith, S.S. Liver disease in patients undergoing head and neck surgery: Incidence and risk for postoperative complications. *Laryngoscope* **2017**, *127*, 102–109. [CrossRef] [PubMed]
45. Piccirillo, J.F.; Lacy, P.D.; Basu, A.; Spitznagel, E.L. Development of a new head and neck cancer-specific comorbidity index. *Arch. Otolaryngol. Head Neck Surg.* **2002**, *128*, 1172–1179. [CrossRef] [PubMed]
46. Siegel, R.; Ward, E.; Brawley, O.; Jemal, A. Cancer statistics, 2011: The impact of eliminating socioeconomic and racial disparities on premature cancer deaths. *CA Cancer J. Clin.* **2011**, *61*, 212–236. [CrossRef] [PubMed]
47. Ward, E.; DeSantis, C.; Robbins, A.; Kohler, B.; Jemal, A. Childhood and adolescent cancer statistics, 2014. *CA Cancer J. Clin.* **2014**, *64*, 83–103. [CrossRef] [PubMed]
48. Dees, E.C.; O'Reilly, S.; Goodman, S.N.; Sartorius, S.; Levine, M.A.; Jones, R.J.; Grochow, L.B.; Donehower, R.C.; Fetting, J.H. A prospective pharmacologic evaluation of age-related toxicity of adjuvant chemotherapy in women with breast cancer. *Cancer Investig.* **2000**, *18*, 521–529. [CrossRef]
49. Gomez, H.; Mas, L.; Casanova, L.; Pen, D.L.; Santillana, S.; Valdivia, S.; Otero, J.; Rodriguez, W.; Carracedo, C.; Vallejos, C. Elderly patients with aggressive non-Hodgkin's lymphoma treated with CHOP chemotherapy plus granulocyte-macrophage colony-stimulating factor: Identification of two age subgroups with differing hematologic toxicity. *J. Clin. Oncol.* **1998**, *16*, 2352–2358. [CrossRef] [PubMed]
50. Schild, S.E.; Stella, P.J.; Geyer, S.M.; Bonner, J.A.; McGinnis, W.L.; Mailliard, J.A.; Brindle, J.; Jatoi, A.; Jett, J.R. The outcome of combined-modality therapy for stage III non-small-cell lung cancer in the elderly. *J. Clin. Oncol.* **2003**, *21*, 3201–3206. [CrossRef] [PubMed]
51. Cheng, C.L.; Lee, C.H.; Chen, P.S.; Li, Y.H.; Lin, S.J.; Yang, Y.H. Validation of acute myocardial infarction cases in the national health insurance research database in Taiwan. *J. Epidemiol.* **2014**, *24*, 500–507. [CrossRef] [PubMed]

3

Reverse Engineering Cancer: Inferring Transcriptional Gene Signatures from Copy Number Aberrations with ICAro

Davide Angeli [1], Maurizio Fanciulli [2,†] and Matteo Pallocca [2,*,†]

[1] Department of Paediatric Haematology, IRCCS Ospedale Pediatrico Bambino Gesù, 00146 Rome, Italy; davide.ang@gmail.com

[2] SAFU Unit, IRCCS Regina Elena National Cancer Institute, 00144 Rome, Italy; maurizio.fanciulli@ifo.gov.it

* Correspondence: matteo.pallocca@ifo.gov.it

† These authors contributed equally.

Abstract: The characterization of a gene product function is a process that involves multiple laboratory techniques in order to silence the gene itself and to understand the resulting cellular phenotype via several omics profiling. When it comes to tumor cells, usually the translation process from in vitro characterization results to human validation is a difficult journey. Here, we present a simple algorithm to extract mRNA signatures from cancer datasets, where a particular gene has been deleted at the genomic level, ICAro. The process is implemented as a two-step workflow. The first one employs several filters in order to select the two patient subsets: the inactivated one, where the target gene is deleted, and the control one, where large genomic rearrangements should be absent. The second step performs a signature extraction via a Differential Expression analysis and a complementary Random Forest approach to provide an additional gene ranking in terms of information loss. We benchmarked the system robustness on a panel of genes frequently deleted in cancers, where we validated the downregulation of target genes and found a correlation with signatures extracted with the L1000 tool, outperforming random sampling for two out of six L1000 classes. Furthermore, we present a use case correlation with a published transcriptomic experiment. In conclusion, deciphering the complex interactions of the tumor environment is a challenge that requires the integration of several experimental techniques in order to create reproducible results. We implemented a tool which could be of use when trying to find mRNA signatures related to a gene loss event to better understand its function or for a gene-loss associated biomarker research.

Keywords: transcriptional signatures; copy number variation; copy number aberration; TCGA mining; cancer CRISPR; firehose; gene signature extraction; gene loss biomarkers; gene inactivation biomarkers; biomarker discovery

---

1. Background

Translational research has been hard at work trying to find a way to characterize genes and gene product functions for decades. One successful approach is the study of particular contexts where the gene expression of interest is perturbed. In the past, biologists mostly tried to characterize gene functions by overexpressing its mRNA, whereas more recently, several tools have been introduced in the field of Cellular and Molecular Biology to erase a gene (or its mRNA). Furthermore, a rapid evolution of induced DNA/RNA ablation techniques have emerged from perfectible approaches including siRNA/shRNA to highly specific ones such as TALEN and CRISPRs/Cas9 [1,2].

An induced gene deletion (or mRNA ablation) event brings about a series of phenotypes, both as direct consequences of the gene/protein absence and as epiphenomena mediated by the cellular environment response of such a relevant change.

The granular study of these phenotypes has been accelerated dramatically by the introduction of omic technologies in basic and translational research. For instance, we can easily take a transcriptome-wide picture of the mRNA status or the profile of a large panel of metabolites. All these data can easily help the investigators to apply the "guilt by association" approach in order to better understand a gene function by looking at the correlated omic response [3]. In spite of the elegant workflow (perturbation → omics → understanding), the process is hindered by a series of issues.

In regards to silencing technologies, while CRISPRs have promised to lead much less off-target effects than shRNAs, they still are a challenging technique for several laboratories worldwide and even show little correlation with RNA interference screens, a worrying scenario since thousands of mechanistic papers on cellular and molecular biology are based on these tools [4]. Furthermore, most of these characterizations are conducted in vitro, where the reproducibility of results is being pointed out as a major issue [5–7].

Several efforts have been made towards also automating and standardizing in vitro results to make them reproducible. Among these proposals, the L1000 connectivity map [8,9] is a clear example of a thorough characterization of the mRNA response of thousands of compounds (shRNA, overexpression, and drugs) in several cell lines.

However, when the whole question shifts to a difficult cellular context such as cancer, the situation worsens. The network of intercellular and intracellular interactions of the tumor macroenvironment is extremely complex and inevitably fails to be modeled by a simple mono-population cell line. In relation to this, organoids are an interesting promise [10], but most medium- and small-sized laboratories worldwide still do not have access to these kinds of models.

On the other hand, one resource that is available to any oncology-based research group is access to public cancer datasets. Only The Cancer Genome Atlas (TCGA) contains several molecular profiles from more than 11,000 patients at the time of the writing [11]. We tried to reason whether we could extract huge amounts of data to make the process of elucidating gene functions in cancer contexts easier and more robust. For this reason, we implemented ICAro (gene signature Inference system from Copy number Aberrations), a framework that enables researchers to extract putative gene signatures from publicly available Cancer Genomic datasets.

This overall idea involves treating cancer as a Cas9 model by using Copy Number Variations (CNVs) and inactivating mutations data on a particular gene target to split the patient dataset in control and inactivated groups. Then, we obtained RNA (RNA-seq) expression levels to extract a gene deletion signature. Here, we show that this method can still be a useful resource as an integrated tool for molecular knowledge mining.

2. Implementation

The algorithm is based on the workflow shown in Figure 1: the main inputs of the model are the gene of interest α and the particular tissue context Σ (chosen from the available TCGA cohort codes, e.g., ACC and COAD). Next, the inactivated and control sample sets are built. In the first step, only samples for which both CNV and mRNA-seq data are present in the TCGA database are included.

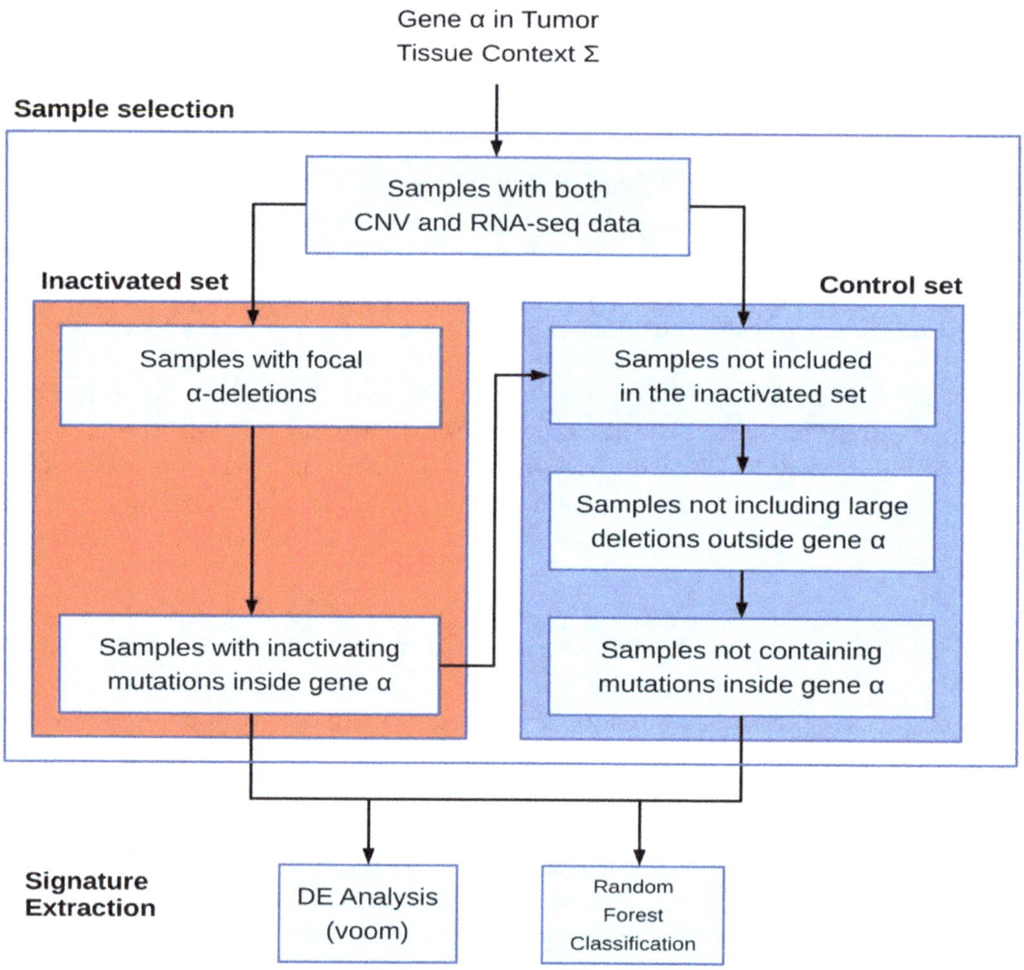

Figure 1. A schematic representation of the ICAro (gene signature Inference system from Copy number Aberrations) workflow. The first part relies on sample filtering based on deletions and inactivating mutations spanning the gene target α in order to build the inactivated and the control sample sets. They are used as input for the signature extraction process, performed via a differential gene expression analysis (the voom function from limma) and a Random Forest classification (randomForest R package).

The inactivated sample selection is performed following two different strategies: in the first one, both deletions and inactivating mutations if provided are used to include samples; in the second one, samples are selected only by inactivating mutations.

The deletion-based filter extracts inactivated samples by selecting CNVs that overlap the gene α location and in which the CNV-GISTIC score [12,13] is lower than -1. An optional filter allows to include only deletions larger than a given threshold. The second filter is based on inactivating mutations and requires an input file containing a list of protein substitution variants in the standard format according to Sequence Variant Nomenclature amino_acid/position/new_amino_acid (e.g., Cys28Ser). Unlike the first filter, it incorporates samples with variations present in the inactivating mutation list. Moreover, the specific format "STOP N" can be added to the list, where N is a number representing the rightmost stop-gain mutation allowing a sample to be included in the set.

The control set is built starting from only samples with both CNV and mRNA-seq data. Other exclusion criteria for the control set include outside the gene α, samples containing CNVs larger than a given threshold (e.g., 1 Mb), or mutations inside the same gene α. With these filters, we tried to minimize the genomic interference of having huge structural rearrangements in the control set.

The downstream analysis is executed only if there are at least five samples in the inactivated set and if the ratio between such a set and the control set is higher than a given threshold (0.05).

RNA-seq raw count data are transformed in count per millions (CPM), and only genes for which CPM is greater than 5 in at least 5 samples are kept.

The second part regarding the signature extraction is performed in two separated methods: the first one is a Differential Expression (DE) strategy in order to fetch up- and downregulated genes with regards to the inactivated set. Secondly, a Random Forest approach (RF) is employed with the aim of building activated and inactivated sets from a binary classifier. From the RF, we extracted a gene ranking list that allows to understand the most discriminatory genes in the classification process and the most likely to be part of our signature.

In the DE approach, the voom function of the limma package is executed on the data and a linear model followed by empirical bayesian statistics are performed in order to find differentially expressed genes between the two sets. On the other hand, Random Forests are built via the randomForest function of the randomForest package which implements the Breiman's random forest algorithm for classification. The preprocessing part is performed via custom Python scripting, whereas the filtered sets are provided as input to an R script that will perform the second step with the voom limma and randomForest [14,15] packages. The data fetch process is automated thanks to the Firebrowse package [16].

The DE output file contains a list of genes with some features, such as the log fold-change and q-value, where the user can observe the putative differentially expressed genes. We appended additional columns to the differential output file in order to give more information on the kind of induction adopted, e.g., two columns with a median expression for each group. The RF output file contains a list of genes ranked by their meanDecreaseGini value, thus having the most important genes in terms of loss of information on top.

The tool is freely available at https://gitlab.com/bioinfo-ire-release/icaro.

3. Results

In order to demonstrate the accuracy of our approach, we extracted 50 pairs of frequently deleted genes (and their matching datasets) from the cBioPortal [17] (Tables S1 and S2) to run the workflow with. Afterwards, from the output signature, we extracted the fold change and the adjusted p-value of the target gene to understand whether we are selecting samples in which the target gene is significantly downregulated. Indeed, almost all of the targets are significantly downregulated (94.0%) and have a strong induction (i.e., $\log_2 FC < -0.58$, meaning a 50% regulation, 93.6%) (Figure 2). We performed a similar benchmarking for the RF results on the same genes. When visualizing the meanDecreaseAccuracy (MDA) and meanDecreaseGini (MDG) of such genes, we observed that only 5/50 (10%) gene-dataset pairs had an MDG higher than 1%, while only 2/50 (4%) pairs showed an MDG over 5% (Figure S1).

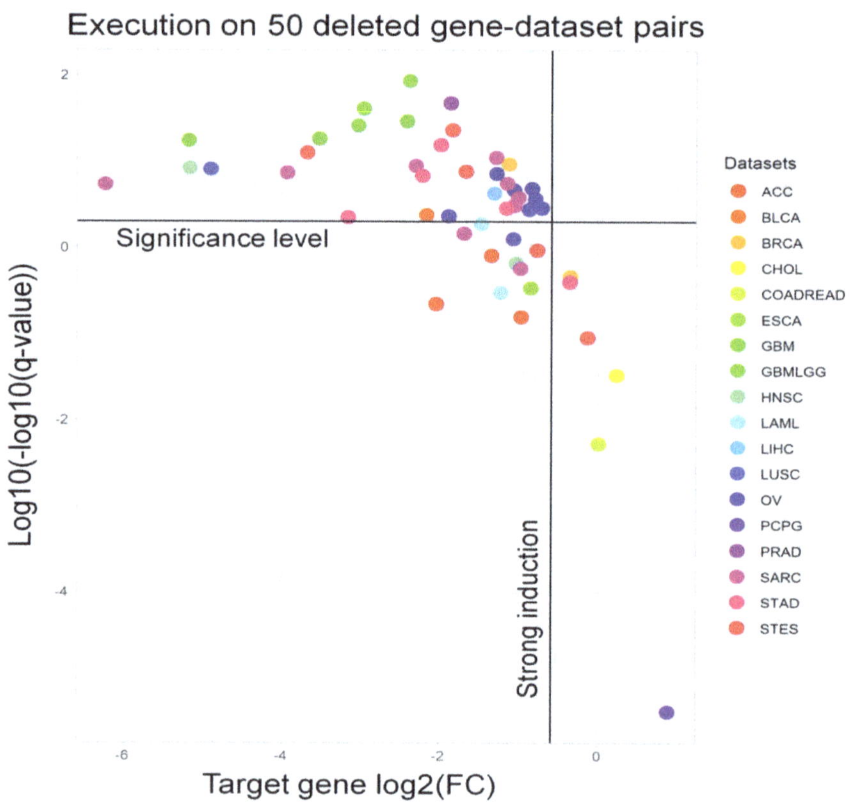

Figure 2. The performance of the ICAro Differential Expression for 50 executions on frequently deleted gene-dataset pairs: Every point represents one ICAro execution on a gene-dataset pair (e.g., TP53 on COADREAD). The different colors represent several TCGA datasets. *X*-axis: log2FC (gene induction), *Y*-axis: transformed *q*-value (statistical significance). Most tests fall in the upper region, meaning that they are significant, and on the center of the *X*-axis, i.e., they are downregulated. The downregulation of deleted genes is a first step towards the in vivo validation of the ICAro process. For a complete key of datasets please refer to Table S1.

We pointed out that inactivated set sizing was the main failure in the workflow. That is, for most datasets, it was difficult to find a high number of patients with focal deletions inside a particular gene. For the RF classification task, it seemed that the deleted gene expression level did not contain a sufficient amount of information in this in vivo setting in order to build a good classifier by itself.

Next, we attempted to demonstrate that the algorithm was able to correlate with other data that were more similar to the typical laboratory approach. The idea involved testing whether the ICAro signature had significant similarities to shRNA knockout perturbations, the routine approach, or other drugs and kinase signatures. To this purpose, we used the aforementioned 50 signatures and we queried L1000 via the Enrichr API [8,9,18] for correlating with the Chemical, Kinase, and Ligand Perturbation. We divided the signatures into up- and downregulated genes; therefore, for each gene-dataset pair, we extracted a L1000 table, 300 in total (Figure 3). On average, every signature correlated with 5 significant terms (adjusted p-value < 0.05, median: 5 terms, and mean: 306 terms). When analyzing the particular sub-signatures, up-signatures tended to poorly overlap (median: 0) while down-signatures had better correlation (median from 2 to 660) (Table S3). This difference is to be clearly attributed to the nature of the model that we tested. In fact, our focus is on deletions; therefore a direct gene downregulation trend will overlap better than an in-trans upregulation event.

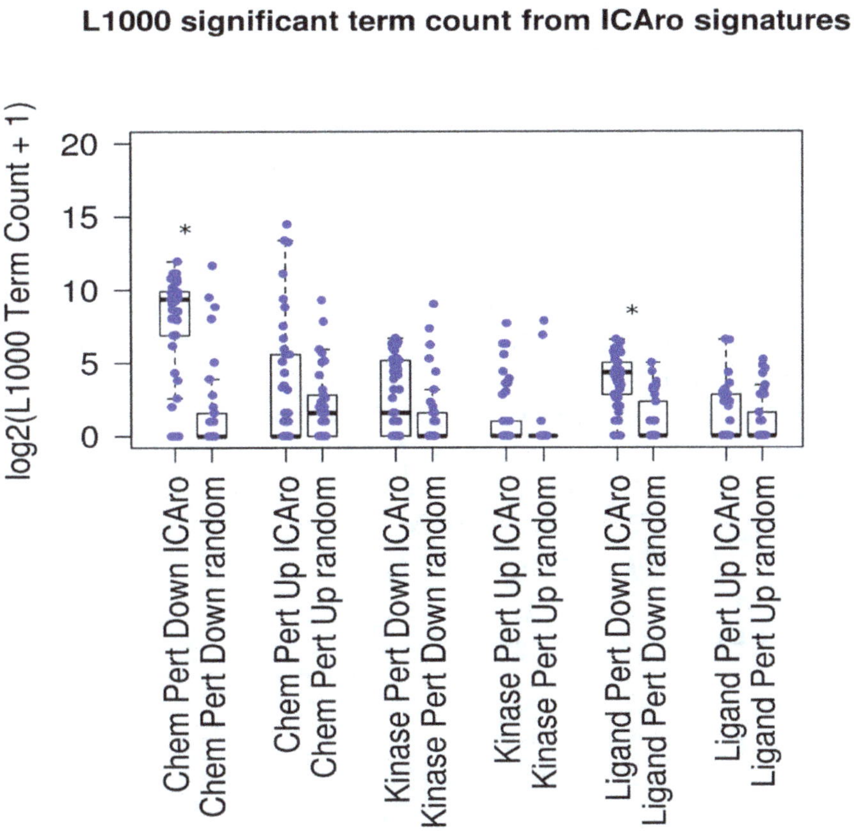

Figure 3. The amount of significant terms for down and up-regulated genes when compared to L1000 signatures: Every point is an ICAro execution with a significant gene set (up or down). Every signature is compared with the amount of significant terms when sampling random gene sets of equal size. Legend: * significant increase between random sampling and ICAro.

In order to show a comparison on the difference between this performance and random distribution, we ran a parallel script, where given N_i, M_i, the number of significant genes from each signature S_i, we extracted N_i, M_i random genes and executed the Enrichr analysis on them. The median number of significant signatures was 0 (adjusted p-value < 0.05, median: 0 terms, and mean: 36 terms), and five out of six classes had a median term number 0 (Figure 3 and Table S3). The mean amount of terms resulted significantly more in 2 out of 6 cases, particularly in the Chemical Perturbation Down and the Ligand Perturbation Down clusters, confirming the aforementioned hypothesis of the ICAro applicability.

As a second validation process, without focusing on frequently deleted genes, we applied the workflow on the genes of interest in tumor genomics, i.e., cancer driver genes. We focused on 459 mutational cancer driver genes (Table S4), deriving from the Integrative Onco Genomics (intOgen) list [19]. Among those, we excluded 23 of them, which were located in sexual chromosomes. Given that we did not separate patients by gender, this would have had a strong bias in the CNV/mRNA separation. The analysis was carried out on 35 datasets (Table S5): only on UCS (Uterine Carcinosarcoma), no results were obtained. For the other datasets, there was a high variability in the number of analyses successfully performed, starting from 2 for CHOL (Cholangiocarcinoma) and DLBC (Diffuse Large B-cell Lymphoma) to 100 for OV (Ovarian serous cystadenocarcinoma), with a mean of 22 successful runs per dataset. From a gene-centered perspective (Table S6), we obtained at least 1 result from 148 genes (34%) and f in which the minimum is 1 for 60 genes and the maximum is

31 for the WNK1 gene, with a mean of 5 analyses for each gene. The main challenge in performing an ICAro analysis is the lack of CNVs on the genes of interest: 59% of analyses failed for this reason. Subsequently, the second main cause for this failure is the absence or the low amount of inactivated mRNA samples: 88% of samples which had passed the previous filters were rejected at this step. Eight analyses were not performed due to a missing control sample. In conclusion, on the whole, only 5% of analyses were successfully performed.

The final step of ICAro modeling features also a Random Forest analysis in addition to the Differential Expression. The aim is to overcome the limitations of linear modeling and to provide a clean gene rank in terms of importance. In order to further describe the relationship among the two analyses, we compared the results of ICAro executions of the aforementioned 50 gene-datasets pairs in terms of the Differential Expression vs. Random Forest results. This profiling presents different scenarios, in which in some cases, the RF approach can massively extend the scope of the DE, that features only a few significant genes (5 out of the top 100 RF genes are significant in DE, Figure 4A). In other cases, the situation is the opposite, and the RF is only an extension of the strong amount of significant DE genes (75 out of the 100 top RF genes are significant in DE, Figure 4B). The full 50 plots are available at the application's webpage.

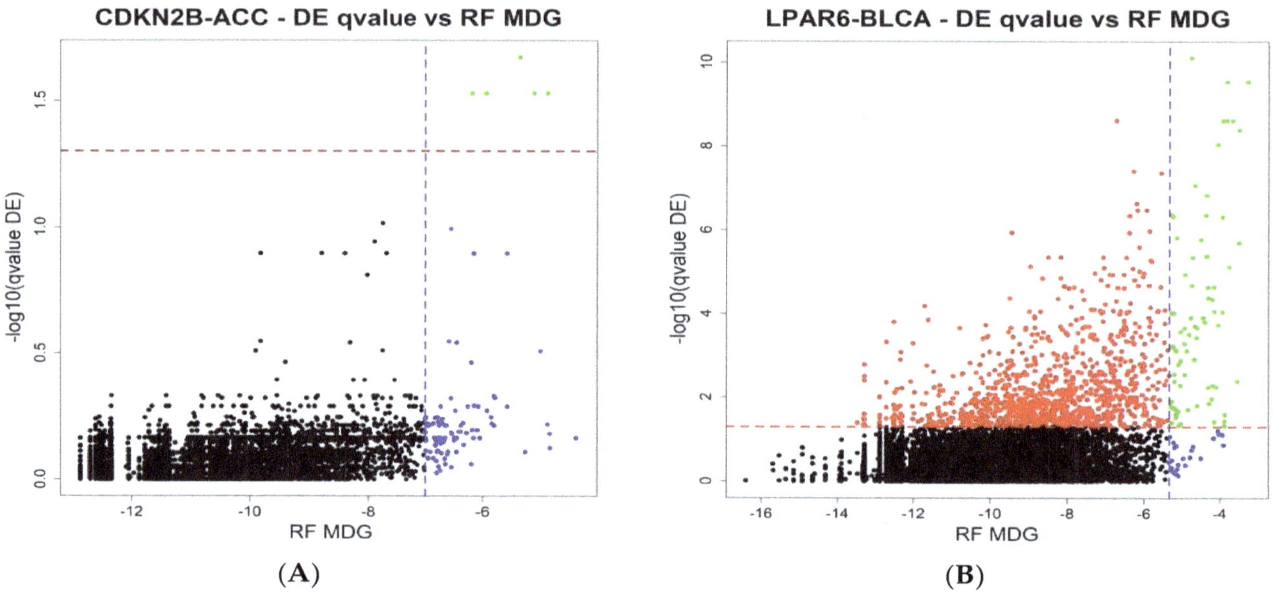

Figure 4. (**A**,**B**) Two representative plots of the Differential Expression against the Random Forest analysis on the ICAro system. Blue line: the top 100 genes from the Random Forest analysis, ranked by the meanDecreaseGini (MDG). Red line: the adjusted *p*-value significance threshold. Left: only a few genes are significantly regulated in the DE analysis, but more can be studied from the top 100 genes on the RF analysis. Right: the opposite situation where most information lies in the differential expression, and just most of the top 100 RF genes are significant in DE terms.

Finally, in order to present the scope and the possible applications of our system, we produced a use case. We exploited a public transcriptomic dataset (GSE76689), a silencing experiment designed to dissect the role of RB1 in Ovarian carcinoma [20]. We reproduced the DE analysis of the paper. Globally, 2 down- and 8 upregulated genes are confirmed to be significant by the system, thus stressing the importance of these mRNAs to discriminate signatures of RB1 loss in Ovarian carcinoma (Table 1). Furthermore, the Random Forest modeling returned 5/10 of the significant genes to be in the top 100 Gini index ranking.

Table 1. The significant genes validated in the GSE76689 dataset from the ICAro system.

Gene	Log2FC siRB1	Log2FC ICAro	adj PVal siRB1	adj P Val ICAro
RB1	−0.83	−1.12	5.73×10^{-4}	1.81×10^{-6}
SH3BP4	−0.64	−0.63	8.21×10^{-4}	3.35×10^{-2}
NUDT21	0.67	0.29	1.22×10^{-3}	4.46×10^{-2}
SLC27A3	0.64	0.40	5.70×10^{-3}	3.45×10^{-2}
C15orf38	0.77	0.42	1.40×10^{-3}	3.82×10^{-2}
ADCY3	0.76	0.49	7.18×10^{-4}	1.78×10^{-2}
TMEM106C	0.66	0.51	2.69×10^{-3}	2.70×10^{-2}
FANCE	0.47	0.57	2.92×10^{-2}	2.36×10^{-3}
WDR34	0.53	0.59	1.31×10^{-2}	4.94×10^{-4}
TCF19	0.49	0.99	2.68×10^{-2}	1.81×10^{-6}

Taken together, these results highlighted that the algorithm is able to extract a few significantly correlated regulation signatures for genes that are frequently deleted in cancer. The workflow performed better than random sampling and could be used by researchers to extract several "parent" signatures from the target gene in a tumor environment. From the cancer gene driver's point-of-view, a small fraction could be queried for gene signatures thanks to ICAro. Finally, it can be exploited to select a subset of genes of interest in a mRNA profiling experiment.

4. Discussion

The intricate patterns of transcriptional networks are complex to decipher for the biomedical researcher, and in our experience, researchers struggle to find evidence to confirm a regulatory hypothesis. This is one of the main reasons that led us to develop a simple algorithm to help investigators in the field of Cancer Transcriptomics.

The other motivation comes from our experience in handling NGS data and bioinformatic analysis of a medium-sized genomic facility. Translational projects are often designed to start with a whole transcriptomic or a whole epigenomic experiment (e.g., RNA-seq and ChIP-seq), intended to be the hypothesis driver for further investigations. As a matter of fact, the process risks to be interrupted when bioinformaticians present researchers with enormous lists of genes and ontologies. We impute this matter to three main factors: the lack of computational biologists in research groups, the intrinsic difficulty of summarizing large quantity of data, and a slow validation process due to the high number of possible targets as starting points. ICAro comes as an aid for the latter issues, providing hints on mRNA targets that could indeed be validated in vivo.

Many confounding factors are not taken into account in the patient partitioning. These are, for instance, patient stratification by demographic data. This is an issue of many algorithmic signatures of the transcriptomic field that do not seem to care even if they are designed to stratify patients into clinical settings [21,22]. In our case, the scarcity of the inactivated set, usually falling below the count of 5, prevents us in further dividing the patient strata.

In addition, most TCGA mutation datasets do not carry Variant Allele Frequency (VAF) information. For this reason, we may erroneously include a few patients in the inactivation set (that is already suffering from typical smaller size) that carry a stop-gain mutation in only a small fraction of tumor cells (e.g., VAF < 10%). This limitation also applies to CNV data, where the GISTIC threshold output are decided on a sample by sample basis [23]. Furthermore, it should be noted that every sample profiled in the TCGA had a tumor cellularity of at least 80% (recently shifted to 60%) and is not available metadata for which we could correct the CNV/Mutation status.

Our implementation process also lacks some features that we plan to employ in the future. The most obvious one is the lack of a gene amplification study. That is, the possibility to extract a signature when a gene has more copies. This could be a valuable experiment mirroring another frequent laboratory approach such as overexpression models. Another interesting add-on would be appending genomic coordinates of each gene locus to the final output in order to understand whether the differential effect is mostly guided by the CNV itself or by some other regulation pathways. Finally, one more aspect that could be improved in the future is the simple automatization of functional APIs from the result dataset, such as LINCs Cloud and ENRICHR, allowing researchers to better investigate the mechanisms involved.

ICAro testing on a list of mutational cancer driver genes pointed out that the main problem is that less than half of such genes are affected by CNVs, and among the samples with these deletions, only 1 over 12 contains related mRNA experiments, thus preventing us from performing the analysis on a larger set of data.

5. Conclusions

Mining knowledge regarding gene function or seeking inactivation biomarkers is not so trivial tasks. It is for this reason, we developed an automated tool to integrate and mine knowledge from third-level TCGA data. Our testing showed that this workflow is able to extract several transcriptional signatures for a discrete set of genes.

From a biological perspective, the authors are aware that (a) the amount of patients with focal deletions for a given gene will be discrete for the time being, (b) the cancer genomic and transcriptomic background is a disorderly environment very different from engineered cell lines, and (c) it is known that most frequent gene losses have recurrent breakpoints [12]. Nevertheless, we remain confident in the value and feasibility of the presented approach due to the rapid increase in the amount of available high-throughput data and in the vast disappointing failures of in vitro derived models.

We are currently working on an extended version for miRNA signature extraction that will be useful for researchers in the non-coding RNA field. Investigators will fetch via ICAro differential miRNA classes that are up-and downregulated by a particular gene deletion, providing additional insights on miRNA-mRNA interaction.

In a real-life setting, we trust that the ICAro approach would be of value when paired with several other approaches such as in vitro or in vivo knockout models, for instance when understanding biomarkers for the inactivation of a particular gene. In this scenario, it will be useful to implement a novel branch of the workflow to take into account also other emerging large-scale omic approaches such as Reverse-Phase Protein Arrays (RPPA).

Supplementary Materials:
Figure S1: Performance of ICAro Random Forest classification for 50 executions on frequently deleted gene-dataset pairs. MDA: meanDecreaseAccuracy and MDG: meanDecreaseGini, Table S1: The list of gene-dataset pairs used for benchmarking purposes in Figures 2 and 3, Table S2: A full key of TCGA dataset names from Firebrowse at the time of the writing, Table S3: The average number of significant L1000 signature overlaps from the ICAro output and random sampling. The *cpd*, *kpd*, etc. stand for classes abbreviations for Chemical Perturbation Down, etc., Table S4: The list of mutational cancer driver autosomal genes used for testing ICAro on each dataset, Table S5: A dataset-centered summary of the ICAro tests using cancer driver genes. The column *total* contains the genes analyzed for each dataset; *no_cnv* is the number of samples without CNVs on the queried gene; *no_or_few_mrna* is the number of samples for which there are no mRNA data, the samples are less than 5, or the ratio between them and the control samples is less than 0.05; *no_control* is the number of samples without mRNA control data; *success* is the number of analysis successfully performed; and *perc_success* is the percentage of succeeded analysis on the total number of analysis attempted for each dataset, Table S6: A gene-centered summary of the ICAro tests using cancer driver genes. The columns follow the same nomenclature as Table S5 but on a gene-centered analysis.

Author Contributions: M.P. conceived the idea, implemented the beta version of the Python algorithm, and wrote the validating script resulting in Figure 3. D.A. tested and extended the first part of the workflow, implemented the whole automated signature extraction in R, and evaluated the algorithm resulting in Figures 1 and 2. M.F. provided the Molecular Biology supervision of the whole process. M.P., D.A., and M.F. wrote the manuscript. All authors read and approved this version of the manuscript.

Acknowledgments: We thank Tania Merlino for the editorial assistance. We thank the members of our laboratory for critically reading the manuscript. We thank Eng. Sara Errigo for the critical discussion and data visualization support. We acknowledge the CINECA award under the ISCRA initiative for the availability of the high-performance computing resources and support.

Abbreviations

DE	Differential Expression
RF	Random Forest
CNV	Copy Number Variations
CNA	Copy Number Aberration
siRNA	small interfering RNA
shRNA	short hairpin RNA
CPM	count per million
TALEN	Transcription Activator-Like Effector Nucleases
CRISPR	Clustered Regulatory Interspaced Short Palindromic Repeats
VAF	Variant Allele Frequency

References

1. Boettcher, M.; McManus, M.T. Choosing the Right Tool for the Job: RNAi, TALEN, or CRISPR. *Mol. Cell* **2015**, *58*, 575–585. [CrossRef] [PubMed]
2. Unniyampurath, U.; Pilankatta, R.; Krishnan, M.N. RNA interference in the age of CRISPR: Will CRISPR interfere with RNAI? *Int. J. Mol. Sci.* **2016**, *17*, 291. [CrossRef] [PubMed]
3. Lefever, S.; Anckaert, J.; Volders, P.J.; Luypaert, M.; Vandesompele, J.; Mestdagh, P. decodeRNA- predicting non-coding RNA functions using guilt-by-association. *Database (Oxford)* **2017**, *2017*, 1–8. [CrossRef] [PubMed]
4. Morgens, D.W.; Deans, R.M.; Li, A.; Bassik, M.C. Systematic comparison of CRISPR/Cas9 and RNAi screens for essential genes. *Nat. Biotechnol.* **2016**, *34*, 634–636. [CrossRef] [PubMed]
5. Freedman, L.P. Know thy cells: Improving biomedical research reproducibility. *Sci. Transl. Med.* **2015**, *7*, 2015–2017. [CrossRef] [PubMed]
6. Phillips, P.; Lithgow, G.J.; Driscoll, M. A long journey to reproducible results. *Nature* **2017**, *548*, 387–388.
7. Northcott, P.A. Cancer: Keeping it real to kill glioblastoma. *Nature* **2017**, *547*, 291–292. [CrossRef]
8. Subramanian, A.; Narayan, R.; Corsello, S.M.; Peck, D.D.; Natoli, T.E.; Lu, X.; Gould, J.; Davis, J.F.; Tubelli, A.A.; Asiedu, J.K.; et al. Resource A Next Generation Connectivity Map: L1000 Platform Resource A Next Generation Connectivity Map. *Cell* **2017**, *171*, 1437–1452. [CrossRef]
9. Duan, Q.; Flynn, C.; Niepel, M.; Hafner, M.; Muhlich, J.L.; Fernandez, N.F.; Rouillard, A.D.; Tan, C.M.; Chen, E.Y.; Golub, T.R.; et al. LINCS Canvas Browser: Interactive web app to query, browse and interrogate LINCS L1000 gene expression signatures. *Nucleic Acids Res.* **2014**, *42*, 1–12. [CrossRef] [PubMed]
10. Huch, M.; Knoblich, J.A.; Lutolf, M.P.; Martinez-Arias, A. The hope and the hype of organoid research. *Development* **2017**, *144*, 938–941. [CrossRef] [PubMed]
11. The Cancer Genome Atlas. Available online: https://tcga-data.nci.nih.gov (accessed on 27 November 2017).
12. Zack, T.I.; Schumacher, S.E.; Carter, S.L.; Cherniack, A.D.; Saksena, G.; Tabak, B.; Lawrence, M.S.; Zhang, C.Z.; Wala, J.; Mermel, C.H.; et al. Pan-cancer patterns of somatic copy number alteration. *Nat. Genet.* **2013**, *45*, 1134–1140. [CrossRef] [PubMed]
13. Mermel, C.H.; Schumacher, S.E.; Hill, B.; Meyerson, M.L.; Beroukhim, R.; Getz, G. GISTIC2.0 facilitates sensitive and confident localization of the targets of focal somatic copy-number alteration in human cancers. *Genome Biol.* **2011**, *12*, R41. [CrossRef] [PubMed]
14. Robinson, M.D.; McCarthy, D.J.; Smyth, G.K. edgeR: A Bioconductor package for differential expression analysis of digital gene expression data. *Bioinformatics* **2009**, *26*, 139–140. [CrossRef] [PubMed]
15. Ritchie, M.E.; Phipson, B.; Wu, D.; Hu, Y.; Law, C.W.; Shi, W.; Smyth, G.K. Limma powers differential expression analyses for RNA-sequencing and microarray studies. *Nucleic Acids Res.* **2015**, *43*, e47. [CrossRef] [PubMed]

16. Broad Institute TCGA Genome Data Analysis Center. *Analysis-Ready Standardized TCGA Data from Broad GDAC Firehose 2016_01_28 Run*; Broad Institute of MIT and Harvard: Cambridge, MA, USA, 2016.
17. Gao, J.; Aksoy, B.A.; Dogrusoz, U.; Dresdner, G.; Gross, B.; Sumer, S.O.; Sun, Y.; Jacobsen, A.; Sinha, R.; Larsson, E.; et al. Integrative Analysis of Complex Cancer Genomics and Clinical Profiles Using the cBioPortal Complementary Data Sources and Analysis Options. *Sci. Signal.* **2014**, *6*, 1–20.
18. Kuleshov, M.V.; Jones, M.R.; Rouillard, A.D.; Fernandez, N.F.; Duan, Q.; Wang, Z.; Koplev, S.; Jenkins, S.L.; Jagodnik, K.M.; Lachmann, A.; et al. Enrichr: A comprehensive gene set enrichment analysis web server 2016 update. *Nucleic Acids Res.* **2016**, *44*, 90–97. [CrossRef] [PubMed]
19. cBioPortal for Cancer Genomics::FAQ. Available online: http://www.cbioportal.org/faq.jsp (accessed on 27 November 2017).
20. Comisso, E.; Scarola, M.; Rosso, M.A.; Piazza, S.; Marzinotto, S.; Ciani, Y.; Orsaria, M.; Mariuzzi, L.; Schneider, C.; Schoeftner, S.; et al. OCT4 controls mitotic stability and inactivates the RB tumor suppressor pathway to enhance ovarian cancer aggressiveness. *Oncogene* **2017**, *36*, 4253–4266. [CrossRef] [PubMed]
21. Jiang, P.; Gu, S.; Pan, D.; Fu, J.; Sahu, A.; Hu, X. Signatures of T cell dysfunction and exclusion predict cancer immunotherapy response. *Nat. Med.* **2018**, *24*, 1550–1558. [CrossRef] [PubMed]
22. Charoentong, P.; Finotello, F.; Angelova, M.; Mayer, C.; Efremova, M.; Rieder, D.; Hackl, H.; Trajanoski, Z. Pan-cancer Immunogenomic Analyses Reveal Genotype-Immunophenotype Relationships and Predictors of Response to Checkpoint Blockade Resource Pan-cancer Immunogenomic Analyses Reveal Genotype-Immunophenotype Relationships and Predictors of Response to Checkpoint Blockade. *Cell Rep.* **2017**, *18*, 248–262. [PubMed]
23. Tamborero, D.; Rubio-Perez, C.; Deu-Pons, J.; Schroeder, M.P.; Vivancos, A.; Rovira, A.; Tusquets, I.; Albanell, J.; Rodon, J.; Tabernero, J.; et al. Cancer Genome Interpreter annotates the biological and clinical relevance of tumor alterations. *Genome Med.* **2018**, *10*, 1–8. [CrossRef] [PubMed]

4

A Toolbox for Functional Analysis and the Systematic Identification of Diagnostic and Prognostic Gene Expression Signatures Combining Meta-Analysis and Machine Learning

Johannes Vey [1,2,†], Lorenz A. Kapsner [3,†], Maximilian Fuchs [1,4], Philipp Unberath [4], Giulia Veronesi [5] and Meik Kunz [4,*]

1 Functional Genomics and Systems Biology Group, Department of Bioinformatics, University of Würzburg, 97074 Würzburg, Germany; johannes.vey@uni-wuerzburg.de (J.V.); maximilian.fuchs@uni-wuerzburg.de (M.F.)
2 Institute of Medical Biometry and Informatics, University of Heidelberg, Im Neuenheimer Feld 130.3, 69120 Heidelberg, Germany
3 Center of Medical Information and Communication Technology, Erlangen University Hospital, 91054 Erlangen, Germany; lorenz.kapsner@uk-erlangen.de
4 Chair of Medical Informatics, Friedrich-Alexander University of Erlangen-Nürnberg, 91058 Erlangen, Germany; philipp.unberath@fau.de
5 Unit of Thoracic Surgery, Humanitas Research Hospital, Via Manzoni 56, 20089 Rozzano (Milan), Italy; giuliaveronesi1@gmail.com
* Correspondence: meik.kunz@fau.de;
† These authors contributed equally.

Abstract: The identification of biomarker signatures is important for cancer diagnosis and prognosis. However, the detection of clinical reliable signatures is influenced by limited data availability, which may restrict statistical power. Moreover, methods for integration of large sample cohorts and signature identification are limited. We present a step-by-step computational protocol for functional gene expression analysis and the identification of diagnostic and prognostic signatures by combining meta-analysis with machine learning and survival analysis. The novelty of the toolbox lies in its all-in-one functionality, generic design, and modularity. It is exemplified for lung cancer, including a comprehensive evaluation using different validation strategies. However, the protocol is not restricted to specific disease types and can therefore be used by a broad community. The accompanying R package vignette runs in ~1 h and describes the workflow in detail for use by researchers with limited bioinformatics training.

Keywords: Bioinformatics tool; R package; machine learning; meta-analysis; biomarker signature; gene expression analysis; survival analysis; functional analysis

---

1. Introduction

The combination of biomarkers (so-called biomarker signature) allows us to represent the information contained in biological samples and fluids, supporting clinical decisions [1]. Numerous studies demonstrated the clinical usefulness of diagnostic (disease detection) and prognostic (disease outcome) gene-expression signatures derived from microarray analysis [2,3]. For instance, MammaPrint is a 70 gene-expression prognostic signature for powerful disease outcome prediction in breast cancer [4]. The diagnostic miR-Test shows promising results for lung cancer early detection [5].

However, reliable clinical signatures are restricted by dataset availability, which often reduces their statistical power [3,6]. Artificially increasing the number of samples by combining different large cohorts using dataset merging (meta-analysis) is a beneficial solution enabling numerous insights into biological systems [7–10], but methods for biomarker signature identification are currently limited. For instance, the R packages virtualArray [11] and inSilicoMerging [12] allow virtual array merging but are no longer available and are removed from current Bioconductor releases [13]. On the other hand, database tools such as SurvExpress [14] and SurvMicro [3] allow for the assessment of a prognostic signature in cancer. Similarly, the miRpower tool provides survival analysis for miRNA biomarkers using expression data from 2178 breast cancer patients [15] and GOBO based on 1881 breast cancer dataset [16], whereas the Kaplan-Meier Plotter enables outcome analysis for ovarian cancer based on 1287 patients [17]. However, these tools focus on specific diseases and signature types. More importantly, they allow only online analysis, requiring a gene list as input, but not the calculation of signatures from in-house data. These characteristics limit them as stand-alone tools, suggesting new bioinformatics approaches.

Machine learning (ML) approaches have been demonstrated to be useful in medicine. For example, studies report that ML could be used in cancer diagnosis [18] and prognosis [19] as well as prediction of optimal cancer therapies [20]. It can also improve the prediction of heart failure readmissions [21].

Regularized Generalized Linear Models such as L1/L2 regularized and Elastic net regression address overfitting and aim to balance between accuracy and simplicity of a model [22,23]. The Least Absolute Shrinkage and Selection Operator (LASSO) uses L1 regularization, whereas Elastic net implements a mixture of L1 and L2 regularization. Applying these regularization techniques to fit a Generalized Linear Model is widely used for feature selection and is extremely effective when dealing with high dimensional data, which contains a large set of features. The LASSO model allows the shrinkage of the coefficients of the less contributive variables to be exactly zero (the penalty term L1-norm) [22]. Thereby, the tuning parameter lambda controls the strength of the penalization (regularization). The cross-validation calculates the lambda.min value, which reflects the model with the lowest prediction error, whereas the lambda.1se value represents a simpler model but within one standard error of the optimal model. However, the LASSO regression tends to over-regularization and has limited strength in highly correlated data.

The Elastic net balances between LASSO (L1-norm) and ridge penalties (L2-norm) shrinking some coefficients close to zero (like ridge) and some exactly to zero (similar to LASSO) [23]. This model is powerful in datasets with e.g., correlations between variables. For this, the hyper-parameter alpha controls the mixing between the two penalty techniques (alpha = 0 for ridge; alpha = 1 for LASSO) and can be set manually between 0 and 1 to receive a model with the desired size, whereas the parameter lambda fine-tunes the amount of shrinkage [23]. Therefore, the Elastic net is a powerful method for feature selection and can operate with continuous as well as categorical features.

Several statistical methods have been developed for survival data analysis [24,25]. The Cox Proportional Hazard model is the most popular multivariate approach to investigate survival time in medical research [24,26]. It describes the relation between event incidence (hazard function, survival probability) and covariates [24,25].

We previously introduced a sample merging approach that is compatible with current Bioconductor releases [27]. It allows the use of datasets from databases such as Gene Expression Omnibus (GEO), The Cancer Genome Atlas (TCGA), and own experimental data [27], greatly enhancing the number of available datasets for analysis. Starting from this, we developed a protocol for the systematical calculation of diagnostic and prognostic gene signatures that combines (i) meta-analysis (multiple dataset integration) with (ii) functional gene expression analysis and (iii) ML approaches. Our aim was to develop a general framework for functional analysis and signature calculation with high predictive performance that is not restricted to specific disease types and can therefore be used by a broad community.

2. Results

2.1. Meta-Analysis (Dataset Download, Normalization, Merging, Batch Effect Correction)

We demonstrate the workflow of our toolbox by analyzing three lung cancer datasets from microarray profiling downloaded from the GEO database. The datasets GSE18842 (45 non-tumor, 46 tumor samples) and GSE19804 (60 tumor/60 non-tumor samples) were downloaded (getGEO) and are already GCRMA normalized deposited in GEO. For the datasets GSE19188 (91 tumor/ 65 non-tumor samples), we downloaded the raw data (CEL files). The files were imported into the R environment and subsequently GCRMA normalized (resulting "ExpressionSet" object) using the gcrma package version 2.56.0 [28] (Figure S1; datasets from Chip GPL570, Affymetrix Human Genome U133 Plus 2.0). The merged dataset contained 54,675 transcripts and 367 samples (197 tumor/170 non-tumor samples; no gene transcripts were excluded during the merging procedure). The batch effect detection using a gPCA (Top) and the resulting boxplot of the merged dataset after batch effect correction (Bottom) are shown in Figure S2.

2.2. Functional Gene Expression Analysis

The differentially expressed genes (DEG) analysis after batch correction resulted in 699 significantly deregulated transcripts (Table S1; q-value < 0.05, logFC $> 2/< -2$ as standard criterion for selecting significantly deregulated genes [29]). Figure 1 shows the heatmap of the DEGs, illustrating a clear separation of tumor and non-tumor samples in two expression clusters. Many of them are known key players in lung cancer, for instance G Protein-Coupled Receptor Kinase 5 (GRK5) [30], Solute Carrier Family 46 Member 2 (SLC46A2) [31], and Collagen Type XI Alpha 1 Chain (COL11A1) [32] function as oncogenic factors in lung cancer.

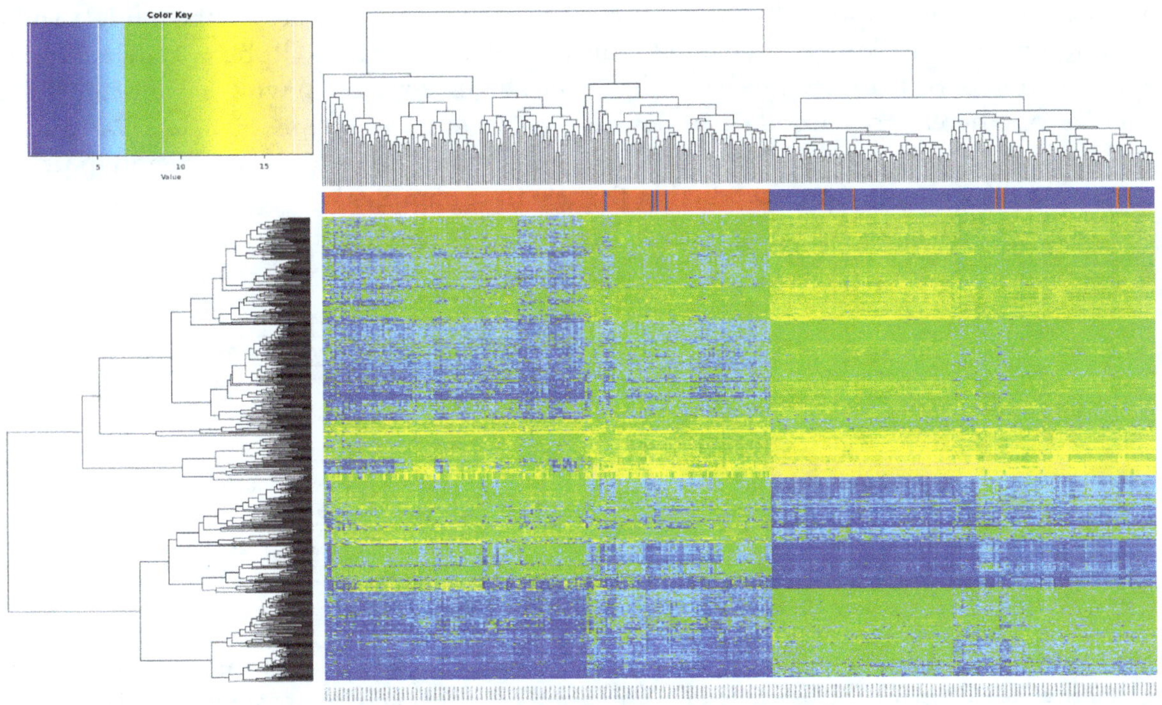

Figure 1. Overview of the differentially expressed genes (DEGs). Heatmap of the 699 DEGs derived from the meta-analysis with the merged datasets GSE18842, GSE19804 and GSE19188 (samples on the x-axis, DEGs on the y-axis; red color represents tumor, blue non-tumor (control) samples).

We further tested the 699 DEGs for enriched Gene Ontology (GO) terms and Kyoto Encyclopedia of Genes and Genomes (KEGG) pathways (Figure 2, enriched GO terms and KEGG pathways after False

Discovery Rate (FDR) control are shown). For instance, the analysis shows enriched functions such as hormone receptor binding and protein serine/threonine kinase activity (Left) and enriched pathways such as Phosphatidylinositol 3-Kinase-Akt (PI3K-Akt) signaling pathway and Mitogen-Activated Protein Kinase (MAPK) signaling pathway (Middle). Moreover, specific pathways depending on the interest of the users can be further investigated. As an example, we show the PI3K-Akt signaling pathway (hsa04151) from the KEGG database including the expression values of the involved DEGs (Figure 2, Right; red: upregulated, green: downregulated).

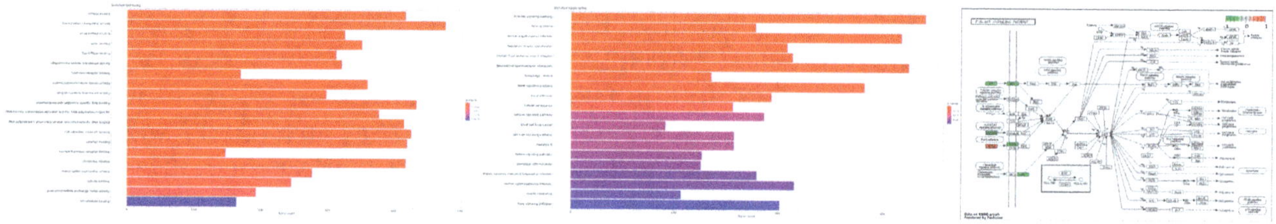

Figure 2. Functional Gene Ontology (GO) term and pathway enrichment analysis. (**Left**) Enriched GO terms including adjusted p-value as color code. (**Middle**) Enriched Kyoto Encyclopedia of Genes and Genomes (KEGG) pathways including adjusted p-value as color code. (**Right**) The phosphatidylinositol 3-kinase (PI3K)-Akt signaling pathway (hsa04151) from the KEGG database including the differentially expressed genes (DEGs) are highlighted considering differential expression.

2.3. Calculation of Diagnostic and Prognostic Signatures

We next analyzed the merged dataset (54,675 transcripts) for a diagnostic signature. We divided the merged dataset into a training dataset (80%; 294 samples) and test dataset (20%, 73 samples). We used a L1/L2 regularized logistic regression to fit a Generalized Linear Model in order to perform a feature selection to include only the potentially most predictive variables (here genes) in the model. The 10-fold cross-validation results in a lambda of 0.009260 and 0.059521 (Figure 3; alpha = 1). The lambda.min identifies a selection of 64 transcript variables (55 unique gene symbols) whose coefficients were not forced to be zero, whereas the lambda.1se identifies a 26 gene transcript signature (24 unique gene symbols) (Table S2). Figure 3 shows the cross-validation error (Left) and the confusion matrix (Right) for the calculated LASSO signatures predicting the test data samples.

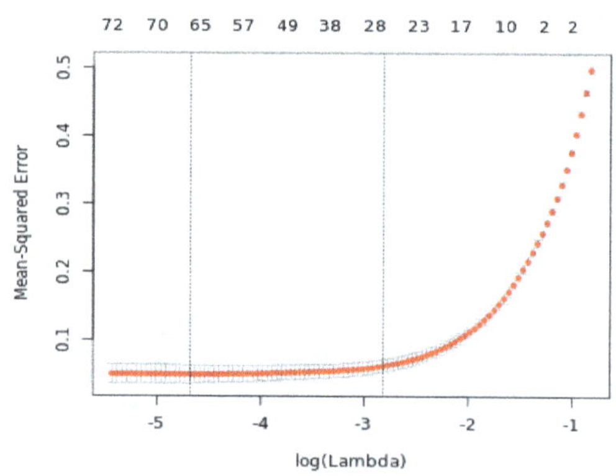

LASSO (λ_{min})		test data	
		0	1
predicted	0	32	2
	1	2	37

LASSO (λ1.se)		test data	
		0	1
predicted	0	34	2
	1	0	37

Figure 3. Mean-Squared error for 10-fold cross-validation according to the log of lambda on the training lung cancer dataset. (**Left**) The cross-validation errors and the upper and lower standard deviation along the lambda values of the Least Absolute Shrinkage and Selection Operator (LASSO) regression model are shown. The vertical dotted lines represent the two selected lambdas. The lambda.min value (left line) minimizes the prediction error (MSE), whereas lambda.1se (right line) gives the most regularized model (most simple model within one standard deviation of the optimal model). Values above the plot show the number of variables included in the model. (**Right**) Confusion matrix depicting the diagnostic potential of the signatures validated on the test dataset (0 = healthy, 1 = tumor).

We further applied the Elastic net regression. The 10-fold cross-validation shows a lambda of 0.010288 and 0.063129 (alpha = 0.9). Notably, we manually set alpha = 0.9 as the grid search for lambda (0 to 0.0001 with 100 intervals) calculates an alpha = 0.1 (lambda = 0.521401), resulting in a signature without an improved predictive performance. The Elastic net regression model identified, for lambda.min, an 80 gene transcript signature (69 unique gene symbols), and for lambda.1se, a 41 transcript signature (36 unique gene symbols) (Table S2). The calculated cross-validation error (Left) and resulting confusion matrix (Right) of the predicted test data samples by the Elastic net model are shown in Figure 4.

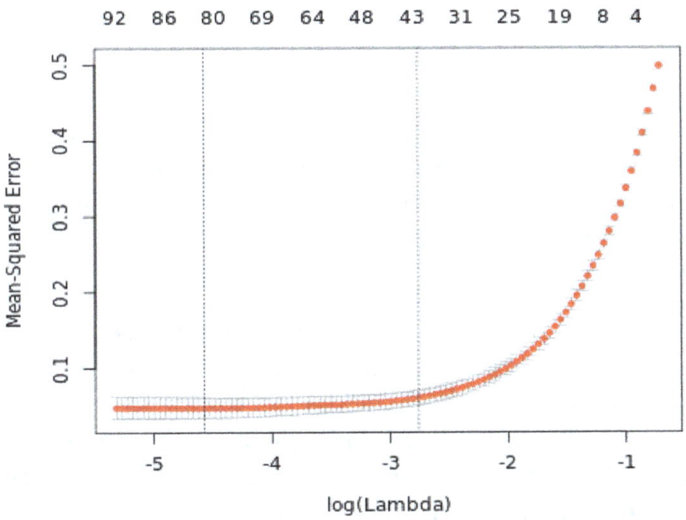

Elastic net (λ_{min})		test data 0	test data 1
predicted	0	32	2
	1	2	37

Elastic net (λ1.se)		test data 0	test data 1
predicted	0	34	2
	1	0	37

Figure 4. Elastic net regression model. (**Left**) The plot displays the 10-fold cross-validation errors and the upper and lower standard deviation along to the lambda values of the Elastic net regression model. The vertical dotted lines represent the two selected lambdas. The lambda.min value (left line) minimizes the prediction error (MSE), whereas lambda.1se (right line) gives the most regularized model (most simple model within one standard deviation of the optimal model). Values above the plot show the number of variables included in the model. (**Right**) Confusion matrix depicting the diagnostic potential of the signatures validated on the test dataset (0 = healthy, 1 = tumor).

To address overfitting and reduce model instability, the framework allows to include further datasets for validation. We validated the gene signatures in three independent datasets (GSE30219, 293 lung/14 non lung cancer samples; GSE102287, 32 lung/34 non lung cancer samples; GSE33356, 60 lung/60 non lung cancer samples; 54,675 genes). The GSE30219 contains <5% non-cancerous samples, whereas the GSE102287 and GSE33356 are more balanced validation datasets. The results of the validation are depicted in Figure 5 (confusion matrices) and Supplementary Table S3 (diagnostic values), showing a high diagnostic power to classify between lung cancer and non-lung cancer samples.

After determining the diagnostic signature, we tested for a relevant prognostic signature. For this, we analyzed the significant influence of the 699 DEGs on the patient survival outcome using a Univariate Cox Proportional Hazard Model (82 patient survival outcome data from GSE19188). The Cox regression analysis revealed 22 DEGs that have a significant influence (effect size) on the patient survival (Table S4; p-value < 0.05). We found known lung cancer drivers such as Lipoprotein Lipase (LPL) [33] and CC Chemokine Receptor 2 (CCL2) [34].

A: Confusion matrix independent dataset GSE30219

LASSO (λ_{min})		test data 0	test data 1
predicted	0	13	30
	1	1	263

LASSO (λ1.se)		test data 0	test data 1
predicted	0	13	4
	1	1	289

Elastic net (λ_{min})		test data 0	test data 1
predicted	0	13	21
	1	1	272

Elastic net (λ1.se)		test data 0	test data 1
predicted	0	13	4
	1	1	289

B: Confusion matrix independent dataset GSE102287

LASSO (λ_{min})		test data 0	test data 1
predicted	0	32	1
	1	2	31

LASSO (λ1.se)		test data 0	test data 1
predicted	0	33	1
	1	1	31

Elastic net (λ_{min})		test data 0	test data 1
predicted	0	32	0
	1	2	32

Elastic net (λ1.se)		test data 0	test data 1
predicted	0	32	1
	1	2	31

C: Confusion matrix independent dataset GSE33356

LASSO (λ_{min})		test data 0	test data 1
predicted	0	60	6
	1	0	54

LASSO (λ1.se)		test data 0	test data 1
predicted	0	59	3
	1	1	57

Elastic net (λ_{min})		test data 0	test data 1
predicted	0	60	8
	1	0	52

Elastic net (λ1.se)		test data 0	test data 1
predicted	0	59	3
	1	1	57

Figure 5. Confusion matrices of the identified diagnostic signatures in independent datasets. The plots illustrate the diagnostic classification using the identified signatures in the independent validation dataset (54,675 genes; 0 = healthy, 1 = tumor). (**A**) GSE30219, 293 lung cancer samples, 14 non lung cancer samples. (**B**) GSE102287, 32 lung cancer samples, 34 non lung cancer samples. (**C**) GSE33356, 60 lung cancer samples, 60 non lung cancer samples.

Next, we trained the prognostic 22 gene classifier using an algorithm comparing the expression profiles between tumor and healthy samples of the merged datasets GSE18842 and GSE19804 (we excluded GSE19188 for classification to avoid selection bias, as it is the dataset for the identification of survival correlated genes). We additionally validated the identified 22 prognostic gene signature in two independent datasets (GSE30219: 278 from 293 patients with survival data, GSE50081: 181 patients with survival data) to evaluate its impact on the patient outcome. Here, we tested whether the 22 gene signature can classify patients with high and low mortality risk. Therefore, we classified the patient samples into high risk and low risk groups using the trained classifier.

The Kaplan-Meier estimators in Figure 6 demonstrate the significant patient classification achieved regarding high and low risk groups for the 22 genes in the validation dataset GSE30219 (Left: p-value = 0.0002166) and GSE50081 (Right: p-value = 0.02919). This indicates that the identified 22 gene classifier reflects a common prognostic signature of dominant tumor factors that can differentiate between high and low risk tumor disease.

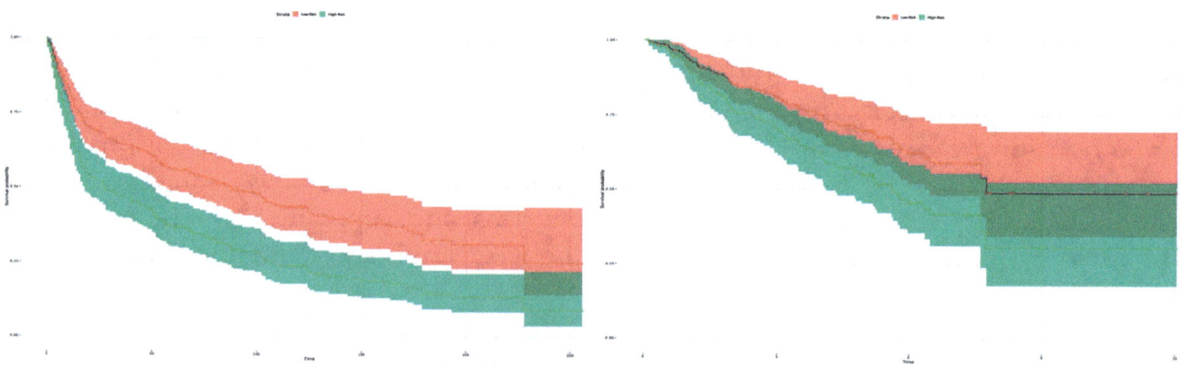

Figure 6. Kaplan-Meier estimators with computed 95% confidence interval to evaluate the patient classification in high and low risk groups deploying the 22 gene signature on two independent datasets. The classification in high and low risk groups is based on the expression profiles between tumor and healthy samples of the merged datasets (GSE18842, GSE19804). (Left) The plot shows a classification in high and low risk groups for the 293 patients from the validation dataset GSE30219 based on the 22 survival correlated genes (p-value = 0.0002166; low risk: 121 samples, high risk: 172 samples, number of events/deaths: 188). (Right) The 22 gene signature can classify the 181 patients in the validation dataset GSE50081 in high and low risk groups (p-value = 0.02919; low risk: 88 samples, high risk: 93 samples, number of events/deaths: 75).

3. Discussion

Our intention was to develop a general and easy to use toolbox that identifies reliable diagnostic and prognostic signatures including the important steps of data augmentation and validation, especially for users with limited bioinformatics resources. It is therefore a step-by-step protocol rather than an improved algorithm or ML method approach.

The tool applies a comparison between the two ML models LASSO and Elastic net, which aim to balance between accuracy and simplicity of a model. LASSO and Elastic net regularization are well-established methods for gene expression analysis, allowing to construct predictive models from datasets with non-linear and large dimensional variable numbers [21]. Especially for generalization of data with additive variable and outcome dimensions or a low number of training datasets they generate predictive results similar to complex ML algorithms [19]. Complex ML approaches such as support vector machines, neural networks, random forest, and gradient boosting algorithms allow unbiased predictive models using complex variable selection and huge datasets but tend to overfitting in the identification of large biomarker combinations [1,19,35]. However, the combinations of biomarkers show better discriminatory power for clinical decision support rather than a single biomarker [1].

The use of ML implies the need for a substantial amount of data in order to train the model, in which the integration of different datasets might be required. However, gene expression analysis often suffers from selection bias, poor sample quality, and poor sample size estimation, influencing the statistical power and validity of downstream analysis [1,36,37]. Combing different gene expression datasets using meta-analysis has been shown to increase statistical power and overcome selection biases including the identification of diagnostic and prognostic biomarkers [7–10,38–40]. However, differentially gene expression selection using meta-analysis is mostly based on univariate p-value statistics which introduces the problem to identify sets of genes with non-redundant information and to find the correct number of genes that describe the data [8]. This limits application for diagnostic and prognostic signatures that integrate several feature selections and covariates such as patient characteristics (e.g., survival) and histology [8]. We overcome this by implementing a meta-analysis for the integration of multiple gene expression datasets into a merging array and then applied ML methods to identify biomarker signatures from datasets with non-linear and large dimensional variable numbers.

Several studies calculate signatures using ML approaches, but often fail during independent validation stages [36]. To overcome overfitting and reduce model instability, we identified a classifier in the training dataset and applied a comprehensive evaluation using different validation strategies—in particular, a split sample, internal validation (cross-validation) and testing in independent datasets. Moreover, we applied a multiple-testing correction using the Benjamini and Hochberg method and set a stringent q-value of 0.05. We recommend using a stringent q-value (can be set by the user) to reduce the false positives and find real biologically deregulated genes but also considering sample size and power estimation approaches based on statistical and clinical significance [1,41]. This strengthens the robustness for the biomarker signature identification capability and validity for clinical usefulness.

In our example, the identified gene signatures from two different ML models show a high diagnostic power and might be promising for the clinic to classify between lung cancer and non-cancer samples. The confusion matrix for the LASSO and Elastic net regression models are similar. Comparing the calculated signatures shows a common set of 12 transcripts (12 unique gene symbols), and similar accuracy and predictive performance. However, this is of course not always the case. For example, studies in breast cancer reported two independent prognostic signatures identified with similar approaches showing only few common genes, which were experimentally validated [42]. This illustrates that different mathematical models should be applied to find the most reliable signature rather than using only one method. Hence, using several methods reduces false positive results even for challenging datasets and avoids misclassification in experimental and clinical testing. This strengthens the validity and clinical usefulness of signatures extracted from large gene expression datasets.

The common gene set contains known cancer markers. For instance, TMEM106B has been shown to be a valuable marker of lung cancer metastasis [43], whereas COL10A1 [44] plays a diagnostic role of circulating extracellular matrix-related proteins. However, LGR4 [45] is known as a diagnostic marker in prostate cancer. This highlights that our analysis approach allows the identification of reliable diagnostic signatures. The next step is then to validate and iteratively refine the marker signature derived from our tool in prospective clinical studies to find an optimal biomarker signature, with the help of more complex ML models.

The significance and novelty of the toolbox lies in its functionality as an „all-in-one tool": it offers an analysis path combining meta-analysis with functional gene expression analysis and robust diagnostic and prognostic signature calculation. The code is implemented in an R package. The four main functions—*sigidentDEG*, *sigidentEnrichment*, *sigidentDiagnostic*, and *sigidentPrognostic*—are wrapper functions around all included smaller functions to execute the analysis steps. However, these can also be run separately, depending on the interests of the users.

The toolbox benefits from its generic design and modularity. We designed it for Affymetrix as a widely used microarray profiling platform [46] and illustrate the generality of the approach using lung cancer gene expression datasets (tumor/healthy) downloaded from the GEO database. The generic design of the tool allows the analysis of different types of gene expression signatures, e.g., mRNA, lncRNA, and miRNA. Furthermore, it supports analysis in front of the high biological complexity of tumors, for instance analysis of tumor subtypes and heterogeneity.

We demonstrated the method's power to be applied to datasets containing a large number of gene probes using the Affymetrix HG-U133 Plus 2.0 platform. However, the merging algorithm is not restricted to this platform, allowing the potential integration of other popular microarray profiling platforms such as HG-U133A, HG-U133B, and HG-U133A 2.0. Moreover, the modularity of the framework allows the future incorporation of additional platforms, such as Illumina, but also other high-throughput data such as genomic, proteomic, metabolomic, and radiomic data. For instance, the Elastic net model shows applicability to genome-scale data such as the identification of genomic markers of drug sensitivity [8,47]. Indeed, the implementation of this complex data requires programming skills and is therefore recommended only for experienced users. Such a broad applicability is in principle possible but was not the intention of the current version of the framework and should be the focus of future work. Further efforts should also focus on the integration of the toolbox into a web application to provide its functionality to users without R programming skills.

Existing tools such as SurvMicro [3] and SurvExpress [14] allow for the online validation of prognostic signatures, but are restricted to datasets from TCGA and limited to cancer. Our toolbox has the advantage to be disease independent and allows the integration of data from TCGA and GEO, but also from in-house experiments.

The framework from Hughey et al. 2015 identifies a diagnostic signature combining meta-analysis with an Elastic net regression [8]. This approach is similar to our method, but our tool calculates prognostic signatures as a further relevant biomarker signature for clinical application. Additionally, the regularization methods LASSO and Elastic net can be applied for the aim of feature selection to identify variables correlated to the desired response variable. The toolbox also integrates an automated method to identify DEGs, including a summary table with gene annotations and functional enrichment analysis. In this way, our method can also be used to perform a functional DEG analysis from merged datasets without the calculation of signatures. In conclusion, the user-friendly R package, the all-in-one functionality, and modularity make the framework useful to a broad community.

4. Materials and Methods

Figure 7 illustrates the workflow of our toolbox. It has been developed and tested on R version 3.6.1 (R Bioconductor version 3.9). We implemented the code into the R package "sigident" (https://gitlab.miracum.org/clearly/sigident), which provides the four main functions—*sigidentDEG*, *sigidentEnrichment*, *sigidentDiagnostic*, and *sigidentPrognostic*. The whole workflow is documented in detail in the R package vignette.

Supplementary Table S5 lists the used R packages. The newly created "sigident" R package integrates a (i) meta-analysis (multiple dataset integration), (ii) functional gene expression analysis, and (iii) the calculation of statistically robust multi-gene signature combinations. As an application example, we used lung cancer datasets from the GEO database (GSE18842, GSE19804, and GSE19188). After merging, we divided the dataset into a training (80%) and test (20%) dataset for the calculation of the diagnostic signature. Moreover, we validated the diagnostic signature in three independent datasets (GSE30219, GSE102287, GSE33356). For the prognostic signature, we performed a survival analysis using the GSE19188 which includes survival information and validated the signature in two independent datasets (GSE30219, GSE50081).

For the meta-analysis (dataset download, normalization, merging) and the functional gene expression analysis (analysis for DEGs, heatmap), we used our previously published sample merging approach, which is based on a modified code of the inSilicoMerging package combined with the limma package [27]. This approach has been developed further in order to integrate it into the "sigident" R package framework. In detail, it uses the R package GEOquery version 2.52.0 for dataset downloading [48], gcrma package version 2.56.0 for CEL file loading, background correction, quantile normalization, and log2-transformation [28], Biobase package version 2.44.0 for integration of standardized data structures [13], gplots package version 3.0.1.1 for graphical representation [49], and the limma package version 3.40.6 for the DEG analysis [50]. We extended the code by detecting batch effects using a guided principal component analysis from the gPCA package version 1.0 [51]. For batch effect correction, we used empirical Bayes framework applying the ComBat function from the sva package version 3.32.1 [52] considering different groups (tumor, ctrl). As a DEG analysis is known to generate false positive results [36], we applied a multiple-testing correction using the Benjamini and Hochberg approach to control the FDR [53]. We used a stringent q-value (adjusted FDR value) of 0.05.

Furthermore, for the DEGs we added a functional gene ontology (GO) and KEGG pathway enrichment analysis using the goana and kegga functions from the limma package (Entrez IDs as input). A further GO and pathway over-representation test is implemented using the clusterProfiler package version 3.12.0 [54] (including FDR control, DEGs are mapped to their Entrez-IDs as input), whereas specific pathways can be further investigated using the pathview package version 1.24.0 [55].

The calculation of statistically robust multi-gene signature combinations focuses on diagnostic and prognostic signatures. For diagnostic signatures, we used the LASSO and Elastic net penalty as implemented in the R package glmnet version 2.0.18 [56]. The hyper-parameter alpha can manually be set to a value between 0 and 1 or can automatically be calculated in combination with the tuning parameter lambda based on cross-validation and a grid search applying the wrapper function train as implemented in the caret package version 6.0.84 [57]. In the case of a fixed value for alpha, lambda is determined by 10-fold cross-validation, and a leave-one-out cross-validation is also possible. For calculation of the Receiver Operating Characteristics (ROC) and the Area Under the Curve (AUC) value of the ML models we used the pROC package version 1.15.3 [58].

For the prognostic signature detection we applied a survival and risk assessment analysis using a Cox Proportional Hazard Model as implemented in the survival R package version 2.44.1.1 [59]. The Cox Proportional Hazard regression analysis identifies genes that have a significant effect size on the survival outcome. To generate a prognostic signature, we applied a classification algorithm that assigns patients in high and low risk groups based on the expression profiles of the identified survival correlated genes between tumor and non-tumor samples. Survival curves were plotted using the survminer package version 0.4.5 [60].

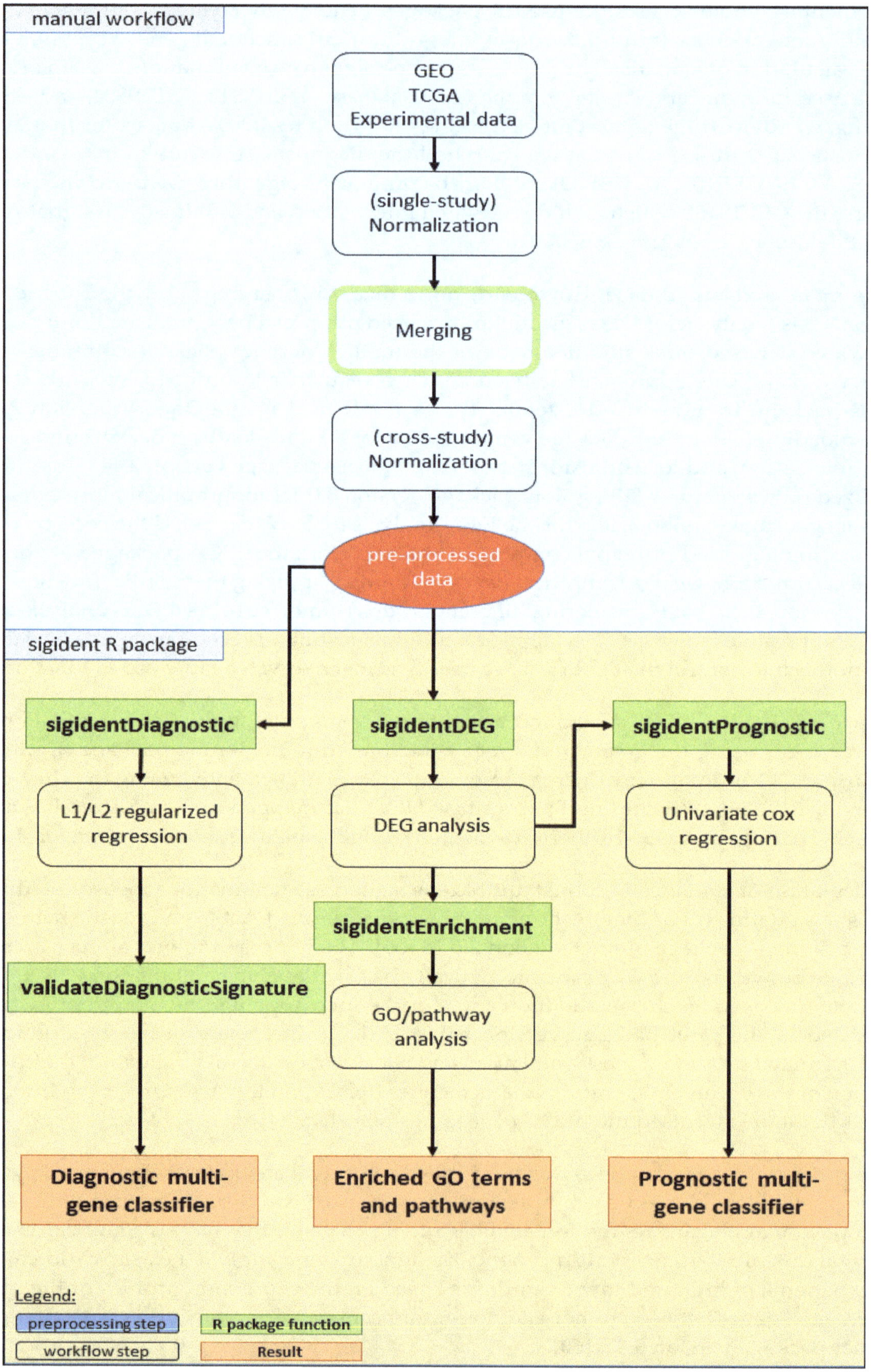

Figure 7. Overview of the workflow of our toolbox. The boxes show the analysis steps, colored rectangles represent the R package functions and results (see legend).

5. Conclusions

We developed an efficient toolbox for the identification of diagnostic and prognostic gene signatures. It is the first R package tool that combines meta-analysis with gene expression analysis and ML approaches for the systematical calculation of statistically robust gene signatures. This helps to reduce study biases and improves the statistical power for the identification of reliable signatures from large sample cohorts. Importantly, the tool is not restricted to a specific disease. We believe that our toolbox will be useful for the research community and opens new windows for an effective analysis of data and a better clinical management of diseases.

Supplementary Materials:
Figure S1. Boxplots of the GCRMA normalized expression data (training and test dataset). The dataset GSE18842 contains 45 non-tumor and 46 tumor samples (Left), the GSE19804 dataset 60 non-tumor and 60 tumor samples (Middle) and the GSE19188 dataset 65 non-tumor and 91 tumor samples (Right). (GCRMA normalized; datasets from Chip GPL570, Affymetrix Human Genome U133 Plus 2.0); Figure S2. Plots for the batch effect detection using the gPCA (training and test dataset). (Top) The merged dataset contains 54,675 transcripts and 367 samples (170 non-tumor (control), 197 tumor samples; no gene transcript were excluded during the merging process). The plots show the gPCA before (Left) and after (Right) batch correction. (Bottom) Boxplots of the merged datasets before (left) and after (right) batch effect removal; Table S1. List of the 699 DEGs. The table lists the 699 DEGs (q-value < 0.05, logFC $> 2/< -2$) in the merged dataset after batch effect correction (517 unique gene symbols of total 699 ID transcripts); Table S2. Overview of the calculated signatures from the LASSO and Elastic net regression models; Table S3. Predictive parameters of the identified diagnostic signatures in the independent dataset. (A) GSE30219, 293 lung cancer samples, 14 non lung cancer samples. (B) GSE102287, 32 lung cancer samples, 34 non lung cancer samples. (C) GSE33356, 60 lung cancer samples, 60 non lung cancer samples. total: 54,675 genes; Table S4. List of the 22 DEGs. The table lists the 22 DEGs that are significantly associated with the survival outcome (affy gene ID according to affy_hg_u133_plus_2; p-value < 0.05; 20 unique genes of total 22 transcripts, two variants of each DLC1 and LPL; HR > 1: poor prognosis, HR < 1: good prognosis, HR $= 1$: no effect); Table S5. Overview of the used R packages (for details see https://gitlab.miracum.org/clearly/sigident).

Author Contributions: J.V. and L.A.K., design of software, data analysis, interpretation of data, and manuscript writing; G.V., corrections and advice on cancer signature; M.F. and P.U., expert analysis and corrections. M.K., conceptualization, methodology, design of the study and software, data analysis, interpretation of data, and manuscript writing. All authors approved the submitted manuscript version.

Acknowledgments: We thank Oisin Roche-Lancaster for native speaker and language corrections. Andreas Pittroff is acknowledged for programming input.

References

1. Borrebaeck, C.A.K. Precision diagnostics: Moving towards protein biomarker signatures of clinical utility in cancer. *Nat. Rev. Cancer* **2017**, *17*, 199–204. [CrossRef] [PubMed]
2. Kunz, M.; Wolf, B.; Schulze, H.; Atlan, D.; Walles, T.; Walles, H.; Dandekar, T. Non-coding rnas in lung cancer: Contribution of bioinformatics analysis to the development of non-invasive diagnostic tools. *Genes* **2016**, *8*, 8. [CrossRef] [PubMed]
3. Aguirre-Gamboa, R.; Trevino, V. Survmicro: Assessment of miRNA-based prognostic signatures for cancer clinical outcomes by multivariate survival analysis. *Bioinformatics* **2014**, *30*, 1630–1632. [CrossRef] [PubMed]
4. Cusumano, P.G.; Generali, D.; Ciruelos, E.; Manso, L.; Ghanem, I.; Lifrange, E.; Jerusalem, G.; Klaase, J.; de Snoo, F.; Stork-Sloots, L.; et al. European inter-institutional impact study of mammaprint. *Breast* **2014**, *23*, 423–428. [CrossRef]
5. Montani, F.; Marzi, M.J.; Dezi, F.; Dama, E.; Carletti, R.M.; Bonizzi, G.; Bertolotti, R.; Bellomi, M.; Rampinelli, C.; Maisonneuve, P.; et al. miR-test: A blood test for lung cancer early detection. *J. Natl. Cancer Inst.* **2015**, *107*. [CrossRef]
6. Taminau, J.; Lazar, C.; Meganck, S.; Nowé, A. Comparison of merging and meta-analysis as alternative approaches for integrative gene expression analysis. *ISRN Bioinform.* **2014**, *2014*, 345601. [CrossRef]
7. Xu, L.; Tan, A.C.; Winslow, R.L.; Geman, D. Merging microarray data from separate breast cancer studies provides a robust prognostic test. *BMC Bioinform.* **2008**, *9*, 125. [CrossRef]
8. Hughey, J.J.; Butte, A.J. Robust meta-analysis of gene expression using the elastic net. *Nucleic Acids Res.* **2015**, *43*, e79. [CrossRef]
9. Ramasamy, A.; Mondry, A.; Holmes, C.C.; Altman, D.G. Key issues in conducting a meta-analysis of gene expression microarray datasets. *PLoS Med.* **2008**, *5*, e184. [CrossRef]

10. Tseng, G.C.; Ghosh, D.; Feingold, E. Comprehensive literature review and statistical considerations for microarray meta-analysis. *Nucleic Acids Res.* **2012**, *40*, 3785–3799. [CrossRef]
11. Heider, A.; Alt, R. virtuAlarray: A R/Bioconductor package to merge raw data from different microarray platforms. *BMC Bioinform.* **2013**, *14*, 75. [CrossRef] [PubMed]
12. Taminau, J.; Meganck, S.; Lazar, C.; Steenhoff, D.; Coletta, A.; Molter, C.; Duque, R.; de Schaetzen, V.; Weiss Solis, D.Y.; Bersini, H.; et al. Unlocking the potential of publicly available microarray data using inSilicoDb and inSilicoMerging R/Bioconductor packages. *BMC Bioinform.* **2012**, *13*, 335. [CrossRef] [PubMed]
13. Huber, W.; Carey, V.J.; Gentleman, R.; Anders, S.; Carlson, M.; Carvalho, B.S.; Bravo, H.C.; Davis, S.; Gatto, L.; Girke, T.; et al. Orchestrating high-throughput genomic analysis with bioconductor. *Nat. Methods* **2015**, *12*, 115–121. [CrossRef] [PubMed]
14. Aguirre-Gamboa, R.; Gomez-Rueda, H.; Martínez-Ledesma, E.; Martínez-Torteya, A.; Chacolla-Huaringa, R.; Rodriguez-Barrientos, A.; Tamez-Peña, J.G.; Treviño, V. Survexpress: An online biomarker validation tool and database for cancer gene expression data using survival analysis. *PLoS ONE* **2013**, *8*, e74250. [CrossRef] [PubMed]
15. Lanczky, A.; Nagy, A.; Bottai, G.; Munkacsy, G.; Szabo, A.; Santarpia, L.; Gyorffy, B. miRpower: A web-tool to validate survival-associated miRNAs utilizing expression data from 2178 breast cancer patients. *Breast Cancer Res. Treat.* **2016**, *160*, 439–446. [CrossRef]
16. Ringner, M.; Fredlund, E.; Hakkinen, J.; Borg, A.; Staaf, J. Gobo: Gene expression-based outcome for breast cancer online. *PLoS ONE* **2011**, *6*, e17911. [CrossRef]
17. Gyorffy, B.; Lanczky, A.; Szallasi, Z. Implementing an online tool for genome-wide validation of survival-associated biomarkers in ovarian-cancer using microarray data from 1287 patients. *Endocr. Relat. Cancer* **2012**, *19*, 197–208. [CrossRef]
18. Schweitzer, S.; Kunz, M.; Kurlbaum, M.; Vey, J.; Kendl, S.; Deutschbein, T.; Hahner, S.; Fassnacht, M.; Dandekar, T.; Kroiss, M. Plasma steroid metabolome profiling for the diagnosis of adrenocortical carcinoma. *Eur. J. Endocrinol.* **2019**, *180*, 117–125. [CrossRef]
19. Beck, A.H.; Sangoi, A.R.; Leung, S.; Marinelli, R.J.; Nielsen, T.O.; van de Vijver, M.J.; West, R.B.; van de Rijn, M.; Koller, D. Systematic analysis of breast cancer morphology uncovers stromal features associated with survival. *Sci. Transl. Med.* **2011**, *3*, 108ra113. [CrossRef]
20. Huang, C.; Mezencev, R.; McDonald, J.F.; Vannberg, F. Open source machine-learning algorithms for the prediction of optimal cancer drug therapies. *PLoS ONE* **2017**, *12*, e0186906. [CrossRef]
21. Mortazavi, B.J.; Downing, N.S.; Bucholz, E.M.; Dharmarajan, K.; Manhapra, A.; Li, S.X.; Negahban, S.N.; Krumholz, H.M. Analysis of machine learning techniques for heart failure readmissions. *Circulation. Cardiovasc. Qual. Outcomes* **2016**, *9*, 629–640. [CrossRef] [PubMed]
22. Tibshirani, R. Regression shrinkage and selection via the lasso. *J. R. Stat. Soc. Ser. B* **1996**, *58*, 267–288. [CrossRef]
23. Zou, H.; Hastie, T. Regularization and variable selection via the elastic net. *J. R. Statist. Soc. B* **2005**, *67*, 301–320. [CrossRef]
24. Bradburn, M.J.; Clark, T.G.; Love, S.B.; Altman, D.G. Survival analysis part II: Multivariate data analysis—An introduction to concepts and methods. *Br. J. Cancer* **2003**, *89*, 431–436. [CrossRef] [PubMed]
25. Clark, T.G.; Bradburn, M.J.; Love, S.B.; Altman, D.G. Survival analysis part I: Basic concepts and first analyses. *Br. J. Cancer* **2003**, *89*, 232–238. [CrossRef]
26. Cox, D.R. Regression models and life-tables. *J. R. Stat. Society. Ser. B* **1972**, *34*, 187–220. [CrossRef]
27. Kunz, M.; Pittroff, A.; Dandekar, T. Systems biology analysis to understand regulatory miRNA networks in lung cancer. In *Computational Cell Biology*; Humana Press: New York, NY, USA, 2018; pp. 235–247.
28. Wu, J.; Gentry, R. Gcrma: Background Adjustment Using Sequence Information. Available online: https://bioc.ism.ac.jp/packages/3.7/bioc/html/gcrma.html (accessed on 27 September 2019).
29. Conesa, A.; Madrigal, P.; Tarazona, S.; Gomez-Cabrero, D.; Cervera, A.; McPherson, A.; Szcześniak, M.W.; Gaffney, D.J.; Elo, L.L.; Zhang, X.; et al. A survey of best practices for RNA-seq data analysis. *Genome Biol.* **2016**, *17*, 13. [CrossRef]
30. Jiang, L.-P.; Fan, S.-Q.; Xiong, Q.-X.; Zhou, Y.-C.; Yang, Z.-Z.; Li, G.-F.; Huang, Y.-C.; Wu, M.-G.; Shen, Q.-S.; Liu, K.; et al. Grk5 functions as an oncogenic factor in non-small-cell lung cancer. *Cell Death Dis.* **2018**, *9*, 295. [CrossRef]

31. Kim, K.Y.; Lee, G.; Yoon, M.; Cho, E.H.; Park, C.-S.; Kim, M.G. Expression analyses revealed thymic stromal co-transporter/Slc46A2 is in stem cell populations and is a putative tumor suppressor. *Mol. Cells* **2015**, *38*, 548–561. [CrossRef]
32. Shen, L.; Yang, M.; Lin, Q.; Zhang, Z.; Zhu, B.; Miao, C. COL11A1 is overexpressed in recurrent non-small cell lung cancer and promotes cell proliferation, migration, invasion and drug resistance. *Oncol. Rep.* **2016**, *36*, 877–885. [CrossRef]
33. Trost, Z.; Sok, M.; Marc, J.; Cerne, D. Increased lipoprotein lipase activity in non-small cell lung cancer tissue predicts shorter patient survival. *Arch. Med Res.* **2009**, *40*, 364–368. [CrossRef] [PubMed]
34. Li, L.; Liu, Y.D.; Zhan, Y.T.; Zhu, Y.H.; Li, Y.; Xie, D.; Guan, X.Y. High levels of CCL2 or CCL4 in the tumor microenvironment predict unfavorable survival in lung adenocarcinoma. *Thorac. Cancer* **2018**, *9*, 775–784. [CrossRef] [PubMed]
35. Chen, T.; Guestrin, C. Xgboost: A scalable tree boosting system. In Proceedings of the 22nd Acm Sigkdd International Conference on Knowledge Discovery and Data Mining, San Francisco, CA, USA, 13–17 August 2016; pp. 785–794.
36. Chibon, F. Cancer gene expression signatures—The rise and fall? *Eur. J. Cancer* **2013**, *49*, 2000–2009. [CrossRef] [PubMed]
37. Ching, T.; Huang, S.; Garmire, L.X. Power analysis and sample size estimation for RNA-seq differential expression. *Rna* **2014**, *20*, 1684–1696. [CrossRef]
38. Wirapati, P.; Sotiriou, C.; Kunkel, S.; Farmer, P.; Pradervand, S.; Haibe-Kains, B.; Desmedt, C.; Ignatiadis, M.; Sengstag, T.; Schutz, F.; et al. Meta-analysis of gene expression profiles in breast cancer: Toward a unified understanding of breast cancer subtyping and prognosis signatures. *Breast Cancer Res.* **2008**, *10*, R65. [CrossRef]
39. Chen, R.; Khatri, P.; Mazur, P.K.; Polin, M.; Zheng, Y.; Vaka, D.; Hoang, C.D.; Shrager, J.; Xu, Y.; Vicent, S.; et al. A meta-analysis of lung cancer gene expression identifies PTK7 as a survival gene in lung adenocarcinoma. *Cancer Res.* **2014**, *74*, 2892–2902. [CrossRef]
40. Sorlie, T.; Tibshirani, R.; Parker, J.; Hastie, T.; Marron, J.S.; Nobel, A.; Deng, S.; Johnsen, H.; Pesich, R.; Geisler, S.; et al. Repeated observation of breast tumor subtypes in independent gene expression data sets. *Proc. Natl. Acad. Sci. USA* **2003**, *100*, 8418–8423. [CrossRef]
41. Jia, B.; Lynn, H.S. A sample size planning approach that considers both statistical significance and clinical significance. *Trials* **2015**, *16*, 213. [CrossRef]
42. Van't Veer, L.J.; Dai, H.; van de Vijver, M.J.; He, Y.D.; Hart, A.A.; Mao, M.; Peterse, H.L.; van der Kooy, K.; Marton, M.J.; Witteveen, A.T.; et al. Gene expression profiling predicts clinical outcome of breast cancer. *Nature* **2002**, *415*, 530–536. [CrossRef]
43. Kundu, S.T.; Grzeskowiak, C.L.; Fradette, J.J.; Gibson, L.A.; Rodriguez, L.B.; Creighton, C.J.; Scott, K.L.; Gibbons, D.L. TMEM106B drives lung cancer metastasis by inducing TFEB-dependent lysosome synthesis and secretion of cathepsins. *Nat. Commun.* **2018**, *9*, 2731. [CrossRef]
44. Andriani, F.; Landoni, E.; Mensah, M.; Facchinetti, F.; Miceli, R.; Tagliabue, E.; Giussani, M.; Callari, M.; de Cecco, L.; Colombo, M.P.; et al. Diagnostic role of circulating extracellular matrix-related proteins in non-small cell lung cancer. *BMC Cancer* **2018**, *18*, 899. [CrossRef] [PubMed]
45. Liang, F.; Yue, J.; Wang, J.; Zhang, L.; Fan, R.; Zhang, H.; Zhang, Q. GPCR48/LGR4 promotes tumorigenesis of prostate cancer via PI3K/Akt signaling pathway. *Med Oncol.* **2015**, *32*, 49. [CrossRef]
46. Zhou, W.; Han, L.; Altman, R.B. Imputing gene expression to maximize platform compatibility. *Bioinformatics* **2016**, *33*, 522–528. [CrossRef] [PubMed]
47. Garnett, M.J.; Edelman, E.J.; Heidorn, S.J.; Greenman, C.D.; Dastur, A.; Lau, K.W.; Greninger, P.; Thompson, I.R.; Luo, X.; Soares, J.; et al. Systematic identification of genomic markers of drug sensitivity in cancer cells. *Nature* **2012**, *483*, 570–575. [CrossRef] [PubMed]
48. Davis, S.; Meltzer, P.S. GEOquery: A bridge between the Gene Expression Omnibus (GEO) and bioconductor. *Bioinformatics* **2007**, *23*, 1846–1847. [CrossRef] [PubMed]
49. Warnes, G.; Bolker, B.; Bonebakker, L.; Gentleman, R.; Liaw, W.; Lumley, T.; Maechler, M.; Magnusson, A.; Moeller, S.; Schwartz, M.; et al. *Gplots: Various R Programming Tools for Plotting Data*; R package version 3.0.1. Available online: https://cran.r-project.org/web/packages/gPCA/index.html (accessed on 27 September 2019).

50. Ritchie, M.E.; Phipson, B.; Wu, D.; Hu, Y.; Law, C.W.; Shi, W.; Smyth, G.K. Limma powers differential expression analyses for RNA-sequencing and microarray studies. *Nucleic Acids Res.* **2015**, *43*, e47. [CrossRef] [PubMed]
51. Reese, S. *Batch Effect Detection via Guided Principal Components Analysis*, R package version 1.0; Available online: https://rdrr.io/cran/gPCA/man/gPCA-package.html (accessed on 27 September 2019).
52. Leek, J.T.; Johnson, W.E.; Parker, H.S.; Jaffe, A.E.; Storey, J.D. The sva package for removing batch effects and other unwanted variation in high-throughput experiments. *Bioinformatics* **2012**, *28*, 882–883. [CrossRef]
53. Benjamini, Y.; Hochberg, Y. Controlling the false discovery rate: A practical and powerful approach to multiple testing. *J. R. Stat. Society. Ser. B* **1995**, *57*, 289–300. [CrossRef]
54. Yu, G.; Wang, L.G.; Han, Y.; He, Q.Y. clusterProfiler: An R package for comparing biological themes among gene clusters. *Omics A J. Integr. Biol.* **2012**, *16*, 284–287. [CrossRef]
55. Luo, W.; Brouwer, C. Pathview: An R/Bioconductor package for pathway-based data integration and visualization. *Bioinformatics* **2013**, *29*, 1830–1831. [CrossRef]
56. Friedman, J.; Hastie, T.; Tibshirani, R. Regularization paths for generalized linear models via coordinate descent. *J. Stat. Softw.* **2010**, *33*, 1–22. [CrossRef] [PubMed]
57. Kuhn, M. *Classification and Regression Training*, R package version 6.0-80; Available online: https://cran.r-project.org/web/packages/caret/index.html (accessed on 27 September 2019).
58. Robin, X.; Turck, N.; Hainard, A.; Tiberti, N.; Lisacek, F.; Sanchez, J.-C.; Müller, M. pROC: An open-source package for R and S+ to analyze and compare ROC curves. *BMC Bioinform.* **2011**, *12*, 77. [CrossRef] [PubMed]
59. Therneau, T. *A Package for Survival Analysis in S*, R package version 2.38; Available online: https://CRAN.R-Proj..Org/Package=Surviv (accessed on 27 September 2019).
60. Alboukadel, K.; Marcin, K. *Survminer: "Drawing Survival Curves Using 'Ggplot2'"*, R package version 0.3.1; Available online: https://cran.r-project.org/web/packages/survminer/index.html (accessed on 27 September 2019).

5

Potential Applications of DNA, RNA and Protein Biomarkers in Diagnosis, Therapy and Prognosis for Colorectal Cancer: A Study from Databases to AI-Assisted Verification

Xueli Zhang [1,2], Xiao-Feng Sun [3,*], Bairong Shen [2,*] and Hong Zhang [1,*]

1 School of Medicine, Institute of Medical Sciences, Örebro University, SE-70182 Örebro, Sweden; zhang.xueli@oru.se
2 Centre for Systems Biology, Soochow University, Suzhou 215006, China
3 Department of Oncology and Clinical and Experimental Medicine, Linköping University, SE-58183 Linköping, Sweden
* Correspondence: xiao-feng.sun@liu.se (X.-F.S.); bairong.shen@suda.edu.cn (B.S.); hong.zhang@oru.se (H.Z.);

Abstract: In order to find out the most valuable biomarkers and pathways for diagnosis, therapy and prognosis in colorectal cancer (CRC) we have collected the published CRC biomarkers and established a CRC biomarker database (CBD: http://sysbio.suda.edu.cn/CBD/index.html). In this study, we analysed the single and multiple DNA, RNA and protein biomarkers as well as their positions in cancer related pathways and protein-protein interaction (PPI) networks to describe their potential applications in diagnosis, therapy and prognosis. CRC biomarkers were collected from the CBD. The RNA and protein biomarkers were matched to their corresponding DNAs by the miRDB database and the PubMed Gene database, respectively. The PPI networks were used to investigate the relationships between protein biomarkers and further detect the multiple biomarkers. The Kyoto Encyclopaedia of Genes and Genomes (KEGG) pathway enrichment analysis and Gene Ontology (GO) annotation were used to analyse biological functions of the biomarkers. AI classification techniques were utilized to further verify the significances of the multiple biomarkers in diagnosis and prognosis for CRC. We showed that a large number of the DNA, RNA and protein biomarkers were associated with the diagnosis, therapy and prognosis in various degrees in the CRC biomarker networks. The CRC biomarkers were closely related to the CRC initiation and progression. Moreover, the biomarkers played critical roles in cellular proliferation, apoptosis and angiogenesis and they were involved in Ras, p53 and PI3K pathways. There were overlaps among the DNA, RNA and protein biomarkers. AI classification verifications showed that the combined multiple protein biomarkers played important roles to accurate early diagnosis and predict outcome for CRC. There were several single and multiple CRC protein biomarkers which were associated with diagnosis, therapy and prognosis in CRC. Further, AI-assisted analysis revealed that multiple biomarkers had potential applications for diagnosis and prognosis in CRC.

Keywords: DNA; RNA; protein; single-biomarkers; multiple-biomarkers; cancer-related pathways; colorectal cancer

1. Introduction

Colorectal cancer (CRC) is one of the most common types of malignancies and third leading cause of cancer-related death [1]. In 2017, there were 135 430 individuals who were diagnosed for CRC and 50 260 dead from CRC only in the United States of the America [2]. Accumulating evidence has shown that the outcome of CRC is clearly dependent on the cancer stage [2,3] and follows the strict rule: early diagnosis with better survival and later diagnosis with worse prognosis [4]. If the CRC patients are diagnosed at stage I cancer the 5-year survival rate is more than 90%, while for the stage IV patients the 5-year survival is around 10% [5]. However, more than 50% of CRC patients are already in stage III + IV at diagnosis [2]. This means that they have already passed the golden diagnostic time: early diagnosis. The rule for better cancer therapy is that it is always more complicated to treat the later stages of the cancers than to treat the early cancer patients [5]. Therefore, we lose the best therapy opportunity for the CRC patients when the golden diagnosis has been missed. Although advanced cancer therapeutic techniques have improved the outcome of cancer patients, the individuals with the same types of cancer respond remarkably differently to the same therapies. A group of cancer may respond very well to the therapy, another group may not respond to the same therapy at all and even some patients will die due to the side effects of the therapy.

Studies have shown that there is great variation among patients concerning cancer therapy and patient survival [6]. During the last decades, the publications concerning genomics, proteomics and molecular pathology have reported a large amount of cancer biomarkers from a plenty of studies from various laboratories. However, there are still huge gaps between the results from the research benches to clinical bedsides. In order to understand how and when the biomarkers can be integrated into clinical practice it is crucial to translate the laboratory results into reality. More accurate early diagnosis and individual therapy will lead us to the better cancer therapy and further improve cancer patient survival [7,8].

Recently, numerous CRC-related biomarkers have been identified and hundreds of these biomarkers have been found to be associated with early diagnosis, therapy and survival of CRC [9]. The knowledge concerning applications of the biomarkers has been considered as one of the most optimal alternative way to improve the diagnosis, therapy and prognosis for CRC [10]. The development of bioinformatics, computer science and computer-assisted biomarker analysis techniques have proven very useful tools for further biomarker investigations [11]. Consequently, several biomarker databases concerning various diseases have been created which provide a large amount of valuable data to further study the functions, interactions and even applications of biomarkers in various diseases [12–15]. However, there is no such public database focusing only on CRC biomarkers and providing comprehensive information and overview of the CRC biomarkers for both basic and clinic studies. With this question in our minds, we have recently established a CRC biomarker database (CBD: http://sysbio.suda.edu.cn/CBD/index.html) [9].

In this study, we used the biomarker data from our CBD database and other public databases to analyse the aspects of the potential applications of DNA, RNA and protein biomarkers focusing in diagnosis, therapy and prognosis for CRC. AI-assisted classification techniques were used to verify the diagnostic and prognostic significances of the single and multiple biomarkers for CRC. We attempted to further clarify the important single and multiple biomarkers as well as biomarker pathways from the laboratory benches to the clinical bedside and to provide more precise criteria in diagnosis, therapy and prognosis and to benefit the CRC patients.

2. Results

2.1. Applications of CRC Biomarkers and Their Interactions in Cancer Diagnosis, Therapy and Prognosis

Applications of CRC biomarkers and their interactions in diagnosis, therapy and prognosis and relationships of the biomarkers to the diagnosis, therapy and prognosis were analysed. As shown in Figure 1A, there were 157 biomarkers which were associated with CRC diagnosis, 152 biomarkers were related to cancer therapy and 707 with cancer prognosis. According to frequency of CRC biomarkers from our database, the sub networks were reconstructed by biomarkers in the high frequency research articles. According to Figure 1B, among the 157 diagnostic biomarkers the most common biomarkers were carcinoembryonic antigen (CEA) and cyclooxygenase-2 (COX-2). For the therapy biomarkers, thymidylate synthase (TS), leucine-rich repeat-containing G protein-coupled receptor 5 (LGR5) and vascular endothelial growth factor (VEGF) were the common ones. CEA most frequently prognostic biomarkers. Interactions among the diagnostic biomarkers, therapeutic biomarkers and prognostic biomarkers were further analysed and the interactions of the multiple functional biomarkers were presented in Figure 1C.

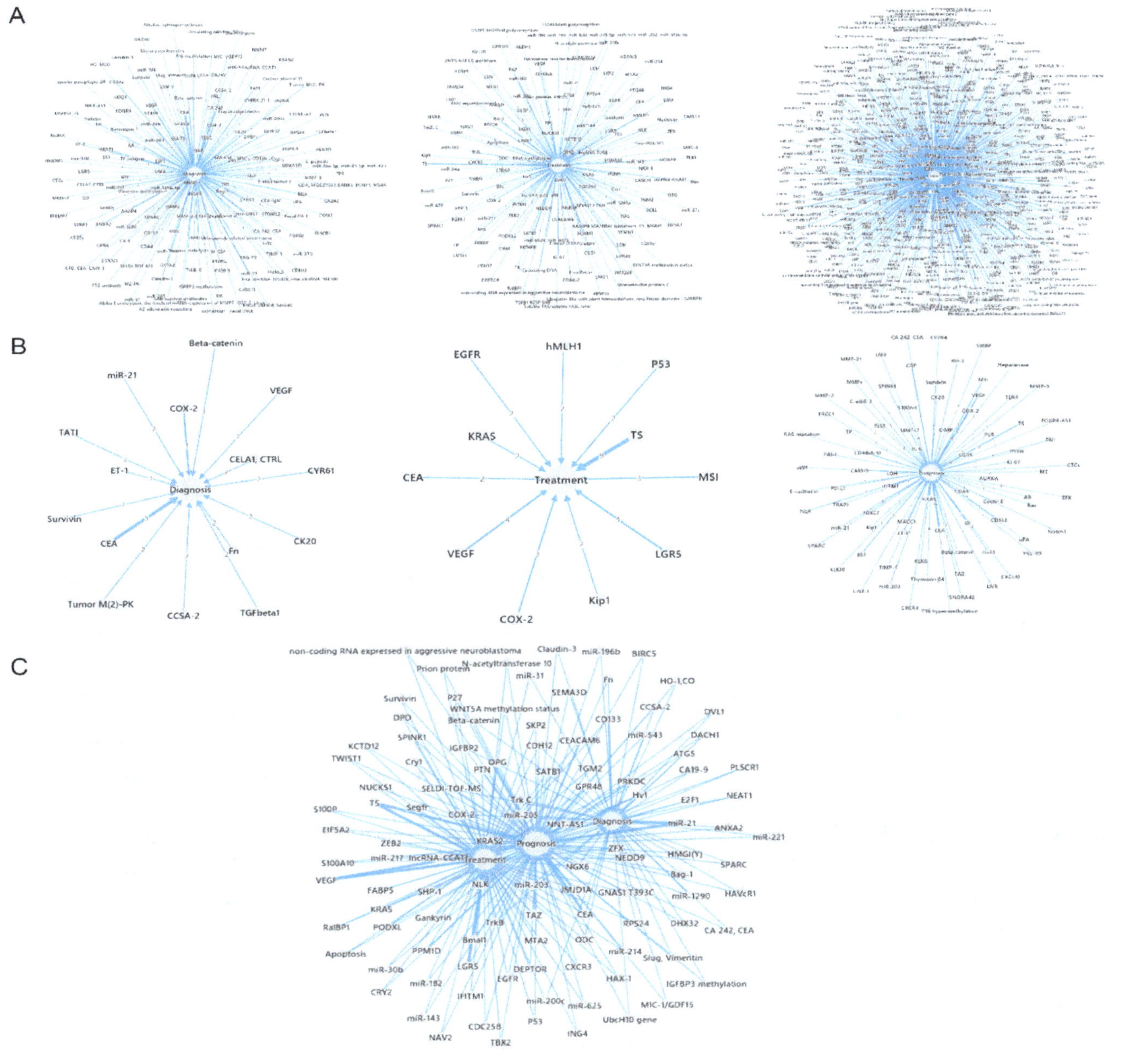

Figure 1. Distributions and interactions of CRC diagnosis, therapy and prognosis biomarkers from the CBD. The numbers mentioned on the lines means the amounts of articles for the correlated biomarkers. (**A**) The CRC biomarkers were classified according to their functions of diagnosis, therapy and prognosis. (**B**) The biomarkers reported by more than 2 articles are presented. (**C**) The interactions of diagnosis, therapy and prognosis biomarkers.

2.2. Applications of PPI Networks for CRC Diagnostic, Therapeutic and Prognostic Protein Biomarkers

As shown in Figure 2, the CRC protein biomarkers were further analysed in the PPI networks for CRC diagnosis, therapy and prognosis. The biomarkers with the highest degree for the diagnosis were TP53, VEGF, IGF1 and CD44 (Figure 2A), for therapy were TP53, PCNA, CDH1 and so forth,

(Figure 2B) and for prognosis were TP53, EGFR, MYC and so forth, (Figure 2C). TP53 was found as the biomarker with highest degree for all CRC diagnosis, therapy and prognosis. EGFR, Ras, CDH1 and BCL2 have been related to both CRC therapy and prognosis. (KRAS protein with therapy and HRAS protein with prognosis) CD44 is associated with both CRC diagnosis and prognosis. Most of the protein biomarkers were associated with CRC prognosis. The top 10 high degree protein biomarkers in each PPI network are selected and presented in Figure 2.

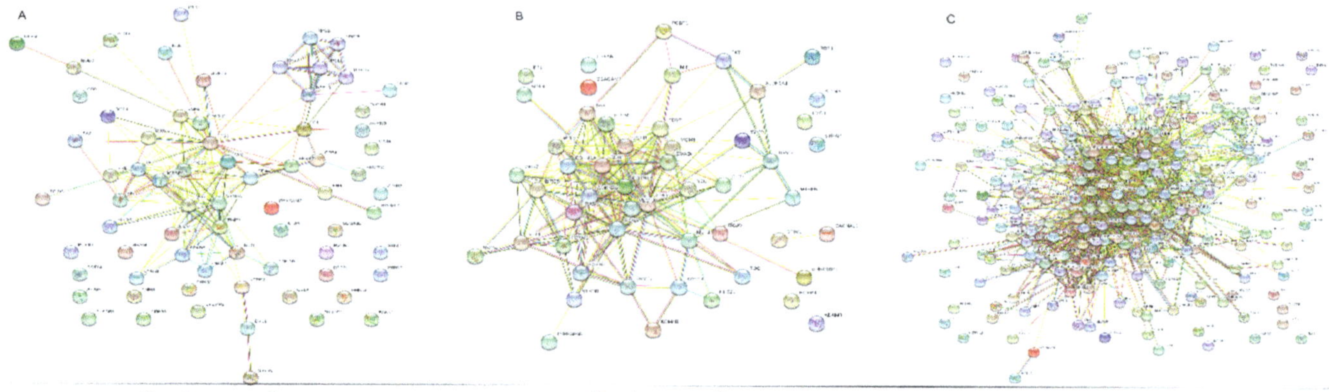

Biomarker	Degree
TP53	27
VEGFA	23
IGF1	20
CD44	16
VIM	15
PTGS2	13
TF	13
CSF2	13
TIMP1	13
AR	11

Biomarker	Degree
TP53	32
PCNA	24
CDH1	23
EGFR	22
VEGFA	22
CDKN2A	20
KRAS	20
BCL2	19
BIRC5	19
CDKN1B	18

Biomarker	Degree
TP53	100
EGFR	69
MYC	68
EGF	63
CDH1	59
BCL2	56
MMP9	56
CTNNB1	55
HRAS	55
CD44	55

Figure 2. PPI networks of CRC protein biomarkers in diagnosis, therapy and prognosis. Distributions of protein biomarkers in diagnosis (**A**), therapy (**B**) and prognosis (**C**) of CRC are displayed. Top 10 most frequent protein biomarkers in related to the diagnosis, therapy and prognosis of the CRC are listed.

We utilized KEGG pathway enrichment to further analyse the top 10 pathways in related to diagnosis, therapy and prognosis in CRC, respectively. Results are shown in Table 1. The top enriched pathways for CRC diagnosis were Ribosome, Pathway in cancer, HIF-1 signalling pathway, Wnt signalling pathway and MicroRNAs in cancer (Table 1A). The pathways for CRC therapy were Pathways in cancer, Bladder cancer, MicroRNAs in cancer, Hepatitis B and Colorectal cancer (Table 1B). Moreover, the pathways for CRC prognosis were MicroRNAs in cancer, bladder cancer, Pathway in cancer, p53 signalling pathway and HTL V-I infection (Table 1C). Pathways in cancer and microRNAs in cancer shared essential roles in CRC diagnosis, therapy and prognosis.

The CRC biomarkers in functional pathways were further analysed by GO analysis and the results showed GO annotation in biological process for diagnosis, therapy and prognosis biomarkers (Table 2). In the CRC diagnosis, phosphorylation was an important functional pathway, such as Positive regulation of phosphorylation, Positive regulation of phosphate metabolic process, Positive regulation of protein phosphorylation and Protein complex subunit organization (Table 2A). For CRC therapy, Negative regulation of cell death, Regulation of apoptotic processes, Response to abiotic stimulus, Regulation of cell death and Negative regulation of apoptotic processes (Table 2B). Regulation of cell proliferation, Response to stress, System development, Positive regulation of cellular processes and Negative regulation of cellular processes seemed playing important roles (Table 2C). Phosphorylation was essential for CRC diagnosis. Regulation of cellular death was critical for CRC therapy. Regulations for cell proliferation and cellular processes were important for CRC prognosis. It seems that different groups of cellular functional pathways play their unique roles for CRC diagnosis, therapy and prognosis, respectively.

Table 1. KEGG pathway enrichment results for CRC protein biomarkers.

Pathway ID	Pathway Description	Counts	FDR
A. KEGG pathway enrichment for diagnosis biomarkers			
03010	Ribosome	6	0.00157
05200	Pathways in cancer	8	0.00213
04066	HIF-1 signalling pathway	5	0.00281
04310	Wnt signalling pathway	5	0.00765
05206	MicroRNAs in cancer	5	0.00803
05131	Shigellosis	3	0.049
B. KEGG pathway enrichment for treatment biomarkers			
05200	Pathways in cancer	15	4.52×10^{-13}
05219	Bladder cancer	7	6.28×10^{-10}
05206	MicroRNAs in cancer	9	8.43×10^{-9}
05161	Hepatitis B	8	1.56×10^{-7}
05210	Colorectal cancer	6	3.78×10^{-7}
04110	Cell cycle	7	9.35×10^{-7}
05218	Melanoma	6	9.35×10^{-7}
05215	Prostate cancer	6	2.7×10^{-6}
05212	Pancreatic cancer	5	1.48×10^{-5}
05220	Chronic myeloid leukaemia	5	2.48×10^{-5}
C. KEGG pathway enrichment for prognosis biomarkers			
05206	MicroRNAs in cancer	23	1.16×10^{-17}
05219	Bladder cancer	13	1.47×10^{-14}
05200	Pathways in cancer	26	3.98×10^{-13}
04115	p53 signalling pathway	12	7.01×10^{-10}
05166	HTLV-I infection	18	3.39×10^{-8}
04060	Cytokine-cytokine receptor interaction	18	5.3×10^{-8}
04151	PI3K-Akt signalling pathway	20	7.36×10^{-8}
05215	Prostate cancer	11	1.15×10^{-7}
05205	Proteoglycans in cancer	16	1.28×10^{-7}

Table 2. GO analysis results in biological process level for CRC protein biomarkers.

Pathway ID	Pathway Description	Counts	FDR
A. GO analysis in biological process level for diagnosis biomarkers			
Go:0042327	Positive regulation of phosphorylation	20	6.22×10^{-9}
Go:0045937	Positive regulation of phosphate metabolic process	21	6.22×10^{-9}
Go:0001934	Positive regulation of protein phosphorylation	19	1.42×10^{-8}
Go:0071822	Protein complex subunit organization	24	1.42×10^{-8}
Go:0042127	Regulation of cell proliferation	24	2.08×10^{-8}
Go:0042981	Regulation of apoptotic process	23	3.65×10^{-8}
Go:0048583	Regulation of response to stimulus	34	4.31×10^{-8}
Go:0043933	Macromolecular complex subunit organization	27	9.8×10^{-8}
Go:0043066	Negative regulation of apoptotic process	18	1.39×10^{-7}
Go:0008284	Positive regulation of cell proliferation	17	4.33×10^{-7}
B. GO analysis in biological process level for treatment biomarkers			
GO:0060548	Negative regulation of cell death	20	7.29×10^{-11}
GO:0042981	Regulation of apoptotic process	21	5.27×10^{-9}
GO:0009628	Response to abiotic stimulus	19	8.77×10^{-9}
GO:0010941	Regulation of cell death	21	8.77×10^{-9}
GO:0043066	Negative regulation of apoptotic process	17	8.77×10^{-9}
GO:0031325	Positive regulation of cellular metabolic process	26	8.79×10^{-8}
GO:0010604	Positive regulation of macromolecule metabolic process	25	1.34×10^{-7}
GO:0009893	Positive regulation of metabolic process	28	1.89×10^{-7}

Table 2. *Cont.*

Pathway ID	Pathway Description	Counts	FDR
GO:0009605	Response to external stimulus	21	3.8×10^{-7}
GO:0048523	Negative regulation of cellular process	29	4.12×10^{-7}
	C. GO analysis in biological process level for prognosis biomarkers		
GO:0042127	Regulation of cell proliferation	76	3.63×10^{-29}
GO:0006950	Response to stress	100	4.56×10^{-21}
GO:0048731	System development	101	1.33×10^{-20}
GO:0048522	Positive regulation of cellular process	111	5.31×10^{-20}
GO:0048523	Negative regulation of cellular process	105	5.31×10^{-20}
GO:0031325	Positive regulation of cellular metabolic process	88	6.82×10^{-20}
GO:0048518	Positive regulation of biological process	119	8.49×10^{-20}
GO:0010604	Positive regulation of macromolecule metabolic process	84	2.55×10^{-19}
GO:0048519	Negative regulation of biological process	107	7.7×10^{-19}
GO:0051247	Positive regulation of protein metabolic process	60	1.19×10^{-18}

However, when we further estimated molecular functions of the CRC biomarkers and their pathways associated with CRC diagnosis, therapy and prognosis with GO analysis the results (Table 3) showed that protein binding, identical protein binding, binding and enzyme binding are the four pathways shared in CRC diagnosis (Table 3A), therapy (Table 3B) and diagnosis (Table 3C). Cellular Component GO analysis for the CRC biomarkers and pathways revealed in Table 4 that CRC diagnosis and prognosis biomarkers shared extracellular space, vesicle, extracellular region and extracellular region part pathways.

Table 3. GO analysis results in molecular function level for CRC protein biomarkers.

Pathway ID	Pathway Description	Counts	FDR
	A. GO Analysis in molecular function level for diagnosis biomarkers		
GO:0005515	Protein binding	44	2.81×10^{-10}
GO:0005102	Receptor binding	20	4.2×10^{-7}
GO:0042802	Identical protein binding	15	0.000526
GO:0005488	Binding	53	0.00127
GO:0001968	Fibronectin binding	3	0.0307
GO:0005539	Glycosaminoglycan binding	6	0.0353
GO:0003735	Structural constituent of ribosome	5	0.0358
GO:0005126	Cytokine receptor binding	6	0.0358
GO:0032403	Protein complex binding	9	0.0358
GO:0019899	Enzyme binding	14	0.0365
	B. GO Analysis in molecular function level for treatment biomarkers		
GO:0005515	Protein binding	36	3.52×10^{-10}
GO:0042802	Identical protein binding	16	8.85×10^{-7}
GO:0046983	Protein dimerization activity	13	1.15×10^{-5}
GO:0005488	Binding	42	0.000317
GO:0019899	Enzyme binding	15	0.000317
GO:0042803	Protein homodimerization activity	10	0.000445
GO:0043566	Structure-specific DNA binding	7	0.00061
GO:0046982	Protein heterodimerization activity	7	0.00061
GO:0030983	Mismatched DNA binding	3	0.000839
GO:0004861	Cyclin-dependent protein serine/threonine kinase inhibitor activity	3	0.00138
	C. GO Analysis in molecular function level for prognosis biomarkers		
GO:0005515	Protein binding	131	4.67×10^{-29}
GO:0005102	Receptor binding	45	1.18×10^{-11}
GO:0044877	Macromolecular complex binding	44	1.98×10^{-11}
GO:0005488	Binding	160	2.91×10^{-9}
GO:0042802	Identical protein binding	35	1.63×10^{-7}
GO:0019899	Enzyme binding	41	5.39×10^{-7}
GO:0032403	Protein complex binding	25	6.42×10^{-7}
GO:0003684	Damaged DNA binding	9	8.98×10^{-6}
GO:0043566	Structure-specific DNA binding	15	1.09×10^{-5}
GO:0019900	Kinase binding	19	9.05×10^{-5}

Table 4. GO analysis results in cellular component level for CRC protein biomarkers.

Pathway ID	Pathway Description	Counts	FDR
	A. GO analysis in cellular component level for diagnosis biomarkers		
GO:0005615	Extracellular space	20	1.49×10^{-6}
GO:0022627	Cytosolic small ribosomal subunit	6	1.49×10^{-6}
GO:0031982	Vesicle	33	1.49×10^{-6}
GO:0031988	Membrane-bounded vesicle	32	2.34×10^{-6}
GO:0005576	Extracellular region	36	2.74×10^{-6}
GO:0044421	Extracellular region part	32	7.96×10^{-6}
GO:0034774	Secretory granule lumen	6	1.67×10^{-5}
GO:0022626	Cytosolic ribosome	6	8.62×10^{-5}
GO:0030141	Secretory granule	9	8.62×10^{-5}
GO:0031093	Platelet alpha granule lumen	5	8.62×10^{-5}
	B. GO analysis in cellular component level for treatment biomarkers		
GO:0005829	Cytosol	24	4.63×10^{-5}
GO:0044428	Nuclear part	26	4.63×10^{-5}
GO:0032991	Macromolecular complex	27	0.000117
GO:0043233	Organelle lumen	26	0.000117
GO:0043234	Protein complex	25	0.000117
GO:0044427	Chromosomal part	11	0.000117
GO:0031981	Nuclear lumen	23	0.000149
GO:0005654	Nucleoplasm	21	0.000153
GO:0005694	Chromosome	11	0.000164
GO:0070013	Intracellular organelle lumen	24	0.000662
	C. GO analysis in cellular component level for prognosis biomarkers		
GO:0005576	Extracellular region	96	1.33×10^{-10}
GO:0005615	Extracellular space	46	1.62×10^{-10}
GO:0044421	Extracellular region part	85	1.96×10^{-10}
GO:0005829	Cytosol	72	6.05×10^{-8}
GO:0005912	Adherens junction	23	1.13×10^{-7}
GO:0005924	Cell-substrate adherens junction	21	2.33×10^{-7}
GO:0043227	Membrane-bounded organelle	163	3.07×10^{-7}
GO:0009986	Cell surface	28	3.94×10^{-7}
GO:0005925	Focal adhesion	20	6.84×10^{-7}
GO:0031982	Vesicle	73	1.04×10^{-6}

2.3. *CRC Biomarkers in Pathway in Cancer and miRNAs in Cancer Pathway*

CRC biomarkers were analysed in association with Pathways in cancer (Figure 3). There were many biomarkers and pathways which are found in the Pathways in cancer which were associated with CRC. However, the most common and important pathways were p53, Ras and PI3K and apoptosis, cell proliferation and angiogenesis pathways.

CRC miRNA biomarkers in the miRNAs in cancer pathway have been closely associated with the Vogelstein's CRC developing model. Different miRNAs and interactions among the miRNAs and a variety of genes, such as APC and K-ras have been involved in CRC initiation and progression process. MiR-135 inhibits APC at CRC initiating level; Let-7, miR-18a and miR-143 inhibit K-ras at CRC progression level; miR-21 and miR-200 involve in the CRC metastasis (Figure 4).

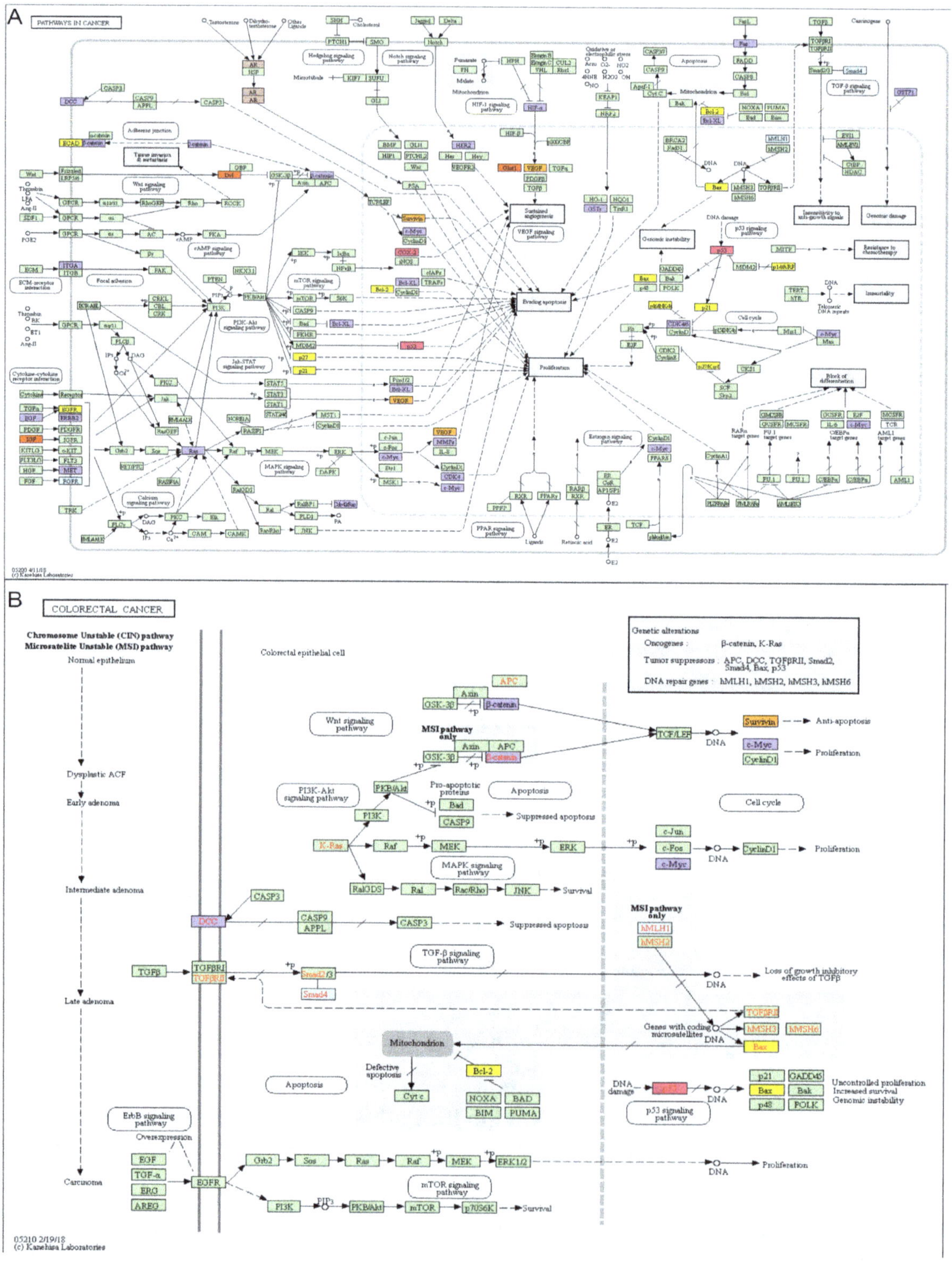

Figure 3. Biomarkers in the Pathways in cancer. (**A**) Various cancer pathways involve in different cancer initiation and progression. (**B**) CRC biomarkers for diagnosis, therapy and prognosis biomarkers in the CBD were mapped in different colours in Pathways in cancer. The CRC biomarkers have been associated with apoptosis, cell proliferation, VEGF signalling pathway and Ras signalling pathway in the Pathways in cancer. Red: diagnosis biomarker; Blue: treatment biomarker; Purple: prognosis biomarker; Orange: diagnosis & treatment biomarker; Yellow: treatment & prognosis biomarker; Pink: diagnosis & treatment & prognosis biomarker.

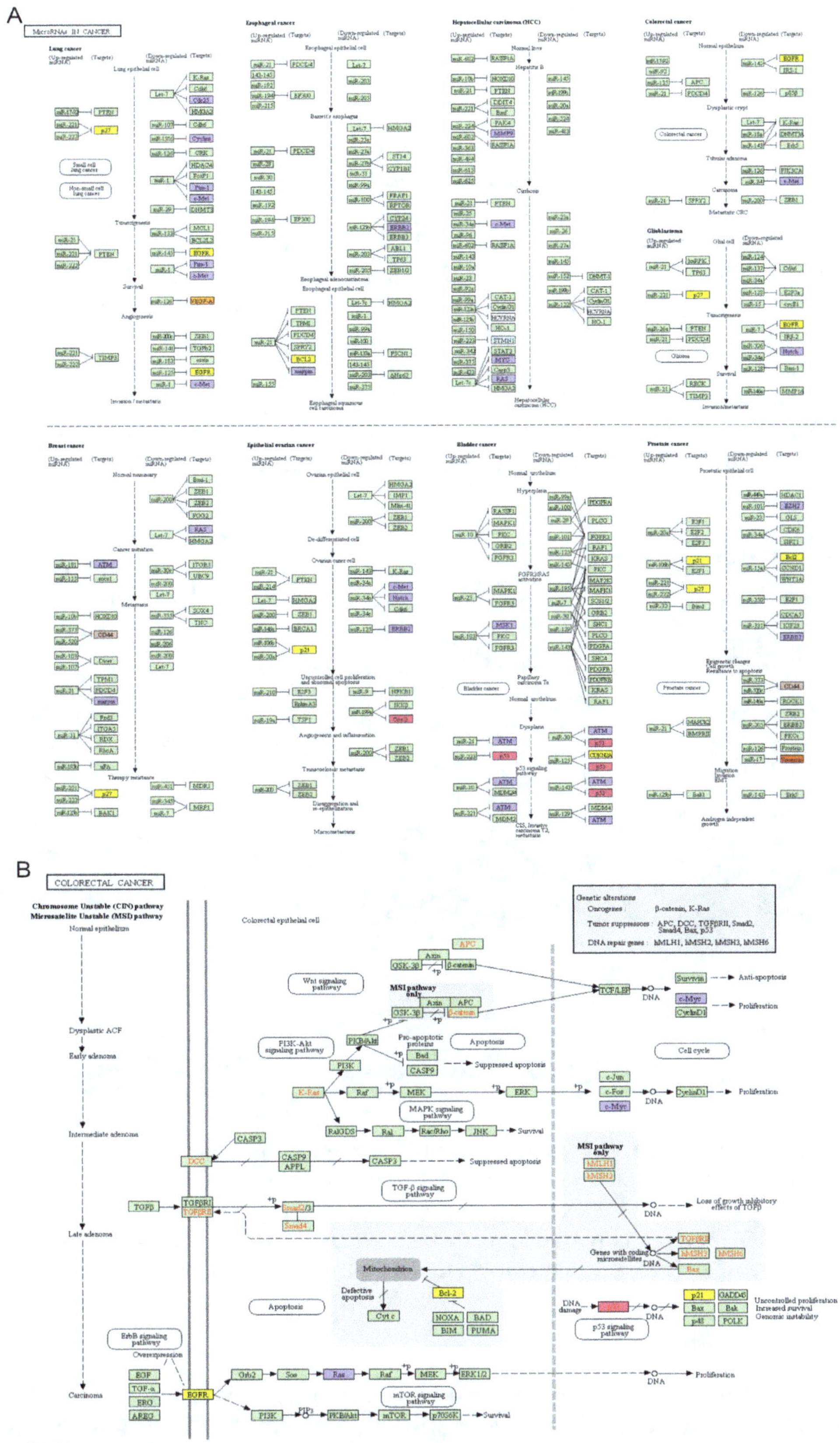

Figure 4. MiRNA in cancers. (**A**) MiRNAs involve in different types of cancers. (**B**) CRC Biomarkers in the miRNAs in cancer pathway. Different miRNAs and interactions among the miRNAs and a variety of genes, such as APC and K-ras have been involved in CRC initiation and progression process.

2.4. *miRNAs and Proteins Biomarkers for CRC Diagnosis, Therapy and Prognosis*

As shown in Figure 5, we analysed miRNA and protein biomarkers concerning CRC diagnosis, therapy and prognosis in our CBD database and found that there are 16 miRNA and 71 protein biomarkers for diagnosis in the CBD database. After standardization through miRBase (http://www.mirbase.org/) and NCBI protein database (https://www.ncbi.nlm.nih.gov/protein), the miRNAs and proteins were converted to their corresponding target DNAs in the miRDB database and NCBI Gene database. 1041 target genes in the miRDB were found for their 18 diagnosis miRNA biomarkers in our CBD and 71 corresponding genes in the NCBI Gene database were found for the 71 diagnostic protein biomarkers in the CBD. The converted DNAs for diagnostic miRNA and protein biomarkers were overlapped in the check points IGFBP3 and PTPRG. For the CRC therapy biomarkers, there were 16 miRNAs and 61 proteins. After the standardization and converting to DNAs, MYA6 was found as the check point for both miRNAs and proteins for CRC therapy. There were 61 miRNAs and 421 proteins were found as the CRC prognostic biomarkers in our CBD database. After the standardization and converting to their corresponding DNAs, 24 check points were found to associate with CRC prognosis between 1187 for miRNAs and 421 for proteins.

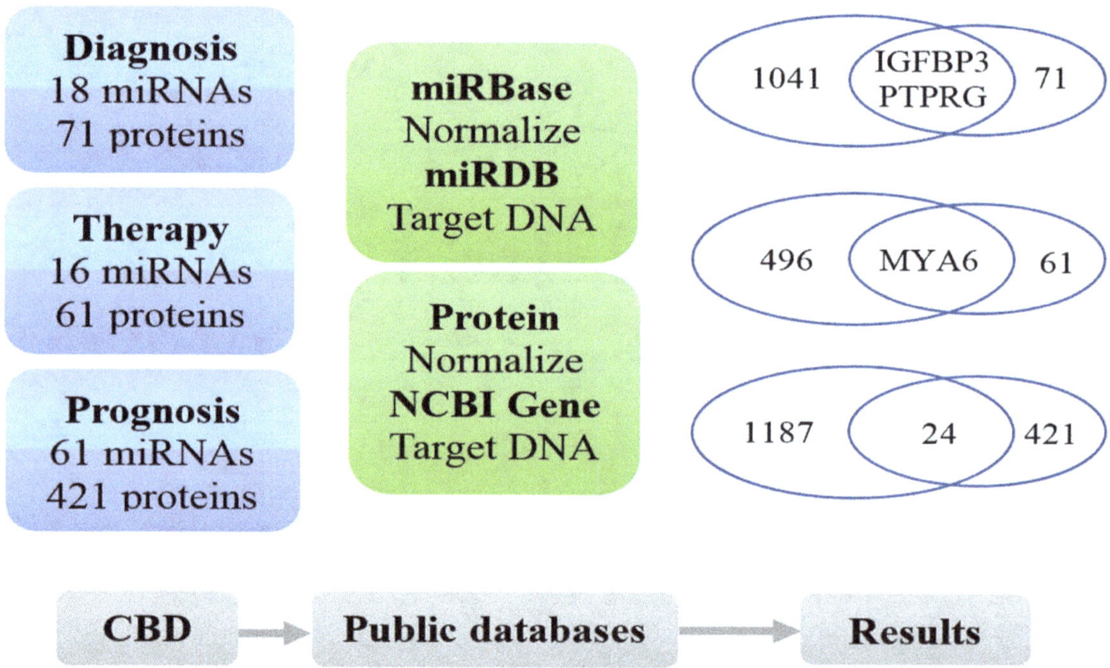

Figure 5. Associations of DNA, RNA and protein biomarkers in diagnosis, therapy and prognosis of CRC. The RNA and protein biomarkers from our CBD were converted to their corresponding genes and the relationships between the overlapping genes were further analysed. There were two genes (IGFBP1 and PTPRG) from both RNA and protein biomarkers which were associated to CRC diagnosis and one gene (MYA6) was related to therapy. However, there were 24 genes which were associated with prognosis.

2.5. *Prognostic DNA Biomarkers in CRC*

For prognosis biomarkers, the protein-miRNA biomarkers overlapping genes are as follows: ATP11A, CASK, CD44, DEK, DUSP5, DYRK2, EIF5A2, EPAS1, HOXB7, KRAS, MACC1, NRCAM, PRRX1, PTEN, RALBP1, S1PR1, SATB1, SLIT2, STAT3, TAGLN2, TBL1XR1, ZEB1, ZEB2, ZFX. After searching in the CBD we find that KRAS gene has been reported as DNA biomarker in CRC [16]. The biological analysis results for these overlapped DNA are shown in Table 5.

Table 5. Biological functional analysis for overlapping DNA transferred by prognosis biomarkers.

Pathway ID	Pathway Description	Counts	FDR
A. KEGG pathway enrichment for overlapping DNA transferred by prognosis biomarkers			
05206	MicroRNAs in cancer	5	0.000171
04068	FoxO signalling pathway	3	0.0466
05200	Pathways in cancer	4	0.0466
B. GO analysis result in biological process level for overlapping DNA transferred by prognosis biomarkers			
GO:0009887	Organ morphogenesis	9	0.00107
GO:0010468	Regulation of gene expression	16	0.00107
GO:0010557	Positive regulation of macromolecule biosynthetic process	11	0.00107
GO:0010628	Positive regulation of gene expression	11	0.00107
GO:2000112	Regulation of cellular macromolecule biosynthetic process	15	0.00107
GO:0031328	Positive regulation of cellular biosynthetic process	11	0.00118
GO:0048514	Blood vessel morphogenesis	6	0.00514
GO:0010556	Regulation of macromolecule biosynthetic process	14	0.00588
GO:0010604	Positive regulation of macromolecule metabolic process	12	0.00608
GO:0001568	Blood vessel development	6	0.00631

In order to find the relationship of the CRC prognostic biomarkers and the prognostic DNA biomarkers in CRC were mapped in PPI network (Figure 6). There were many single genes which were confirmed to be associated in the PPI networks. We showed also 15 significant gene interactions such as KRAS/PTEN and ZEB1/ZEB2 in the PPI networks, which may serve as combined biomarkers.

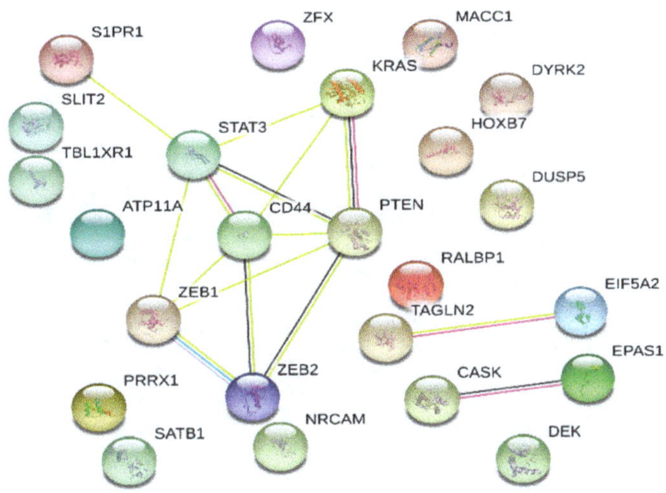

Figure 6. PPI network for the 24 overlapping prognosis genes. There were 13 genes which can been used to predict patients survival. The remaining genes worked in pairs or in groups to predict the prognosis.

2.6. *Verifications of Protein Biomarkers in Diagnosis and Prognosis*

AI-assisted classification techniques were utilized to further verify the significance of the 15 commonly combined multiple biomarkers predicted from PPI networks in diagnosis and prognosis for CRC. In Figure 2 we showed that many biomarkers can be applied in more than one ways along diagnosis, treatment and prognosis. So the diagnostic value for these 15 multiple biomarkers were further analysed. Figure 7 revealed the diagnostic ROC curves and distributions of AUC across biosignatures of the combined multiple protein biomarkers in CRC. The combined multiple protein biomarker of KRAS-PTEN-STAT3-CD44-ZEB1-ZEB2-S1PR1 had the most significant value amount the 15 combined biomarkers and it played the most significant role in CRC diagnosis.

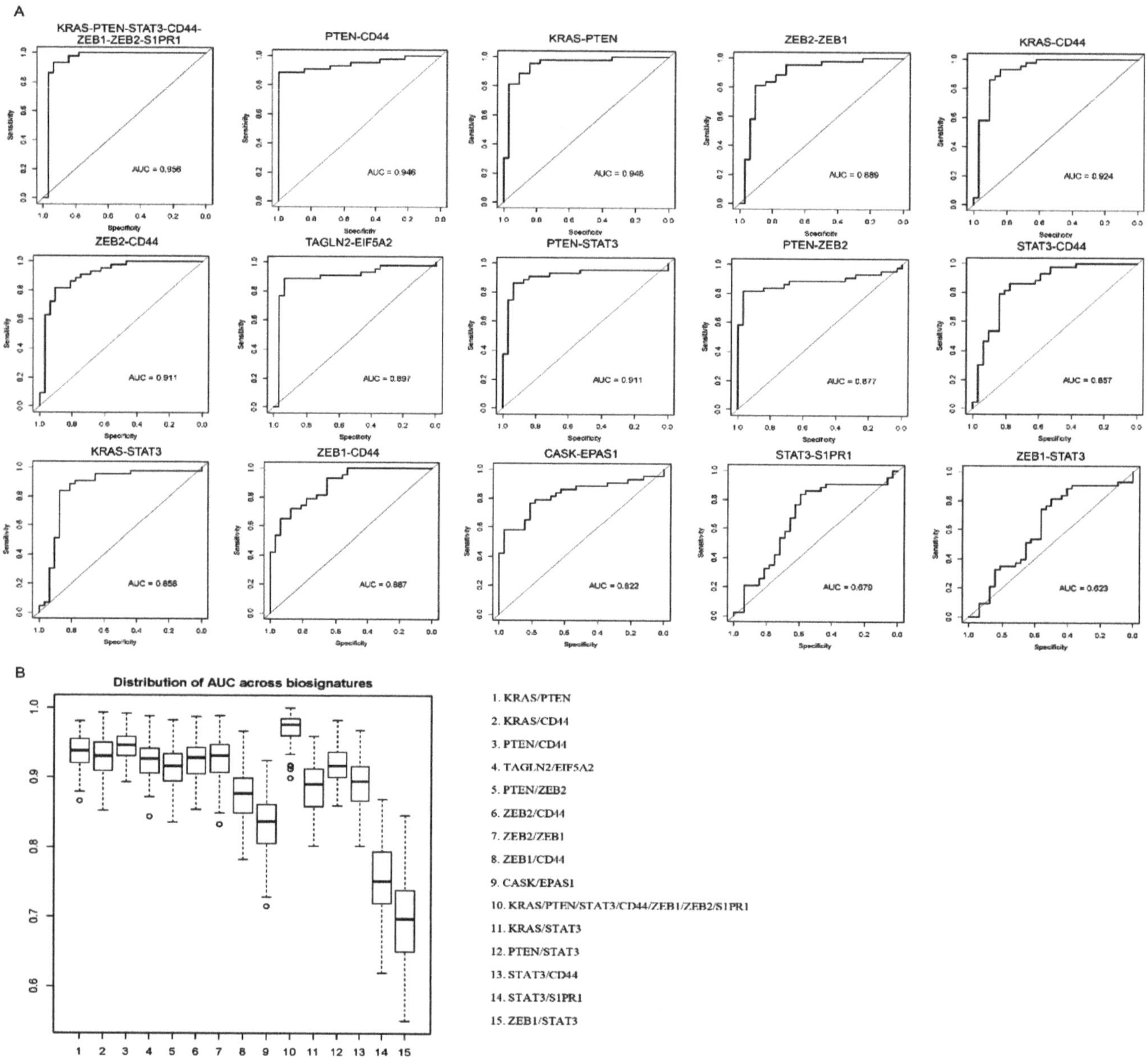

Figure 7. Diagnostic performance of multiple biomarkers for CRC. (**A**) The receiver operating (ROC) curves of all the 15 multiple biomarkers. (**B**) Distributions of AUC across biosignatures. The area under curve (AUC) statistics from 100 random training/testing divisions. The 15 multiple biomarkers were ranked.

AI-assisted prognosis analysis showed that five of the 15 combined had statistical significance to predict CRC prognosis. Of these, 5 biosignatures were significant at a level of 0.05 using the log-rank test. After multiplicity correction using the Holm FWER correction, a single biosignature was significant, the PTEN-ZEB2 pair. Its corresponding Log rank Score is 9.31. Further analyses revealed that the CRC patients with lower S1PR1 levels had better prognosis and those with higher S1PR1 levels had worse prognosis, independent of PTEN and STAT3 (Figure 8).

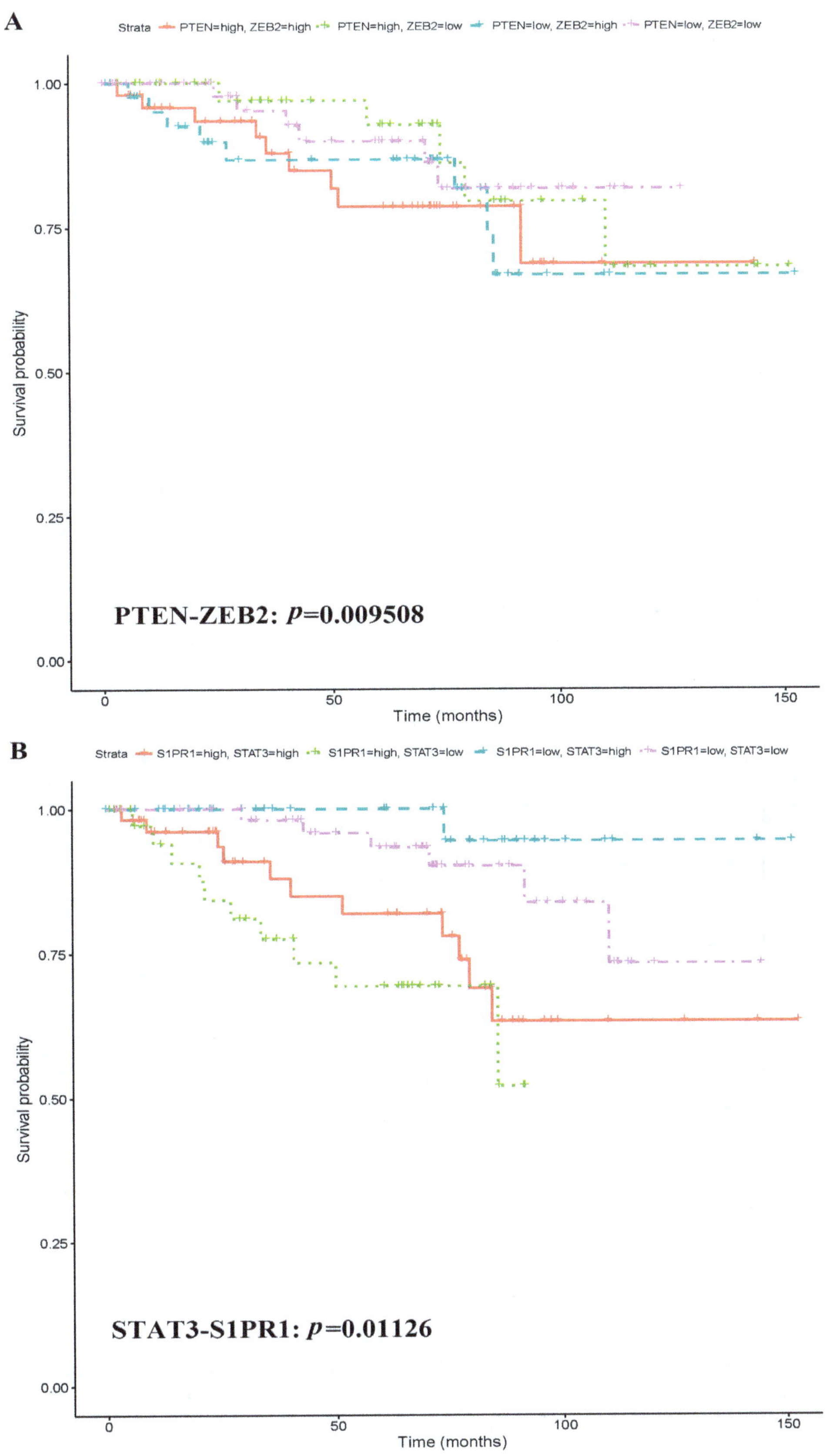

Figure 8. *Cont.*

C

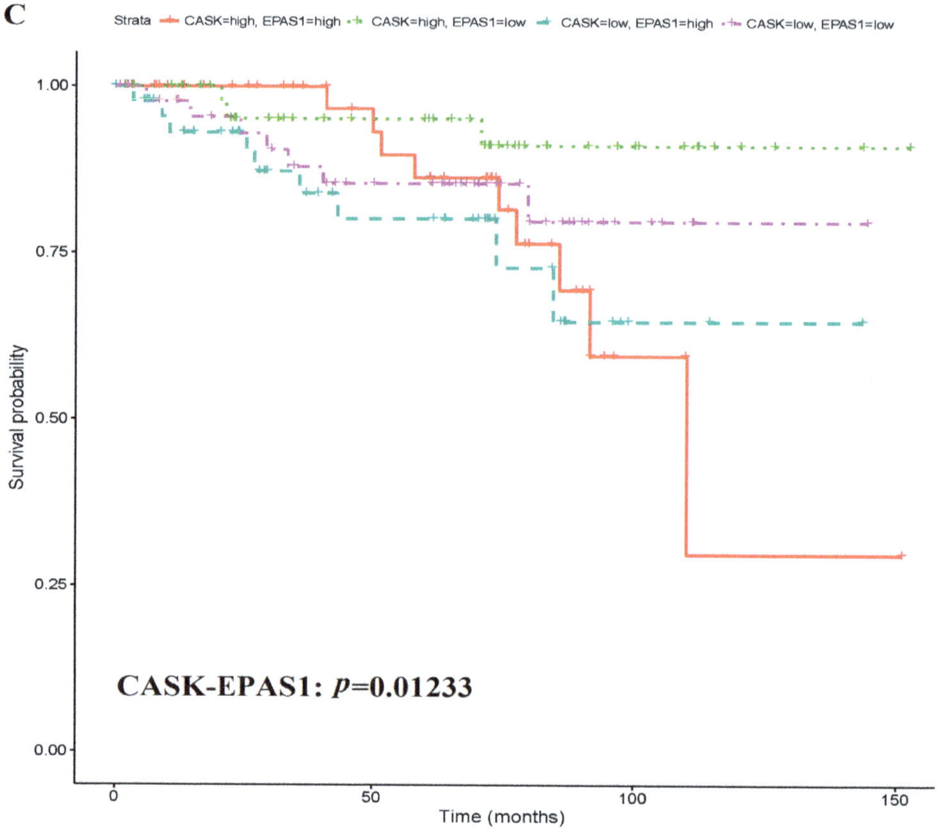

D

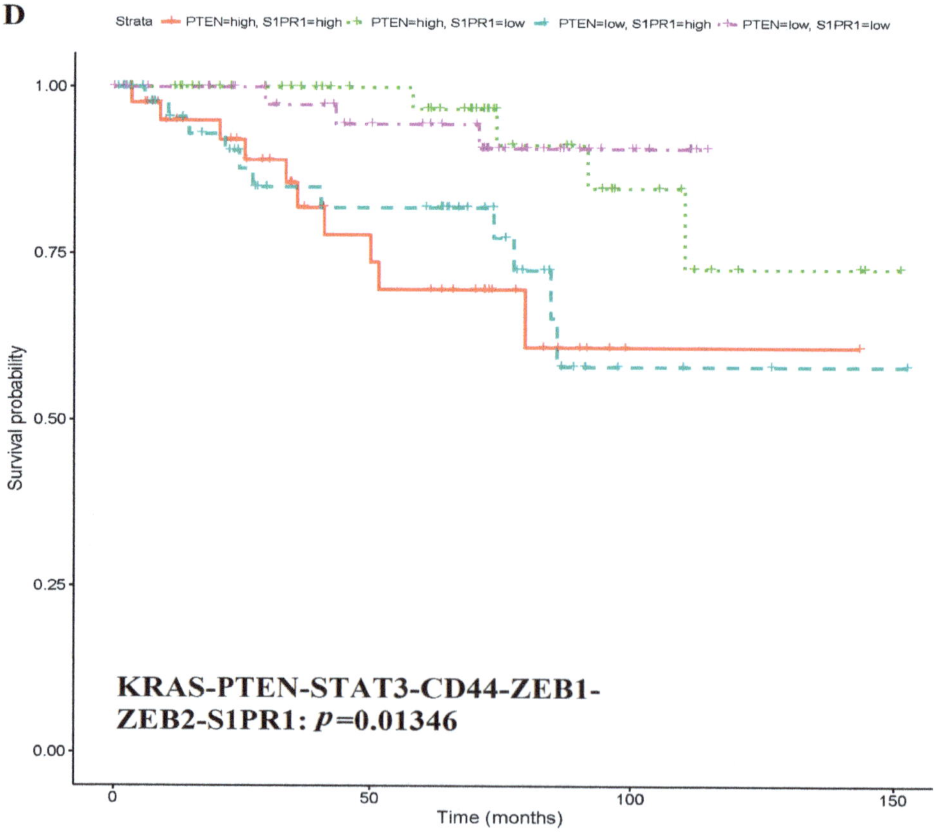

Figure 8. *Cont.*

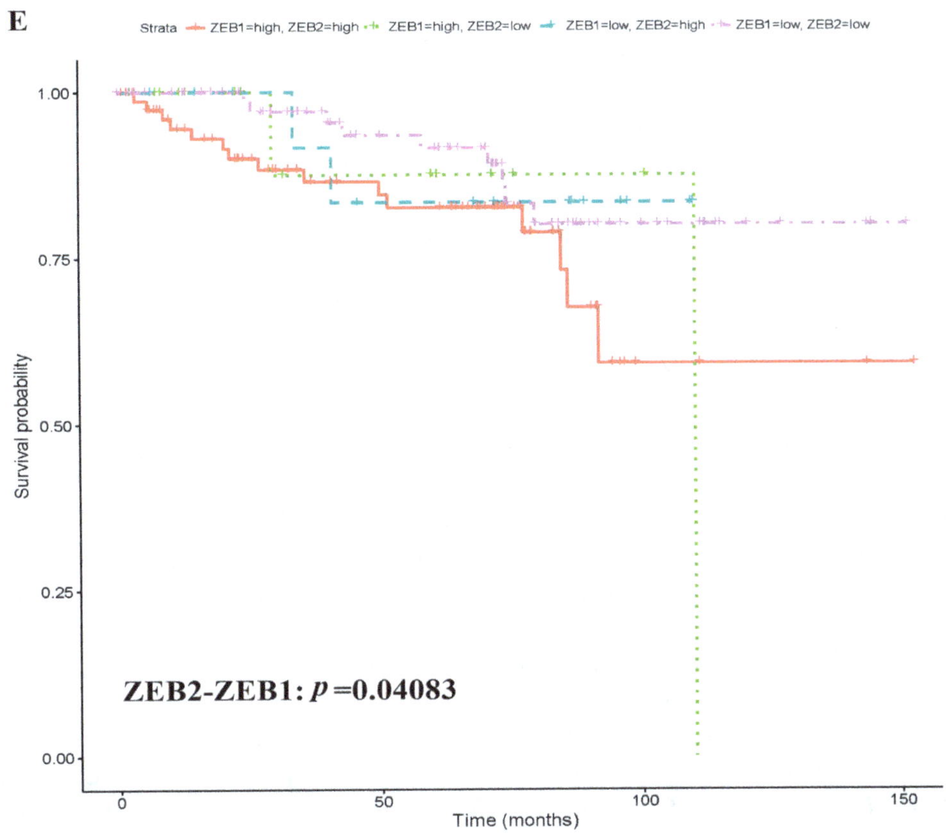

Figure 8. Kaplan-Meier survival curves of five multiple biomarkers with significant prognosis value. (**A**) Kaplan-Meier survival curves of multiple biomarker combined by PTEN and ZEB2. (**B**) Kaplan-Meier survival curves of multiple biomarker combined by STAT3 and S1PR1. (**C**) Kaplan-Meier survival curves of multiple biomarker combined by CASK and EPAS1. (**D**) Kaplan-Meier survival curves of multiple biomarker combined by KRAS, PTEN, STAT3, CD44, ZEB1, ZEB2 and S1PR1. (**E**) Kaplan-Meier survival curves of multiple biomarker combined by ZEB2 and ZEB1.

3. Discussion

In the CBD database [9] we have collected all the reported CRC biomarkers from the PubMed, which has provided a useful platform for CRC researchers to further investigate the effects of the biomarkers in early diagnosis, beneficial therapy and improved prediction for CRC patient survival. In this study, the potential applications of CRC biomarkers and their interactions in cancer diagnosis, therapy and prognosis and relationships of the biomarkers among the diagnosis and prognosis were further analysed and verified by AI-assisted techniques. We found there were several single and multiple functional biomarkers which are important in diagnosis, therapy and prognosis for CRC.

Although accumulating evidence concerning studies of biomarkers in cancers have been focused on cancer diagnosis, therapy and prognosis there are only few biomarkers which have been clinically utilized for early diagnosis, selecting the suitable cancer patients for better therapy and predicting prognosis. In this study, the applications of the CRC biomarkers in diagnosis, therapy and prognosis were investigated at cellular, molecular and pathway levels to further understand the biological and molecular process of the biomarkers. GO analysis showed that various biological processes, such as molecular functions and cellular composition of the protein biomarkers are involved in CRC diagnosis, therapy and prognosis. Protein phosphorylation and cell proliferation have been associated with the CRC diagnosis. Cell death and apoptosis are related to the CRC therapy and cell proliferation and biological process to the CRC prognosis. We provided clear evidence from molecular pathways and cell biology levels that the CRC biomarkers can be utilized to early diagnosis, better therapy and predicting patients outcome.

CRC biomarkers in various molecule networks and biological pathways are important for CRC. In this study, we showed the top enriched pathways in diagnosis, therapy and prognosis with the KEGG enrichment analysis. The Pathways in cancer and miRNA in cancer pathway are the most common pathways for the CRC biomarkers. As expected, the CRC biomarkers have been mainly working for the molecular binding and there are the similar pathways for the molecular binding function of CRC protein biomarkers. In the biological processes, most of annotated pathways are positive regulators for diagnosis and prognosis biomarkers and negative regulators for therapy biomarkers, indicating that protein biomarkers play different roles in CRC diagnosis, therapy and prognosis.

Proteins are the major consistency of CRC biomarkers and biological functions are always implemented by several different proteins. In this study, we collected all the protein biomarkers from our CBD [9] and drew PPI networks concerning diagnosis, therapy and prognosis, respectively. Most of the protein biomarkers were connected to the PPI networks. There were several protein biomarkers which acted as essential hubs in all the three PPI networks, such as TP53, EGFR, CDH11 and BCL2. GO analysis showed that these proteins played an important role in positive regulation of intracellular transportation, cellular protein localization and cell-cell adhesion, which provided the evidence that our future study should focus on such hub proteins as the biomarkers for CRC.

Potential applications of the CRC protein biomarkers in PPI networks for diagnostic, therapeutic and prognostic biomarkers were further analysed and we found that the most frequent protein biomarkers were associated with CRC prognosis. However, the roles of CRC protein biomarkers for diagnosis, therapy and prognosis can be overlapped with multiple functions, such as TP53 in CRC therapy and prognosis [17–19], Ras [20], BCL2 [21], CD44 [22], CEA [23] in CRC prognosis. The similar results from gene expression and PPI data analysis for accurate prediction have been found in leukaemia [24]. The molecular functions in protein networks of the protein biomarkers decided whether the protein biomarkers play a single or multiple roles in CRC. High degree protein biomarkers from our CRC database [9] were found to associate with p53, Ras, PI3K, apoptosis, proliferation and angiogenesis, which are the essential pathways in CRC formation, diagnosis, therapy and prognosis. We further analysed the CRC protein biomarkers from our database by KEGG pathway enrichment concerning diagnosis, therapy and prognosis, respectively. The diagnosis, therapy and prognosis protein biomarkers have been found to share the same pathways, such as pathway in cancer and microRNAs in cancer. Moreover, the CRC diagnosis protein biomarkers were enriched in the Wnt signalling pathway. The therapy-associated protein biomarkers were found in the colorectal cancer pathway and prognosis protein biomarkers in p53 signalling pathway, indicating that there are single and multiple cancer pathways which may play various role in CRC diagnosis, therapy and prognosis.

Various miRNAs and their interactions with different genes, such as APC and KRAS, have been involved in CRC initiation, development and progression processes. The miRNAs have been considered as important players in the tumorigenesis. A number of miRNAs have been identified with miRNA microarrays as potential biomarkers for cancers [25–27]. Different miRNAs and genes are involved in various CRC progression, such as miR-135 with APC and miR-21 with PDCD4 in the CRC initiation (Figure 4). In addition, miRNAs in cancer pathway has been related to cancer initiation, development and progression of several cancer types (Figure 4). In this study, we showed that different miRNAs played different roles in the CRC development and progression by suing NCBI, miRBase, miRDB, KEGG, GO Consortium and STRING databases which contain a huge amount of genomics and proteomics data. Systematic and integrated analyses of the CRC biomarkers in the miRNAs in cancer pathway provided an evidence the multiple miRNA biomarkers should play more critical roles in diagnosis, therapy and prognosis of CRC. Under CRC progression from the normal epithelial cells to primary and metastatic cancer cells, there are up-regulated and down-regulated miRNAs which are involved in this molecular process, such as the up-regulated miRNA-135 inhibiting expression of APC gene to block the process from the normal cells to dysplastic cells. EGFR as a therapy and prognosis biomarker and c-Met as a prognosis biomarker have both down-regulated under the CRC progression. EGFR is regulated by miR-145, which has been reported as a biomarker for acute pulmonary embolism [28], bipolar mania [29], temporal lobe epilepsy [30], breast cancer [31] and lung cancer [32]. C-Met is regulated by miR-34, which is a known biomarker in CRC, [33] indicating that different miRNAs may involve in a variety of cancer types and cancer progression in various cancer types may be regulated by the same miRNAs.

There were many protein biomarkers which were regulated by various miRNAs that identified as biomarkers for CRC. Moreover, further analyses of the relationship between protein and miRNA biomarkers showed that DNA was considered as the connection between protein miRNA biomarkers. Multiple biomarkers played better roles in the diagnosis [34–36], therapy [37,38] and prognosis [39–41] for CRC although there was disagreement concerning combination of two biomarkers [35].

In this study, we utilized AI-assisted classification techniques to further verify the significance of both the single and multiple protein biomarkers in diagnosis and prognosis for CRC. The multiple biomarkers revealed strongly statistical significance to precise diagnosis and predict prognosis in CRC and a more optimal and precise tool to investigate cancer biomarkers.

4. Materials and Methods

4.1. Data Collection and Construction of the CRC Biomarker Application Networks

870 CRC biomarkers were collected from the published articles indexed in PubMed to construct a CBD database [8]. In this study, we selected the CRC biomarkers concerning diagnosis, therapy and prognosis to produce the CRC biomarker application networks and further analyse significant importance of the biomarkers from our CBD in the diagnosis, therapy and prognosis biomarkers for CRC. The gene expression data collected from Gene Expression Omnibus (GEO) database: Series GSE87211, Platform GPL13497 were used to test the prognosis and diagnosis value of multiple biomarkers, which contains 203 rectal tumour samples and 160 control samples and was obtained from Affymetrix Human Genome arrays [42].

4.2. Systematic Analysis for the CRC Protein Biomarkers

In order to perform a systematic analysis for protein biomarkers, all the 583 CRC protein biomarkers from the CBD were collected to construct the protein-protein interaction (PPI) networks using the STRING database (https://string-db.org/). The relationship between the biomarkers and diagnosis, therapy and prognosis were further investigated. The pathway enrichment analysis was conducted with the Kyoto Encyclopaedia of Genes and Genomes (KEGG) database (http://www.genome.jp/kegg/) to further cluster these protein biomarkers at pathway levels. The Gene Ontology Consortium database (GO: http://www.geneontology.org/) was used to annotate the CRC protein biomarkers into corresponding pathways at three levels: biological process, cellular component and molecular function. The enriched pathways were ranked according to the false discovery rate (FDR) and gene counts.

4.3. Overlapping Analysis of miRNA and Protein Biomarkers

In order to make comprehensive overlapping analysis of the CRC biomarker, both miRNA and protein biomarkers were matched to their corresponding genes. The miRDB database (http://www.mirdb.org/) was utilized to assign the miRNA biomarkers to their gene targets (the genes with more than 95 target prediction score were selected). The algorithm for the prediction score (S) of each gene is as following:

$$S = 100 \times (1 - \prod ni = 1Pi)$$

where n represents the number of predicted target gene sites number and Pi is statistical significance of gene sites calculated by support vector machines (SVMs) [43]. For each target gene, higher predicted score represents greater statistical confidence.

The NCBI Gene database (https://www.ncbi.nlm.nih.gov/gene) was used to match the protein biomarkers to their coding genes. The biological functions of the overlap between the genes matching the miRNA and protein biomarkers were further investigated. The STRING PPI network was utilized to analyse the relationships among the overlapping genes and to search for multiple biomarkers. The biological functions of the biomarkers were studied with KEGG pathway enrichment analysis and GO annotation.

4.4. AI-assisted Verification

Tissue samples were classified as cancerous according to a binary classification model. The tissue classes were normal mucosa (0) and tumour (1) tissues. The tissue class Y was modelled according to logistic regression,

$$\log\left(\frac{E(Y)}{1 - E(Y)}\right) = \beta_0 + \sum_{j=1}^{J} \beta_j x_j$$

where $p = E(Y)$ is the expected proportion belonging to the tumour class and parameter β_j corresponds to biomarker j.

Altogether, 15 models (multiple biomarkers found in PPI network) were considered, one for each of the candidate biosignatures. For each candidate, we randomly divided the data set into a training and testing set according to an 80/20 division. We then fit the model to the training set and evaluated the predictive performance on the testing set according to the area under the curve (AUC), a measure of a model's ability to discriminate between classes. To evaluate the stability of each model, we replicated the above procedure 100 times to generate 100 AUC statistics for each model.

Associated with these samples were censored survival times, with the event death due to tumour being recorded. We modelled time of death due to tumour according to a Cox Proportional Hazards Model using the list of 15 biosignatures. The corresponding Kaplan-Meier survival curve test were used to estimate the statistical significances of the multiple biomarkers in CRC prognosis. When the p-values < 0.05, the results were considered as statistically significant.

The statistical package R (3.4.3) was used to analyses gene expression data. R-package GEOquery (2.46.15) was used to access data from the GEO repository. R-package pROC (1.10.0) was used to calculate AUCs. R-package survival was used to fit proportional hazards models. R-packages ggplot2 (2.2.1) and survminer (0.4.2) were used to produce Kaplan-Meier curves.

5. Conclusions

In this study, we showed the potential applications of the CRC biomarkers in diagnosis, therapy and prognosis for CRC. We reported that there were many single biomarkers which were associated with the early diagnosis, better therapy and predict prognosis in CRC. However, the combinations of multiple biomarkers and pathways might play more critical roles in diagnosis, therapy and prognosis for CRC than the single biomarkers. Therefore, the applications of multiple biomarkers and pathways could provide more precise criteria as valuable tools for early diagnosis, benefiting therapy and predicting prognosis for CRC patients.

Author Contributions: X.Z. executed and drafted the manuscript. X.-F.S., B.S. and H.Z. supervised the study and edited the manuscript. All authors read and approved the final manuscript.

Acknowledgments: The authors are grateful to the staff in our research groups who involved in the study for their valuable contributions and discussions. The authors also thank Stephen T.A. Rush for his help in the bioinformatics AI-assisted analysis and linguistics revision.

References

1. Siegel, R.L.; Miller, K.D.; Jemal, A. Cancer statistics, 2018. *CA Cancer J. Clin.* **2018**, *68*, 7–30. [CrossRef] [PubMed]
2. Siegel, R.L.; Miller, K.D.; Fedewa, S.A.; Ahnen, D.J.; Meester, R.G.S.; Barzi, A. Colorectal cancer statistics, 2017. *CA Cancer J. Clin.* **2017**, *67*, 177–193. [CrossRef] [PubMed]
3. Shah, R.; Jones, E.; Vidart, V.; Kuppen, P.J.; Conti, J.A.; Francis, N.K. Biomarkers for early detection of colorectal cancer and polyps: Systematic review. *Cancer Epidemiol. Biomark. Prev.* **2014**, *23*, 1712–1728. [CrossRef] [PubMed]

4. SEER. Available online: http://seer.cancer.gov/statfacts/html/colorect.html (accessed on 31 January 2019).
5. Brenner, H.; Kloor, M.; Pox, C.P. Colorectal cancer. *Lancet* **2014**, *383*, 1490–1502. [CrossRef]
6. Center, M.M.; Jemal, A.; Smith, R.A.; Ward, E. Worldwide variations in colorectal cancer. *CA Cancer J. Clin.* **2009**, *59*, 366–378. [CrossRef] [PubMed]
7. Shin, S.H.; Bode, A.M.; Dong, Z. Precision medicine: The foundation of future cancer therapeutics. *NPJ Precis. Oncol.* **2017**, *1*, 12. [CrossRef] [PubMed]
8. Henry, N.L.; Hayes, D.F. Cancer biomarkers. *Mol. Oncol.* **2012**, *6*, 140–146. [CrossRef] [PubMed]
9. Zhang, X.; Sun, X.F.; Cao, Y.; Ye, B.; Peng, Q.; Liu, X.; Shen, B.; Zhang, H. CBD: A biomarker database for colorectal cancer. *Database* **2018**. [CrossRef]
10. Schirripa, M.; Lenz, H.J. Biomarker in Colorectal Cancer. *Cancer J.* **2016**, *22*, 156–164. [CrossRef]
11. Lin, Y.; Qian, F.; Shen, L.; Chen, F.; Chen, J.; Shen, B. Computer-aided biomarker discovery for precision medicine: Data resources, models and applications. *Brief. Bioinform.* **2017**. [CrossRef]
12. Lobdell, D.T.; Mendola, P. Development of a biomarkers database for the National Children's Study. *Toxicol. Appl. Pharmacol.* **2005**, *206*, 269–273. [CrossRef] [PubMed]
13. Yerlikaya, S.; Broger, T.; MacLean, E.; Pai, M.; Denkinger, C.M. A tuberculosis biomarker database: The key to novel TB diagnostics. *Int. J. Infect. Dis.* **2017**, *56*, 253–257. [CrossRef] [PubMed]
14. Yang, I.S.; Ryu, C.; Cho, K.J.; Kim, J.K.; Ong, S.H.; Mitchell, W.P.; Kim, B.S.; Oh, H.B.; Kim, K.H. IDBD: Infectious disease biomarker database. *Nucleic Acids Res.* **2008**, *36*, D455–D460. [CrossRef]
15. Dai, H.J.; Wu, J.C.; Lin, W.S.; Reyes, A.J.; Dela Rosa, M.A.; Syed-Abdul, S.; Tsai, R.T.; Hsu, W.L. LiverCancerMarkerRIF: A liver cancer biomarker interactive curation system combining text mining and expert annotations. *Database* **2014**. [CrossRef] [PubMed]
16. Osumi, H.; Shinozaki, E.; Suenaga, M.; Matsusaka, S.; Konishi, T.; Akiyoshi, T.; Fujimoto, Y.; Nagayama, S.; Fukunaga, Y.; Ueno, M.; et al. RAS mutation is a prognostic biomarker in colorectal cancer patients with metastasectomy. *Int. J. Cancer* **2016**, *139*, 803–811. [CrossRef] [PubMed]
17. Sun, X.F.; Carstensen, J.M.; Zhang, H.; Stal, O.; Wingren, S.; Hatschek, T.; Nordenskjold, B. Prognostic significance of cytoplasmic p53 oncoprotein in colorectal adenocarcinoma. *Lancet* **1992**, *340*, 1369–1373. [CrossRef]
18. Wang, M.J.; Ping, J.; Li, Y.; Adell, G.; Arbman, G.; Nodin, B.; Meng, W.J.; Zhang, H.; Yu, Y.Y.; Wang, C.; et al. The prognostic factors and multiple biomarkers in young patients with colorectal cancer. *Sci Rep.* **2015**, *5*, 10645. [CrossRef] [PubMed]
19. Pathak, S.; Meng, W.J.; Nandy, S.K.; Ping, J.; Bisgin, A.; Helmfors, L.; Waldmann, P.; Sun, X.F. Radiation and SN38 treatments modulate the expression of microRNAs, cytokines and chemokines in colon cancer cells in a p53-directed manner. *Oncotarget* **2015**, *6*, 44758–44780. [CrossRef]
20. Sun, X.F.; Ekberg, H.; Zhang, H.; Carstensen, J.M.; Nordenskjold, B. Overexpression of ras is an independent prognostic factor in colorectal adenocarcinoma. *APMIS* **1998**, *106*, 657–664. [CrossRef]
21. Sun, X.F.; Bartik, Z.; Zhang, H. Bcl-2 expression is a prognostic factor in the subgroups of patients with colorectal cancer. *Int. J. Oncol.* **2003**, *23*, 1439–1443. [CrossRef]
22. Iseki, Y.; Shibutani, M.; Maeda, K.; Nagahara, H.; Ikeya, T.; Hirakawa, K. Significance of E-cadherin and CD44 expression in patients with unresectable metastatic colorectal cancer. *Oncol. Lett.* **2017**, *14*, 1025–1034. [CrossRef] [PubMed]
23. Ning, S.; Wei, W.; Li, J.; Hou, B.; Zhong, J.; Xie, Y.; Liu, H.; Mo, X.; Chen, J.; Zhang, L. Clinical significance and diagnostic capacity of serum TK1, CEA, CA 19-9 and CA 72-4 levels in gastric and colorectal cancer patients. *J. Cancer* **2018**, *9*, 494–501. [CrossRef] [PubMed]
24. Yuan, X.; Chen, J.; Lin, Y.; Li, Y.; Xu, L.; Chen, L.; Hua, H.; Shen, B. Network Biomarkers Constructed from Gene Expression and Protein-Protein Interaction Data for Accurate Prediction of Leukemia. *J. Cancer* **2017**, *8*, 278–286. [CrossRef]
25. McGuire, A.; Brown, J.A.; Kerin, M.J. Metastatic breast cancer: The potential of miRNA for diagnosis and treatment monitoring. *Cancer Metastasis. Rev.* **2015**, *34*, 145–155. [CrossRef] [PubMed]
26. Shin, V.Y.; Chu, K.M. MiRNA as potential biomarkers and therapeutic targets for gastric cancer. *World J. Gastroenterol.* **2014**, *20*, 10432–10439. [CrossRef] [PubMed]
27. De Robertis, M.; Poeta, M.L.; Signori, E.; Fazio, V.M. Current understanding and clinical utility of miRNAs regulation of colon cancer stem cells. *Semin. Cancer Biol.* **2018**. [CrossRef] [PubMed]

28. Xiao, J.; Jing, Z.C.; Ellinor, P.T.; Liang, D.; Zhang, H.; Liu, Y.; Chen, X.; Pan, L.; Lyon, R.; Liu, Y.; et al. MicroRNA-134 as a potential plasma biomarker for the diagnosis of acute pulmonary embolism. *J. Transl. Med.* **2011**, *9*, 159. [CrossRef]
29. Rong, H.; Liu, T.B.; Yang, K.J.; Yang, H.C.; Wu, D.H.; Liao, C.P.; Hong, F.; Yang, H.Z.; Wan, F.; Ye, X.Y.; et al. MicroRNA-134 plasma levels before and after treatment for bipolar mania. *J. Psychiatr. Res.* **2011**, *45*, 92–95. [CrossRef]
30. Wang, X.; Luo, Y.; Liu, S.; Tan, L.; Wang, S.; Man, R. MicroRNA-134 plasma levels before and after treatment with valproic acid for epilepsy patients. *Oncotarget* **2017**, *8*, 72748–72754. [CrossRef]
31. O'Brien, K.; Lowry, M.C.; Corcoran, C.; Martinez, V.G.; Daly, M.; Rani, S.; Gallagher, W.M.; Radomski, M.W.; MacLeod, R.A.; O'Driscoll, L. miR-134 in extracellular vesicles reduces triple-negative breast cancer aggression and increases drug sensitivity. *Oncotarget* **2015**, *6*, 32774–32789. [CrossRef]
32. Wang, T.; Lv, M.; Shen, S.; Zhou, S.; Wang, P.; Chen, Y.; Liu, B.; Yu, L.; Hou, Y. Cell-free microRNA expression profiles in malignant effusion associated with patient survival in non-small cell lung cancer. *PLoS ONE* **2012**, *7*, e43268. [CrossRef]
33. Lu, G.; Sun, Y.; An, S.; Xin, S.; Ren, X.; Zhang, D.; Wu, P.; Liao, W.; Ding, Y.; Liang, L. MicroRNA-34a targets FMNL2 and E2F5 and suppresses the progression of colorectal cancer. *Exp. Mol. Pathol.* **2015**, *99*, 173–179. [CrossRef] [PubMed]
34. Zhu, M.; Huang, Z.; Zhu, D.; Zhou, X.; Shan, X.; Qi, L.W.; Wu, L.; Cheng, W.; Zhu, J.; Zhang, L.; et al. A panel of microRNA signature in serum for colorectal cancer diagnosis. *Oncotarget* **2017**, *8*, 17081–17091. [CrossRef] [PubMed]
35. Carpelan-Holmstrom, M.A.; Haglund, C.H.; Roberts, P.J. Differences in serum tumor markers between colon and rectal cancer. Comparison of CA 242 and carcinoembryonic antigen. *Dis. Colon Rectum.* **1996**, *39*, 799–805. [CrossRef] [PubMed]
36. Han, M.; Liew, C.T.; Zhang, H.W.; Chao, S.; Zheng, R.; Yip, K.T.; Song, Z.Y.; Li, H.M.; Geng, X.P.; Zhu, L.X.; et al. Novel blood-based, five-gene biomarker set for the detection of colorectal cancer. *Clin. Cancer Res.* **2008**, *14*, 455–460. [CrossRef] [PubMed]
37. Komuro, Y.; Watanabe, T.; Tsurita, G.; Muto, T.; Nagawa, H. Evaluating the combination of molecular prognostic factors in tumor radiosensitivity in rectal cancer. *Hepatogastroenterology* **2005**, *52*, 666–671.
38. Nakajima, T.E.; Yamada, Y.; Shimoda, T.; Matsubara, J.; Kato, K.; Hamaguchi, T.; Shimada, Y.; Okayama, Y.; Oka, T.; Shirao, K. Combination of O6-methylguanine-DNA methyltransferase and thymidylate synthase for the prediction of fluoropyrimidine efficacy. *Eur. J. Cancer* **2008**, *44*, 400–407. [CrossRef]
39. Chen, H.; Sun, X.; Ge, W.; Qian, Y.; Bai, R.; Zheng, S. A seven-gene signature predicts overall survival of patients with colorectal cancer. *Oncotarget* **2017**, *8*, 95054–95065. [CrossRef]
40. Ge, J.; Chen, Z.; Li, R.; Lu, T.; Xiao, G. Upregulation of microRNA-196a and microRNA-196b cooperatively correlate with aggressive progression and unfavorable prognosis in patients with colorectal cancer. *Cancer Cell Int.* **2014**, *14*, 128. [CrossRef]
41. Tatsuta, S.; Tanaka, S.; Haruma, K.; Yoshihara, M.; Sumii, K.; Kajiyama, G.; Shimamoto, F. Combined expression of urokinase-type plasminogen activator and proliferating cell nuclear antigen at the deepest invasive portion correlates with colorectal cancer prognosis. *Int. J. Oncol.* **1997**, *10*, 125–129. [CrossRef]
42. Hu, Y.; Gaedcke, J.; Emons, G.; Beissbarth, T.; Grade, M.; Jo, P.; Yeager, M.; Chanock, S.J.; Wolff, H.; Camps, J.; et al. Colorectal cancer susceptibility loci as predictive markers of rectal cancer prognosis after surgery. *Genes Chromosomes Cancer* **2018**, *57*, 140–149. [CrossRef] [PubMed]
43. Wang, X. Improving microRNA target prediction by modeling with unambiguously identified microRNA-target pairs from CLIP-ligation studies. *Bioinformatics* **2016**, *32*, 1316–1322. [CrossRef] [PubMed]

6

A Systematic Pan-Cancer Analysis of Genetic Heterogeneity Reveals Associations with Epigenetic Modifiers

Mafalda Ramos de Matos [1], Ioana Posa [1], Filipa Sofia Carvalho [1], Vanessa Alexandra Morais [1], Ana Rita Grosso [1,2,*] and Sérgio Fernandes de Almeida [1,*]

1 Instituto de Medicina Molecular João Lobo Antunes, Faculdade de Medicina da Universidade de Lisboa, 1649-028 Lisboa, Portugal; mafaldarmatos@msn.com (M.R.d.M.); ioana.posa@gmail.com (I.P.); filipa.carvalho@medicina.ulisboa.pt (F.S.C.); vmorais@medicina.ulisboa.pt (V.A.M.)

2 UCIBIO, Departamento de Ciências da Vida, Faculdade de Ciências e Tecnologia, Universidade NOVA de Lisboa, 2829-516 Caparica, Portugal

* Correspondence: argrosso@fct.unl.pt (A.R.G.); sergioalmeida@medicina.ulisboa.pt (S.F.d.A.)

Abstract: Intratumor genetic heterogeneity (ITH) is the main obstacle to effective cancer treatment and a major mechanism of drug resistance. It results from the continuous evolution of different clones of a tumor over time. However, the molecular features underlying the emergence of genetically-distinct subclonal cell populations remain elusive. Here, we conducted an exhaustive characterization of ITH across 2807 tumor samples from 16 cancer types. Integration of ITH scores and somatic variants detected in each tumor sample revealed that mutations in epigenetic modifier genes are associated with higher ITH levels. In particular, genes that regulate genome-wide histone and DNA methylation emerged as being determinant of high ITH. Indeed, the knockout of histone methyltransferase SETD2 or DNA methyltransferase DNMT3A using the CRISPR/Cas9 system on cancer cells led to significant expansion of genetically-distinct clones and culminated in highly heterogeneous cell populations. The ITH scores observed in knockout cells recapitulated the heterogeneity levels observed in patient tumor samples and correlated with a better mitochondrial bioenergetic performance under stress conditions. Our work provides new insights into tumor development, and discloses new drivers of ITH, which may be useful as either predictive biomarkers or therapeutic targets to improve cancer treatment.

Keywords: cancer; intratumor heterogeneity; genomic instability; epigenetics; mitochondrial metabolism

---

1. Introduction

The expansion of genetically-distinct cell populations within a tumor creates a subclonal architecture that varies dynamically throughout cancer progression [1]. This acquired cancer trait, termed intratumor heterogeneity (ITH), is the substrate for Darwinian evolution to act upon, selecting subclones carrying phenotypes that favor tumor progression [2]. The outgrowth of such subclones impacts cancer development, drug resistance and tumor relapse [3–6]. Despite the key role ITH plays in cancer, important questions regarding its magnitude, origin and genetic drivers across different cancer types remain largely unanswered. By facilitating the emergence of nucleotide sequence mutations, copy-number alterations, chromosomal translocations or aneuploidies, genomic instability has been regarded as the major source of ITH [4,7–9]. However, discrepancies in the rates of genomic instability and ITH observed in previous comprehensive studies [3] suggest that additional events congregate to increase genetic heterogeneity in tumors.

Besides mutations, cancer cells invariably present with some degree of epigenetic alterations that contribute to the acquisition of the cancer hallmarks [10,11]. Indeed, there is evidence that epigenomic reprogramming plays a seminal role in tumorigenesis by creating a progenitor-like cell state that facilitates expression of driver mutations and tumor initiation [12]. High-resolution genome-sequencing efforts have identified driver mutations in genes that regulate the epigenome, namely, genome-wide chromatin and DNA methylation [13,14]. For instance, acute monocytic leukemias frequently (20.5%) carry mutations in the de novo DNA methyltransferase gene *DNMT3A*, displaying aberrant genome-wide DNA methylation profiles [15]. Ten percent of kidney renal clear cell carcinomas (KIRC) have mutations in *SETD2*, the methyltransferase responsible for trimethylation of Lys36 in histone H3 (H3K36me3), which is necessary for accurate gene expression and DNA repair [16–19]. H3K36me3 is also involved in targeting DNMT3A to chromatin [20], highlighting the finely tuned epigenetic interplay between histone and DNA methylation that is needed for normal cell function and is frequently disrupted in cancer cells.

While epigenetic deregulation in cancer arises primarily as a consequence of DNA mutations, the view that altered epigenomes may also change DNA mutation rates highlights reciprocal interactions that contribute to cancer development [14,21]. Accordingly, epigenomic disruption should favor the development of genetically-diverse tumor cell populations, fueling ITH [21]. In fact, a possible relationship between genomic and epigenomic alterations during clonal evolution of tumors has recently been suggested in esophageal squamous cell carcinoma and glioma, where high concordance was observed between the evolution of genetic and epigenetic diversification [22,23]. In this study, we reasoned that analysis of whole-exome datasets of The Cancer Genome Atlas (TCGA) would disclose patterns of covariation between specific epigenetic modifier genes and ITH levels. Our integrative pan-cancer characterization of somatic variants and ITH identified mutations in epigenetic modifier genes that display an association with increased clonal evolution across several cancer types. Experimental ablation of specific *loci* provided direct evidence that loss of *SETD2* or *DNMT3A* drives the emergence of genetically-distinct subclonal cell populations. Knockout cells showed increased mitochondrial bioenergetic performance under stress conditions, a phenotypic trait that fosters the Darwinian selection of clones. Our results provide an unprecedented pan-cancer portrait of the major determinants of ITH and an experimental validation of the role of specific epigenetic modifier genes, laying a foundation for more effective cancer prognoses and treatment.

2. Results

2.1. Genomic Instability Does Not Predict ITH in Many Cancer Types

To estimate correlations between genomic instability and ITH in different cancers, we examined 2807 tumor whole-exome sequences from 16 cancer types of TCGA. We assigned an overall genomic instability score to each tumor, defined as the number of somatic point mutations and small insertions and deletions (INDELs) ranging from 1 to 100 bp in length. The ITH score was obtained using the mutant-allele tumor heterogeneity (MATH) method (Figure 1A and Table S1) [24]. MATH evaluates the variability of the mutant-allele fractions among all tumor-specific mutated *loci*. Therefore, homogeneous tumors with high mutation incidence have a narrower distribution of mutant-allele fractions than heterogeneous tumors. In agreement with previous reports [3], we found that the degree of genomic instability is highly variable across tumors types (Figure 1A). Notably, high levels of genomic instability were not positively correlated with ITH in several tumors (Figure 1B). Individual analysis of each cancer type revealed that only thyroid carcinoma (THCA), pancreatic adenocarcinoma (PAAD) and kidney renal clear cell carcinoma (KIRC) exhibited a statistically significant positive correlation between genomic instability and ITH (Figure 1B). Moreover, we found a significant negative correlation between these two features in kidney renal papillary cell carcinoma (KIRP) and adrenocortical carcinoma (ACC) (Figure 1B). This finding suggests that factors other than increased mutability determine the development and expansion of genetically-distinct subclonal cell populations within a tumor.

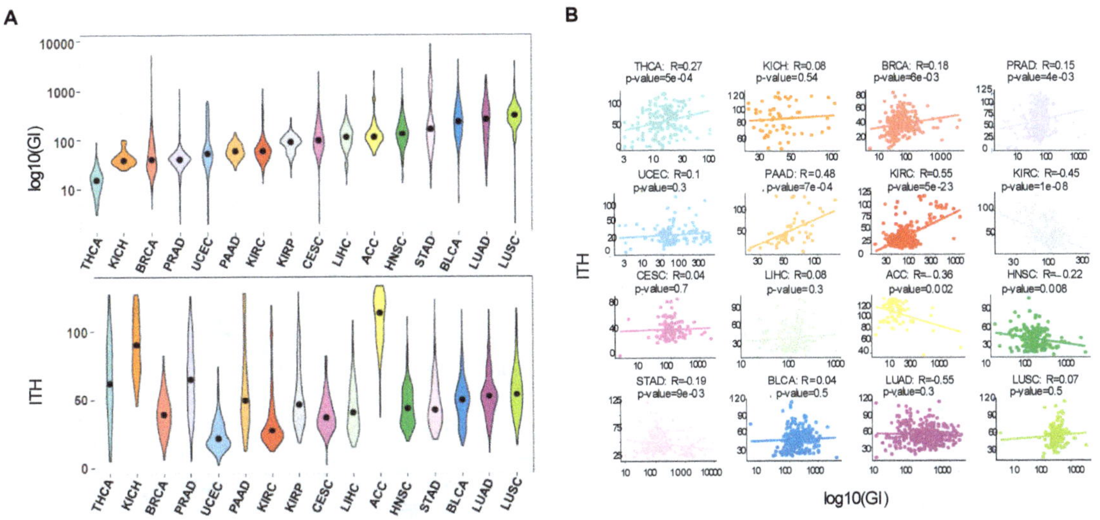

Figure 1. Pan-cancer correlations reveal that genomic instability does not predict ITH. (**A**) Distribution of genomic instability (log10 transformed) and ITH across 16 TCGA cancer types: THCA (thyroid carcinoma), KICH (kidney Chromophobe), BRCA (breast invasive carcinoma), PRAD (prostate adenocarcinoma), UCEC (uterine Corpus Endometrial Carcinoma), PAAD (pancreatic adenocarcinoma), KIRC (kidney renal clear cell carcinoma), KIRP (kidney renal papillary cell carcinoma), CESC (cervical squamous cell carcinoma and endocervical adenocarcinoma), LIHC (liver hepatocellular carcinoma), ACC (adrenocortical carcinoma), HNSC (head and neck squamous cell carcinoma), STAD (stomach adenocarcinoma), BLCA (bladder urothelial carcinoma), LUAD (lung adenocarcinoma), LUSC (lung squamous cell carcinoma). Cancers are ordered according to genomic instability levels. (**B**) Pearson correlation between genomic instability (log10 transformed) and ITH for each cancer type. Each point represents one patient and the line shows the fitted linear model.

2.2. Mutations in Epigenetic Modifier Genes Are Strong Determinants of ITH

To investigate whether epigenomic deregulation drives the development of tumors with high levels of ITH, we focused our analysis on KIRC, the cancer type with the highest frequency of mutations in epigenetic modifiers (Figure 2A). The important role of epigenomic deregulation in the development and progression of KIRC is illustrated by the finding that patients with mutations in epigenetic modifiers have worse overall survival compared to those without mutations in these genes ($p < 0.05$, log-rank test; Figure 2B). To investigate how epigenomic deregulation compares with other specific cellular processes in influencing ITH in KIRC, we analyzed significantly mutated genes grouped in broad functional categories as previously described [25]. The linear model revealed that mutations in epigenetic modifiers are the most strongly associated with high ITH in KIRC, amongst all categories of genes analyzed (Figure 2C). Moreover, the presence of mutations in epigenetic modifier genes correlates positively with increased ITH across different cancer types (Figure 2D and Table S2). Next, we aimed at identifying the individual genes that, when mutated, more accurately predict ITH. To this end, we used generalized linear models previously applied to infer the association of genetic alterations with other phenotypic variables [26]. The strongest predictor of high ITH in both KIRC alone or across several cancer types was the presence of mutations in *SETD2*, *DNMT1* and *DNTM3A* (Figure 2E). Importantly, we could model 32% of variability in KIRC ITH using only mutations in *SETD2*, *DNMT1* and *DNTM3A* (Figure 2F). The optimal model showed a significant correlation between the observed and predicted ITH levels based on the tumor mutation profiles (Figure 2F,G). These data suggest that epigenomic deregulation is an important determinant of ITH and identify mutations in *SETD2*, *DNMT1* and *DNTM3A* as candidate drivers of ITH.

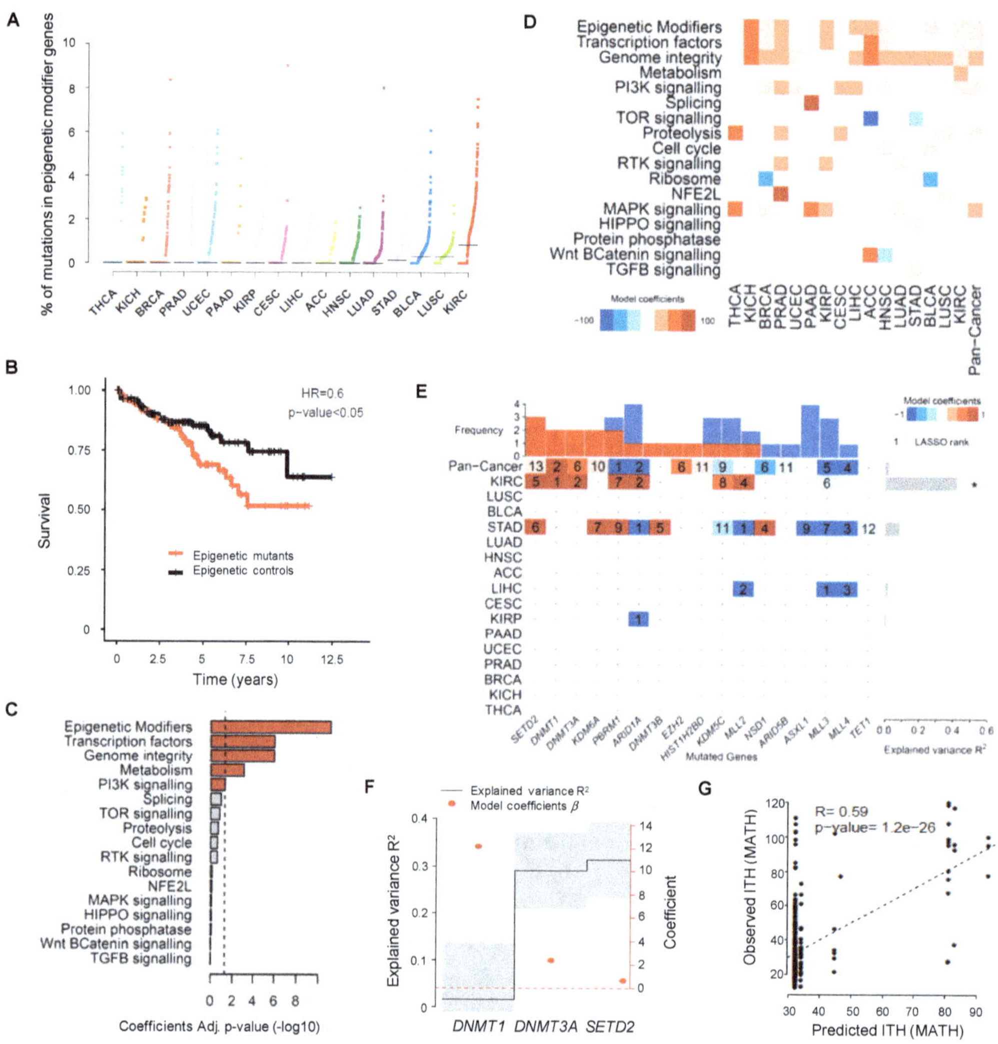

Figure 2. Driver mutations of pan-cancer ITH. (**A**) Pan-cancer analysis of the percentage of somatic mutations in epigenetic modifier genes across 16 TCGA cancer types. The vertical axis shows the percentage of mutations in epigenetic modifier genes whereas the different cancer types are ordered on the horizontal axis from the lowest to the highest percentage of mutations in these genes. (**B**) Kaplan-Meier plot comparing the survival of KIRC patients segregated according to the presence (red) or absence (black) of mutations in epigenetic modifiers. The log-rank test was used for statistical analysis. (**C**) Statistical significance (−log 10 Benjamini-Hochberg Adj. p-value) of the linear model coefficients estimated for each gene group in KIRC. The vertical dashed line corresponds to the significance level (BH adj. p-value of 0.05). (**D**) Heatmap of the linear model coefficients estimated for each cancer type and gene group. Only statistically significant coefficients are represented (BH adj. p-value < 0.05). (**E**) Heatmap of driver mutations of ITH across several cancer types depicted by a LASSO penalized model. LASSO-selected coefficients are colored according to the effect of each standardized covariate in the optimal model. The numbers on each tile denote the order in which variables are included indicating their relative importance. The top bar plot indicates the frequency at which each driver-gene mutation occurs in the ITH fitted model. The right bar plot shows the explained variance. An asterisk (*) denotes models where the explained variance (R^2) is greater than zero by a margin of more than one standard deviation. (**F**) Variance explained by selected driver genes (black line ± 1 standard deviation) ordered by their occurrence in a LASSO penalized model for ITH in KIRC using only the mutated genes *DNMT1*, *DNMT3A* and *SETD2*. The optimal model maximizes the explained variance R2. The right axis indicates the effect of each standardized covariate in the optimal model (red dots). (**G**) Scatter plot of predicted and observed ITH for KIRC (Estimate and statistical significance of the Pearson correlation are presented).

2.3. Knockout of SETD2 or DNMT3A Expands the Clonal Diversity of Cancer Cell Populations

We next sought to experimentally validate the role of *SETD2, DNMT1* and *DNMT3A* mutations in driving the emergence of genetically-distinct subclonal cell populations. The mutations found in these genes were predicted as deleterious causing loss of function (Table S3). To recapitulate this phenotype, we employed CRISPR/Cas9 system to specifically knockout each of these genes in KIRC Caki-2 cell lines. Insertion of small INDELs at the target sites was confirmed by DNA sequencing and efficiency of gene knockout evaluated by measuring protein levels (Figure 3A). Decreased H3K36me3 levels were used as a surrogate for SETD2 depletion (Figure 3A). Importantly, knockout of DNMT1 rendered KIRC cells senescent (Figure 3B), in contrast to DNMT3A and SETD2 depletion, which were well tolerated and did not significantly affect cell proliferation (Figure 3C). This finding suggests that additional compensatory mutations are required to allow the proliferation of *DNMT1* mutant cells within tumors. Alternatively, *DNMT1* mutant clones could be selected during tumor evolution due their ability to promote carcinogenesis through the senescence-associated secretory phenotype [27–29].

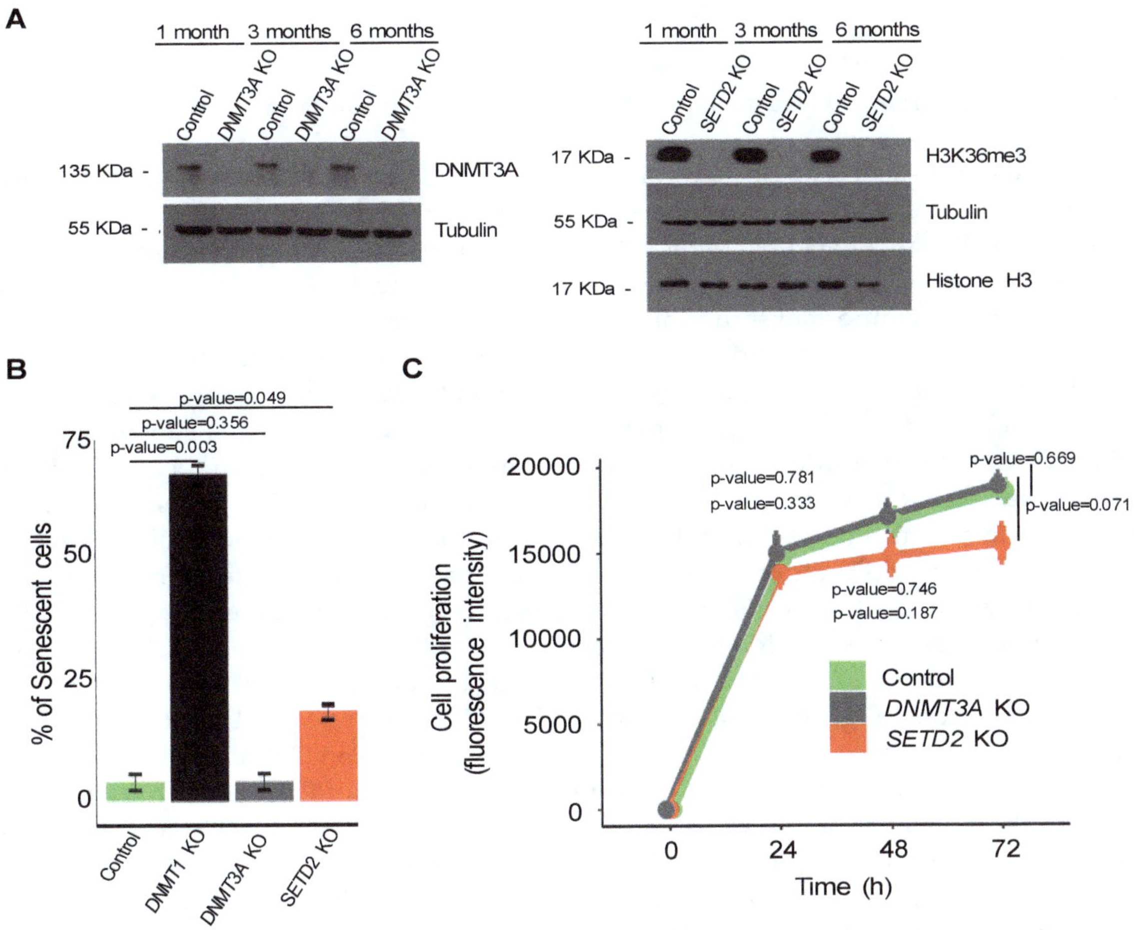

Figure 3. CRISPR/Cas9 knockout of candidate ITH-driver genes in cancer cells. (**A**) The levels of DNMT3A and H3K36me3 were estimated by western blot 1, 3 and 6 months after knockout. (**B**) The percentage of senescent cells in control and mutant conditions (*SETD2, DNMT1* and *DNMT3A* knockouts) was assessed by β-galactosidase staining (error bars indicate SEM; $n = 3$ counting regions of 150 cells/condition in triplicate; Student t-test). (**C**) The proliferation rate of the indicated cells was measured by AlamarBlue dye reduction at the indicated time points. All data are presented as mean (four technical replicates in the same experiment) ± SEM.

To investigate whether loss of *DNMT3A* or *SETD2* drives the acquisition of genetically-heterogeneous cell populations over time, we performed whole-exome sequencing of control and knockout cells cultured during 1, 3 and 6 months (Figure 4A). ITH levels of three different cell populations per experimental condition (control, *SETD2* and *DNMT3A* knockout) were measured at each time point using MATH. Compared to control cells, loss of either *SETD2* or *DNMT3A* resulted in significantly increased and comparable levels of ITH after just one month (Figure 4B and Table S4). However, while ITH rose for up to three months after *SETD2* depletion, it remained constant through time in *DNMT3A* knockout cells (Figure 4B). Bayesian cluster analysis of mutations using PyClone [30] identified 25 mutation clusters that are distributed in each cell population at a frequency that permits segregation according to the knockout gene (Figure 4C). ITH scores observed in *SETD2* and *DNMT3A* knockout cell lines were not significantly different from those determined in TCGA samples carrying *SETD2* and *DNMT3A* mutations, respectively (Figure 4D). This finding reveals that the clonal dynamics of cancer cells grown in vitro recapitulates the in vivo scenario. Altogether, these data suggest that loss of *SETD2* or *DNMT3A* drives specific patterns of clonal evolution that culminate in tumors with increased levels of ITH.

2.4. *Epigenomic Deregulation Drives Favorable Metabolic Phenotypic Variation*

The increased ITH observed knockout of *SETD2* or *DNMT3A* knockout suggests that new clones carrying phenotypic traits that confer selective advantage within the cell populations have expanded and were selected. In cancer cells, mitochondria play important roles in energy production, redox and calcium homeostasis, transcriptional regulation and cell death [31]. Changes in mitochondrial metabolism constitute an important source of variability for natural selection to act upon [32,33]. To test whether epigenomic deregulation drives altered mitochondrial metabolic functions, we evaluated the ability of cells to adapt to shifts in energy demands by measuring mitochondrial respiration rates using an oxygen electrode on the Seahorse platform. In this assay, the oxygen consumption rate was measured before and after the addition of inhibitors to derive parameters of mitochondrial respiration in baseline and stress conditions (Figure 5A). Basal mitochondrial respiration in knockout and parental cells was equally efficient (Figure 5B), indicating that no major intrinsic metabolic alterations were caused upon loss of either *SETD2* or *DNMT3A*. We then measured the maximal respiratory capacity and spare capacity rate (SCR) of cells challenged with the mitochondrial uncoupler FCCP and the Complex I and Complex III specific inhibitors rotenone and antimycin A, respectively. Both parameters were significantly increased in *SETD2* and *DNMT3A* knockout cells when compared to parental cells under similar conditions (Figure 5C,D). Analysis of *SETD2* and *DNMT3A* knockout cells revealed mutations in genes involved in mitochondria biogenesis and function (Table S5); however, inspection of mitochondria network in knockout cells using fluorescence confocal microscopy did not reveal any major alterations (Figure 5E). These data rule out altered morphology as a causing factor for the observed increase in the spare capacity rate. Instead, our data suggest that gain-of-function mutations in genes involved in mitochondrial function drive higher spare capacity rates in knockout cells. Such an association between epigenetics, altered nuclear DNA expression and mitochondrial function has already been demonstrated in previous studies [34]. Altogether, these data provide direct experimental evidence for the emergence of favorable characteristics in *SETD2* and *DNMT3A* depleted cells that may foster the increased number of genetically-distinct clones within the cell population.

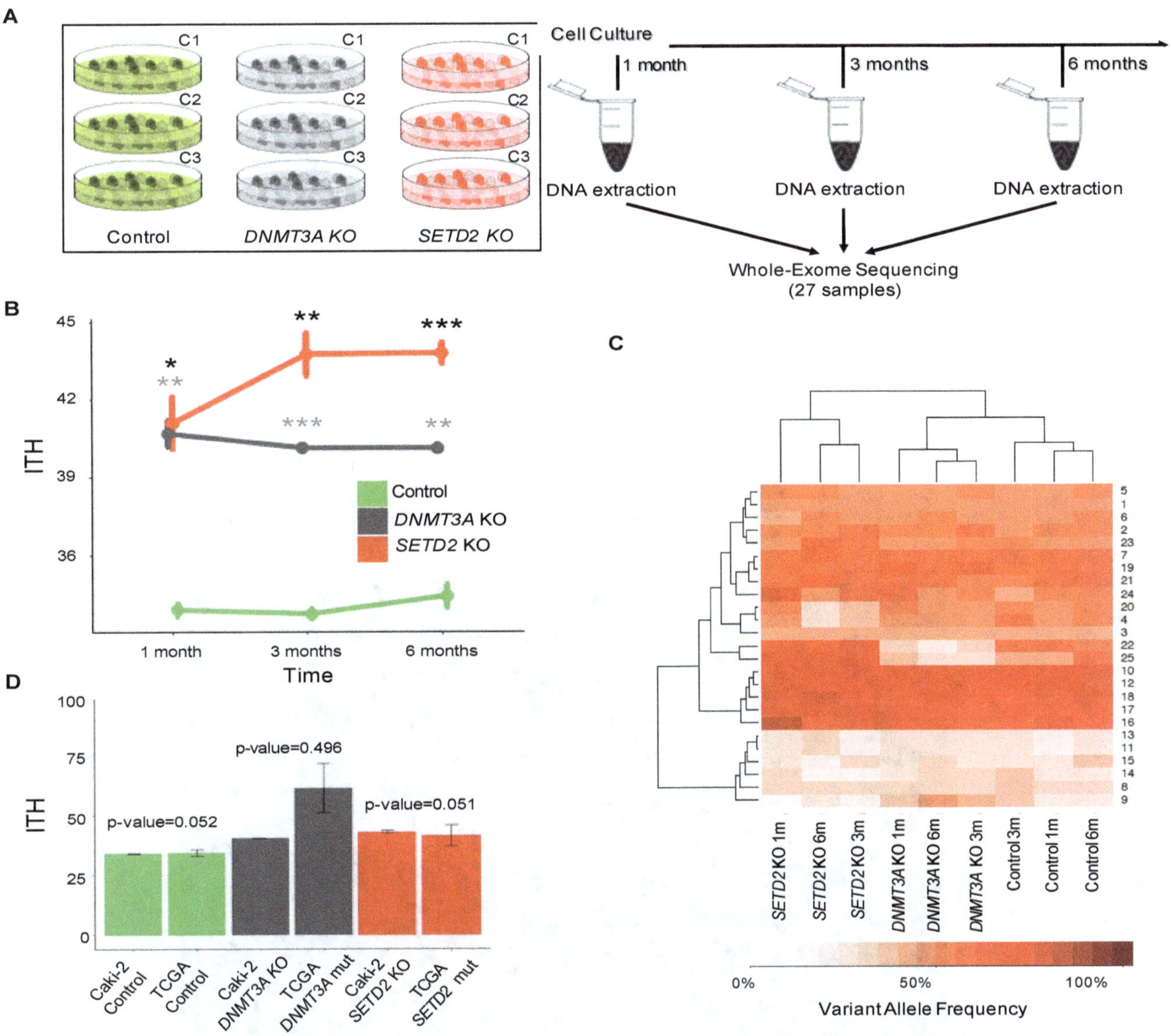

Figure 4. *SETD2* and *DNMT3A* knockout drive ITH. (**A**) Schematic representation of the experimental setup. Control and knockout cells were cultured during the indicated time periods before DNA extraction and whole-exome sequencing (WES). ITH was inspected after three independent clonal expansions (C1–C3) for each knockout at each time point. (**B**) ITH levels of *SETD2* and *DNMT3A* knockout cells after 1, 3 and 6 months. WES data of the indicated conditions were used to calculate ITH, as described in the Methods. Data from three independent clonal expansions analyzed per group are presented as mean ± SEM. Statistical analysis was a two-tailed Student's *t*-test (* $p < 0.05$, ** $p < 0.01$, *** $p < 0.001$). (**C**) Hierarchical cluster analysis of the mean variant allele frequency estimated with PyClone in control, *SETD2* and *DNMT3A* knockout cells. (**D**) Distribution and comparison of the ITH levels across KIRC patients from TCGA and Caki-2 cell lines for the indicated conditions (control, *SETD2* and *DNMT3A* knockouts). The bar graph displays mean ITH values and s.e.m. (standard error of the mean). Statistical analysis was performed with Wilcox-test but no statistical significance was observed between TCGA patients and each cell line.

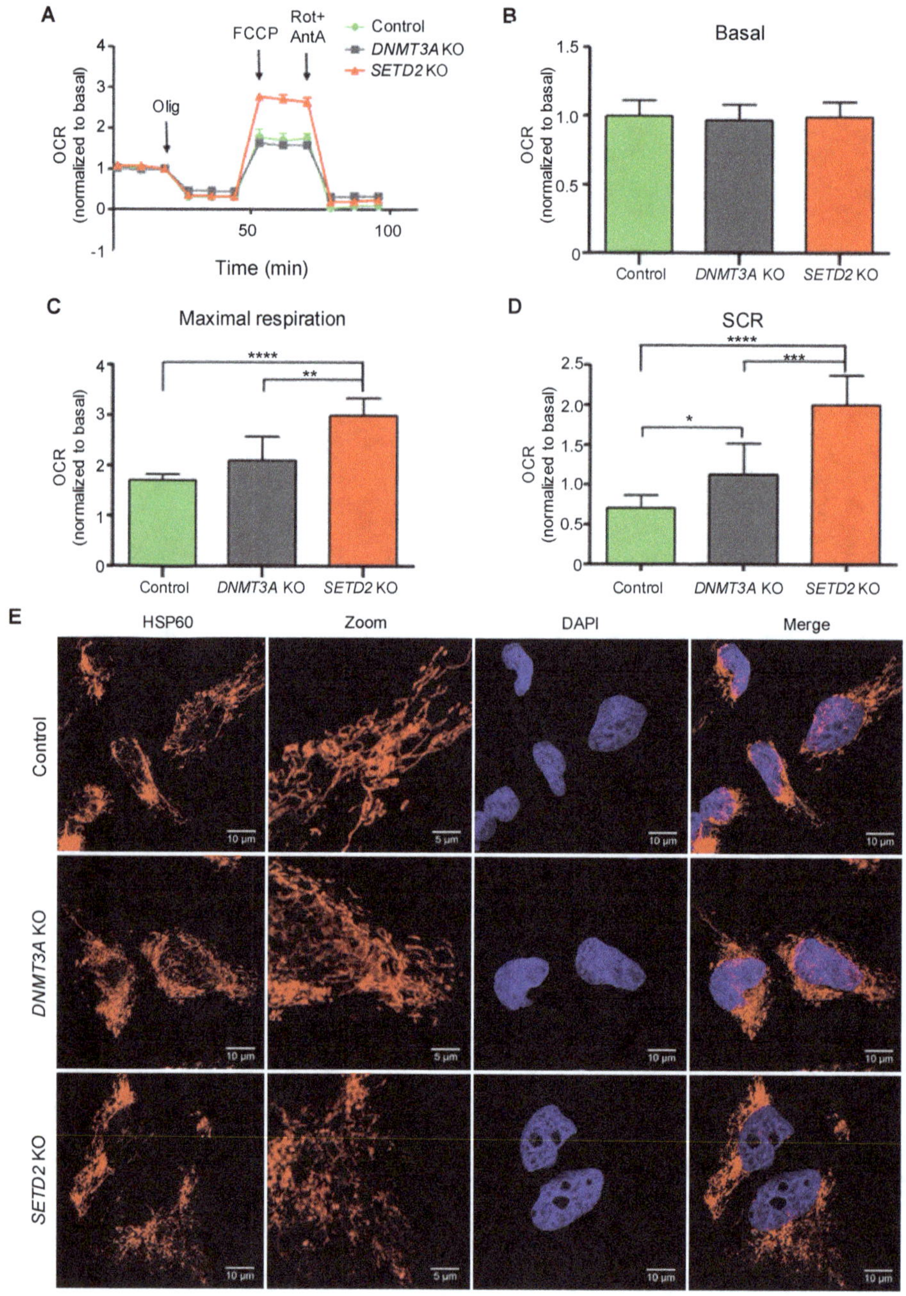

Figure 5. *SETD2* and *DNMT3A* knockout increase bioenergetic performance. Oxygen Consumption Rates (OCR) trace and respiration parameters were measured in control, *SETD2* and *DNMT3A* knockout cells. Seahorse extracellular flux measurements of OCR was normalized to basal respiration (**A**). Basal respiration (**B**), maximal respiration (**C**) and spare capacity rate (SCR) (**D**) of Caki-2 cell lines were obtain by OCR values representative of 3 independent experiments in which each data point represents replicates of three to five wells each cell line. Statistical analysis was performed using the unpaired Student's *t*-test, where * $p < 0.05$; ** $p < 0.01$; *** $p < 0.001$; **** $p < 0.0001$, data were represented as the mean ± SD. Olig: Oligomycin; FCCP; carbonyl cyanide-4-(trifluoromethoxy)phenylhydrazone; Rot+AntA; Rotenone+Antimycin A. (**E**) Mitochondria morphology of Caki-2 control, *DNMT3A* KO and *SETD2* KO cell lines. Cells were fixed and stained with the mitochondrial marker Hsp60 (red) and with the nucleus marker DAPI (blue). Cells were imaged on an inverted Zeiss LSM 880 microscope. Fiji software was used to calculate scale bar (10 μm or 5 μm for zoom-in). Selected image is representative of three independent experiments.

3. Discussion

Tumors evolve through multiple rounds of clonal expansion, diversification and selection that enable the acquisition of metabolic and bioenergetic phenotypes better adapted to the local microenvironment. Such evolutionary adaptation also accounts for therapeutic failure as drug-resistant tumor clones may be selected during therapy. High ITH is the substrate for this Darwinian model of cancer evolution and therapeutic resistance, and hence, highlights the need for further understanding of drivers and mechanisms of clonal evolution. Despite the major discrepancies observed in their covariance rates [3], genomic instability is still considered a major source of ITH [4,7–9]. In this study we show that genomic instability is not positively correlated with ITH in most cancer types. In fact, there is a significant negative correlation in some cancers, suggesting that additional processes must congregate to drive genetic heterogeneity. Our results are in agreement with previous studies, where ITH was associated with different forms of instability [35]. Recently, high concordance was observed between the evolution of genetic and epigenetic diversification in esophageal squamous cell carcinoma and in glioma, disclosing possible relationships between genomic and epigenomic alterations during the clonal evolution of tumors [22,23]. An interesting hypothesis linking DNA mutations and epigenetics in cancer is that altered DNA methylation or chromatin modifications may accelerate mutation rates. Examples of such relationship were already described. For example, abnormal DNA hypomethylation near guanine quadruplexes (G4s)-rich regions is a common signature for many DNA breakpoints associated with somatic copy-number alterations [36]. This finding suggests that DNA hypomethylation in genomic regions enriched for G4s acts as a mutagenic factor in cancer. Additionally, the genome organization into heterochromatin and euchromatin-like domains is a dominant determinant of mutation rates, as illustrated by the finding that H3K9me3 levels alone can predict over 40% of somatic mutation *loci* in human cancer samples [37]. Conversely, we and others have shown that H3K36me3 protects active coding sequences of the genome from error-prone DNA double-strand break repair mechanisms by promoting homologous recombination [17,38,39]. Together, these data establish a strong association between epigenomic deregulation—namely, DNA and histone methylation and genomic mutations, which we show play important roles during clonal evolution and genetic diversification of tumors. In fact, we found that mutations in epigenetic modifier genes are the strongest determinants of ITH amongst a panel of 17 distinct cellular pathways. Particularly, we identified and validated mutations in the methyltransferase genes *SETD2* and *DNMT3A* as potent drivers of ITH. Other epigenetic modifiers were also associated with high levels of ITH in KIRC (e.g., *PBRM1* or *KDM5C*), but correlated with lower heterogeneity in a pan-cancer analysis or in other cancer types. Our findings add direct experimental evidence to previous studies implicating SETD2 loss-of-function in mechanisms that generate ITH [40,41].

As tumor cells adapt to the environment, they acquire distinctive bioenergetic features to take advantage of available fuels. For instance, tumor cells growing in an environment rich in adipocytes could use fatty acids as a major energy source [33]. This remarkable versatility arises from clonal evolution, during which genetic heterogeneity would eventually impact the function of metabolic enzymes [32,33]. We thus reasoned that the increased ITH observed upon *SETD2* or *DNMT3A* knockout likely underpins phenotypic variations in mitochondrial metabolism upon which natural selection could act. In agreement with this, we observed that both *SETD2* and *DNMT3A* depleted cell populations have increased bioenergetic performance under stress conditions, a phenotype that was accompanied by mutations in genes involved in mitochondria function.

4. Materials and Methods

4.1. Cell Culture

Caki-2 cells (Cell Line Services, Eppelheim, Germany) that do not have *SETD2* mutations were selected as a cellular model of KIRC. Caki-2 and human embryonic kidney (HEK) 293T (ATCC, Manassas, VA, USA) cells were grown as monolayers in Dulbecco's modified Eagle medium (DMEM,

Invitrogen, Carlsbad, CA, USA), supplemented with 10% (*v/v*) FBS, 1% (*v/v*) nonessential amino acids, 1% (*v/v*) L-glutamine and 100U/mL penicillin-streptomycin and maintained at 37 °C in a humidified atmosphere with 5% CO_2.

4.2. Gene Knockout by CRISPR/Cas9

To establish knockout cell lines, we used the genome editing one vector system (lentiCRISPR-v2) (Addgene #52961). sgRNAs were designed by GenScript and the potential off-target effects was confirmed using the CRISPR tool (http://crispr.mit.edu). The following sgRNA sequences were selected: *DNMT1* CRISPR guide RNA 1: CTAGACGTCCATTCAC TTCC; *DNMT3A* CRISPR guide RNA 2: TGGCGCTCCTCCTTGCCACG and *SETD2* CRISPR guide RNA 1: AGTTCTTCTCGGTGTCCAAA. As a control we used a pCas-Scramble CRISPR Vector (SantaCruz, sc-418922). Recombinant lentiviruses were produced by co-transfecting HEK293T cells with each lentiCRISPR-v2 expression plasmid together with packaging plasmid pCMV-dR8.91 (Addgene) and the envelope plasmid pCMV-VSV-G (Addgene #8454) using Lipofectamine™ 3000 (Thermo Fisher Scientific, Waltham, MA, USA) as a transfection reagent and Opti-MEM (Invitrogen), according to the manufacturer's instructions. Infectious lentiviruses were collected 48 h after transfection. The supernatant was filtered through 0.45 μm filters (GE Healthcare, Chicago, IL, USA) and concentrated by ultra-centrifugation at 25,000 rpm, 4 °C for 90 min. Cells were infected with lentivirus at approximately 60% confluence. After 24 h, cells were incubated with 5 μg/mL of puromycin (InvivoGen, San Diego, CA, USA) for 2 days. To identify KO clones, infected cells were single-cell cloned in 96-well plates. Several clones from 96-well plates were selected and the presence of DNMT1, DNMT3A and SETD2 was verified by western blot and Sanger sequencing. Genomic DNA was extracted from each clone and a segment surrounding the *DNMT1*, *DNMT3A* and *SETD2* edited region was amplified with specific primers (Table S6). Target sites and specificity were validated using the UCSC Genome Browser (https://genome.ucsc.edu/).

4.3. Western Blot

Whole cell protein extracts were prepared by cell lysis with SDS-PAGE buffer (80 mM Tris-HCL pH 6.8, 16% glycerol, 4.5% SDS, 450 mM DTT, 0.01% bromophenol blue) with 200 U/mL benzonase (Sigma-Aldrich, St. Louis, MO, USA), 50 μM MgCl2 and were boiled for 5 min. Equal amounts of protein extracts were resolved by SDS-polyacrylamide gel electrophoresis (SDS-PAGE) and transferred to a nitrocellulose membrane. After 1 h blocking with 5% non-fat dry milk in 1× PBS, 0.1% Tween20 at room temperature, membranes were incubated with antibodies as follows: anti-DNMT1 (2 μg/mL, Active Motif, Carlsbad, CA, USA), anti-DNMT3A (1:1000, Cell Signaling), anti-H3K36me3 (1:500, Abcam, Cambridge, UK), α-tubulin (1:15,000, Sigma-Aldrich) and anti-histone H3 (1:1000, Abcam). Detection was performed with the appropriate secondary antibodies (Bio-Rad, Hercules, CA, USA) and enhanced luminescence substrate (Pierce ECL, Thermo Fisher Scientific, Waltham, MA, USA). Details of antibodies used are mentioned in Table S6.

4.4. Cell Senescence and Proliferation Assays

Senescent cells were identified by β-galactosidase staining in low-density culture. Caki-2 cells (controls and KOs) were seeded in 6-well plates at 10×10^4 cells/cm^2. In the next day, cells were washed with PBS 1×, fixed for 5 min (RT) in 2% formaldehyde/0.2% glutaraldehyde, washed, and incubated at 37 °C (with no CO_2) with senescence cells histochemical staining kit (Sigma-Aldrich, CS0030) according to manufacturer's recommendations for 12 h. Blue-stained cells and total number of cells was counted under the phase contrast microscope (Leica DM2500, Leica Biosystems, Wetzlar, Germany).

Cellular proliferation for human cancer cell lines (controls and KOs) was measured every 24 h for four days, using AlamarBlue™ (Thermo Fisher Scientific). Briefly, 10×10^4 cells/well were seeded on 96-well plates in a final volume of 100 μL per well. This is a reliable method for measuring cell viability, using the metabolic activity of cells to reduce resazurin (oxidized form: 7-hydroxy-3H-phenoxazin-3-1-10-oxide) to resorufin. The fluorescence of these two forms is measured at 560 nm as excitation wavelength and at 590 nm emission wavelength was measured every 24 h for 72 h, using a microplate reader (Microplate Reader TECAN Infinite M200, Tecan, Mannedorf, Switserland).

4.5. Mitochondria Oxygen Consumption Rate

Mitochondria oxygen consumption rate (OCR) was measured with the XF24 Extracellular Flux Analyzer (Seahorse Bioscience, Agilent, Santa Clara, CA, USA), according to the standard protocol. Briefly, at least 3 months after each knockout, cells were seeded one day prior to the assay in a 24-well XF plates at a density of 2×10^5 cell/well and incubated overnight at 37 °C, 5% CO_2. Twenty-four hours later, cells were incubated with Seahorse XF Base medium supplemented with 10 mM glucose, 2 mM L-glutamine and 1mM sodium pyruvate at pH 7.4 and calibrated for 1 h at 37 °C in the absence of CO_2. Hydration of the sensor cartridge was performed one day prior to the assay at 37 °C in the absence of CO_2. OCR was evaluated in a time course set-up where the following compounds were sequentially injected in the following order: oligomycin (1 μM final concentration), carbonyl cyanide-4-(trifluoromethoxy)phenylhydrazone (FCCP) (0.5 μM final concentration), and rotenone plus antimycin A (0.5 μM final concentration). Rates were normalized to protein concentration measured according to the Bradford method (Bio-Rad, Hercules, CA, USA). Three to five wells from each cell line were measure in a total of $n = 3$ experimental assays. Values for each parameter were calculated as the difference of OCR measures after and before injection:

a. Non-mitochondrial respiration was calculated as the average of OCR measurements after rotenone and antimycin A injection;
b. Basal respiration is calculated as the difference between non-mitochondrial respiration and the third point of baseline cellular oxygen consumption;
c. Maximal respiration corresponds to the difference between the average OCR value after FCCP injection and the non-mitochondria respiration;
d. Spare capacity rate (SCR) is the difference between maximal and basal respiration values.

4.6. Determination of Mitochondrial Morphology

Caki-2 control, Caki-2 DNMT3A and Caki-2 SETD2 cells were seeded on 13 mm coverslips. Twenty-four hours post seeding, cells were washed three times in PBS, fixed in 4% paraformaldehyde for 20 min, washed three times in PBS, permeabilized in 0.1% Triton X-100 in PBS for 10 min, followed by three washes in PBS. Cells were blocked in blocking buffer (0.2% gelatin, 2% fetal bovine serum, 2% BSA, 0.3% bovine serum albumin, 0.3% Triton X-100 in PBS) with 5% goat serum (DAKO) for 1 h. Cells were stained using the primary antibody mouse anti-hsp60 at 1/250 dilution (BD Bioscience) for 2 h. After 3 washes in PBS, cells were incubated with the secondary antibody Alexa Fluor 568 goat anti-mouse at 1/500 dilution (Life Technologies, Carlsbad, CA, USA) for 1 h and with DAPI at 1/10,000 dilution for 10 min. Images were visualized with a confocal laser point-scanning microscope Zeiss LSM 880 with airyscan through an objective of 63× 1.40 oil dipping lens (Zeiss, Oberkochen, Germany). Images were acquired using the ZEN software package (Zeiss) and analyzed in open source Fiji software (https://fiji.sc/).

4.7. Pan-Cancer Data Sets

WES data published in the context of TCGA was downloaded from Broad Institute MAF dashboard https://confluence.broadinstitute.org/display/GDAC/MAF+Dashboard, released (14 April 2017). A total of 2807 patients corresponding to 16 different carcinomas were analyzed: 71 adrenocortical carcinoma (ACC), 270 bladder urothelial carcinoma (BLCA), 228 breast invasive carcinoma (BRCA), 101 cervical squamous cell carcinoma (CESC), 196 head and neck squamous cell carcinoma (HNSC), 167 liver hepatocellular carcinoma (LIHC), 324 lung adenocarcinoma (LUAD),

118 lung squamous cell carcinoma (LUSC), 58 kidney chromophobe (KICH), 274 kidney renal clear cell carcinoma (KIRC), 149 kidney renal papillary cell carcinoma (KIRP), 46 pancreatic adenocarcinoma (PAAD), 349 prostate adenocarcinoma (PRAD), 181 stomach adenocarcinoma (STAD), 163 thyroid carcinoma (THCA), 112 uterine corpus endometrial carcinoma (UCEC). None of the patients were subjected to neoadjuvant therapies (neither chemotherapy or radiotherapy or immunotherapy) before tumor resection. A complete list of samples is given in Table S1. The effect mutations were predicted using cBioportal (Table S3) [42].

4.8. Pan-Cancer Characterization of Genomic Instability and Intratumor Heterogeneity

Genomic instability and ITH were determined using all the somatic point mutations and INDELs downloaded from the Broad Institute MAF dashboard. Genomic instability was calculated as the absolute number of mutations and INDEL observed in each tumor sample. The ITH defined as the genetic heterogeneity was measured considering the same somatic mutations and using the mutant-allele tumor heterogeneity (MATH) approach [24] (see Supplementary Methods for details). Briefly, for each individual tumor we: (1) obtained the mutant-allele fraction (MAF) values of the somatic mutations (the fraction of DNA that shows the mutated allele at a locus), (2) calculated the center (median) and the width of the distribution (median absolute deviation, MAD); (3) multiplied the median by a factor of 1.4826, so that the expected MAD of a normally distributed variable is equal to its standard deviation; (4) calculated the MATH value as the percentage ratio of the MAD to the median distribution of MAFs among the tumor's genomic *loci* (MATH = 100 × MAD/median). Correlation between genomic instability and ITH was determined using Pearson method as implemented in cor.test function of R package [43].

4.9. Pan-Cancer Discovery of Driver-Gene Mutations of ITH

To identify driver-gene mutations, a binary matrix was produced representing the presence/absence of mutations for each gene on each tumor sample, eliminating the bias introduced by hypermutated genes. First, mutated genes were classified according to cancer specific pathways previously defined: epigenetic modifiers, transcription factors/regulators, genome integrity, RTK signaling, cell cycle, MAPK signaling, PI(3)K signaling, TGF-β signaling, Wnt/β-catenin signaling, proteolysis, splicing, HIPPO signaling, metabolism, NFE2L, protein phosphatase, ribosome, TOR [25]. By doing this, we reduced noise from passenger mutations and discover which group of genes is the major contributor of ITH in a wide range of carcinomas. Then, we applied a linear model per cancer type, extracting: explained variance, estimated coefficients, Benjamin-Hochberg adjusted p-values for the fitted model and for each estimated coefficient (Table S2). Second, to identify specific gene driver-events we used generalized linear models previously applied to infer association of genetic alterations with other variables [26] (see Supplementary Methods for details). Briefly, ITH for each individual cancer type and all cancers was modelled by Lasso regression as implemented in glmnet R package [44]. Significance of the explained variance by each model was determined for values greater than zero by a margin of more than one standard deviation. Finally, the fitted models were evaluated by comparing the observed and predicted ITH levels based on the tumor mutation profiles and assessing the Pearson correlation.

4.10. Whole-Exome Sequencing from Human Cancer Cell Lines

The genomic DNA from cells was prepared using the QIAamp DNA Mini Kit (Qiagen, Hilden, Germany) following the manufacturer's instructions and the quality and quantity of purified DNA was assessed by NanoDrop™ 2000 (Thermo Fisher Scientific) and gel electrophoresis. Genomic DNA was extracted from control, DNMT3A and SETD2 KOs carcinoma cell lines following 1, 3 and 6 months in culture and then used for WES. Whole-exome capture libraries were constructed using 100 ng of DNA from Caki-2 cells (controls and KOs) sequenced as paired-end 151-bp sequence tags with coverage of 30×. Samples were barcoded and prepared for sequencing by GATC Biotech AG (www.gatc-biotech.com) using Illumina protocols. Integrity and quantity of the starting material was determined by appropriate methods (e.g., volume measurement, gel electrophoresis and fluorimeter measurements). Library preparation incorporated adaptor sequences and indexing compatible for Illumina sequencing technology, using proprietary methods of GATC Biotech. Enrichment was performed using Agilents SureSelectXT Human All Exon V6 technology. The quality of the final library was assessed by determination of size distribution and by quantification, following GATC Biotech protocols. Sequencing was carried out on the Illumina HiSeq platform. Delivered raw data is the result of a primary analysis using Illumina CASAVA software (http://cancan.cshl.edu/labmembers/gordon/fastq_illumina_filter/).

4.11. Variant Calling from Whole-Exome Sequencing

Whole-exome sequence data processing and analysis were performed by RubioSeq software (http://rubioseq.bioinfo.cnio.es/) using default parameters for somatic variation analysis [45]. Briefly, sequencing data were first checked by FastQC for quality control checks on raw sequence data and then aligned to the human reference genome (GRCh37/hg19) using Burrows-Wheeler alignment (BWA) [46]. Reads unmapped by BWA were realigned using BFAST [47]. Sequenced samples presented 71% of bases in the targeted exome above 30× coverage (see Supplementary Methods for details and Table S7). For variant calling we used GATK Unified Genotyper v2 [48] applying the "Discovery" genotyping mode and default parameters for filtering. The GATK QUAL field was employed for ranking selected somatic variants. Mutations were filtered to ensure that each variant had at least 5 reads supporting the mutant allele and coverage of $\geq$30. Single-nucleotide variants reported in dbSNP150 were filtered out from VCF output files, unless they were also present in COSMICv85 [49]. Only single nucleotide variants were used for downstream analyses. The filtered variants were annotated with SnpEff (VEP) [50]. Finally, to remove the germinal variants (i.e., present in the original cell population) we filtered out variants present in the earliest replicate (1 month) from each experiment (individual knockouts or control) and with MAF equal to 1.

4.12. Assessing ITH and Subclones Number from Whole-Exome Sequencing

The ITH from control and knockout cell lines was determined using the mutant-allele tumor heterogeneity (MATH) approach [24]. A Bayesian clustering approach was also used to infer clonal population structures present in control and knockout cell lines as implemented in Pyclone [30] (see Supplementary Methods for details). Pyclone analysis was performed jointly on all samples using variants supported at least by 50 reads and with copy number information estimated by RubioSeq and processed using CopyWriteR Bioconductor package [51].

4.13. Statistical Analysis and Graphical Representation

Figures were produced using ggplot R package [52] and default packages from R environment [43] and also Graph Pad Prism5 Software (https://www.graphpad.com/scientific-software/prism/). The statistical significance of differences between groups was evaluated using unpaired Student's *t*-test and Mann-Whitney-Wilcoxon test (* $p < 0.05$; ** $p < 0.01$; *** $p < 0.001$; **** $p < 0.0001$). Results are depicted either as mean $\pm$ standard deviation (SD) or median $\pm$ SD, of minimum 3 independent replicates. Survival was analyzed by Kaplan-Meier curve comparison using a log-rank test and with a multivariate Cox proportional hazards analysis as implemented in the survival R package [53]. Statistical significance was determined using p-value < 0.05 as cut-off.

5. Conclusions

Our pan-cancer analyses revealed that mutations in epigenetic modifiers, namely *SETD2* and *DNMT3A*, are major determinants of ITH. These genes are recurrently mutated in several cancer types. For instance, *SETD2* mutations are found in 10% of KIRC [16], 9% of non-small cell lung carcinomas [54], 15% of pediatric high-grade gliomas and 8% of adult high-grade gliomas [55], whereas mutations in

DNMT3A are observed in over 20% acute monocytic leukemias [15]. These numbers illustrate the broad significance of our findings, which provide an unprecedented pan-cancer portrait of the major determinants of ITH. Our experimental validation of the role of specific epigenetic modifier genes in driving ITH reveals novel biomarkers and/or therapeutic targets that may contribute to more effective cancer prognoses and treatment.

Supplementary Materials:
Method S1: Pan-Cancer Data Sets, Method S2: Intratumor heterogeneity score using mutant-allele tumor heterogeneity (MATH) score, Method S3: Identification of deregulated cancer pathways associated with ITH, Method S4: Pan-cancer discovery of driver-gene mutations of ITH, Method S5: Whole-exome sequencing and variant calling for human cancer cell lines, Method S6: Clonality analyses. This file contains the description of the computational methods used in this study, Table S1: Clinical data and genomic features (genomic instability and MATH values) for samples from 16 different TCGA cancer types, Table S2: Linear models associating mutations in functional groups and ITH for each cancer type, Table S3: Predicted effect of DNMT1, DNMT3A and SETD2 mutations in KIRC samples from cBioportal, Table S4: ITH values (MATH) estimated for control, DNTM3A and SETD2 KO cell lines, Table S5: Mutations generated after SETD2 and DNMT3A knockouts (not present in controls), including the mutations with GO terms associated with mitochondria, Table S6: Material and Methods Table (e.g., plasmids, gRNAs, antibodies, primers and other products), Table S7: Read length, total reads and mapped reads for each condition.

Author Contributions: M.R.d.M., I.P. and A.R.G. analyzed TCGA and WES data. M.R.d.M. established the knockout cell lines. M.R.d.M., A.R.G. and S.F.d.A. designed the study, interpreted data and wrote the manuscript. F.S.C. and V.A.M. measured mitochondria oxygen consumption rates and analyzed mitochondria morphology. All authors read and approved the final manuscript.

Acknowledgments: We thank Claus Azzalin, João Barata and Afonso Almeida for helpful discussions. We thank all members of the SAlmeida and VMorais labs for their comments and technical assistance. We are also indebted to the IMM Bioimaging facility for excellent technical support.

References

1. Burrell, R.A.; McGranahan, N.; Bartek, J.; Swanton, C. The causes and consequences of genetic heterogeneity in cancer evolution. *Nature* **2013**, 338–345. [CrossRef]
2. Gerlinger, M.; McGranahan, N.; Dewhurst, S.M.; Burrell, R.A.; Tomlinson, I.; Swanton, C. Cancer: Evolution Within a Lifetime. *Annu. Rev. Genet.* **2014**, *48*, 215–236. [CrossRef]
3. McGranahan, N.; Swanton, C. Clonal Heterogeneity and Tumor Evolution: Past, Present, and the Future. *Cell* **2017**, 613–628. [CrossRef] [PubMed]
4. Andor, N.; Graham, T.A.; Jansen, M.; Xia, L.C.; Aktipis, C.A.; Petritsch, C.; Ji, H.P.; Maley, C.C. Pan-cancer analysis of the extent and consequences of intratumor heterogeneity. *Nat. Med.* **2016**, *22*, 105–113. [CrossRef] [PubMed]
5. Waclaw, B.; Bozic, I.; Pittman, M.E.; Hruban, R.H.; Vogelstein, B.; Nowak, M.A. A spatial model predicts that dispersal and cell turnover limit intratumour heterogeneity. *Nature* **2015**, *525*, 261–264. [CrossRef]
6. Cleary, A.S.; Leonard, T.L.; Gestl, S.A.; Gunther, E.J. Tumour cell heterogeneity maintained by cooperating subclones in Wnt-driven mammary cancers. *Nature* **2014**, *508*, 113–117. [CrossRef]
7. Turner, K.M.; Deshpande, V.; Beyter, D.; Koga, T.; Rusert, J.; Lee, C.; Li, B.; Arden, K.; Ren, B.; Nathanson, D.A.; et al. Extrachromosomal oncogene amplification drives tumour evolution and genetic heterogeneity. *Nature* **2017**, *543*, 122–125. [CrossRef] [PubMed]
8. Laughney, A.M.; Elizalde, S.; Genovese, G.; Bakhoum, S.F. Dynamics of Tumor Heterogeneity Derived from Clonal Karyotypic Evolution. *Cell Rep.* **2015**, *12*, 809–820. [CrossRef]
9. Sotillo, R.; Schvartzman, J.M.; Socci, N.D.; Benezra, R. Mad2-induced chromosome instability leads to lung tumour relapse after oncogene withdrawal. *Nature* **2010**, *464*, 436–440. [CrossRef]
10. Hanahan, D.; Weinberg, R.A. Hallmarks of cancer: The next generation. *Cell* **2011**, 646–674. [CrossRef]
11. Berdasco, M.; Esteller, M. Aberrant Epigenetic Landscape in Cancer: How Cellular Identity Goes Awry. *Dev. Cell* **2010**, 698–711. [CrossRef] [PubMed]
12. Kaufman, C.K.; Mosimann, C.; Fan, Z.P.; Yang, S.; Thomas, A.J.; Ablain, J.; Tan, J.L.; Fogley, R.D.; van Rooijen, E.; Hagedorn, E.J.; et al. A zebrafish melanoma model reveals emergence of neural crest identity during melanoma initiation. *Science* **2016**, *351*. [CrossRef] [PubMed]

13. Plass, C.; Pfister, S.M.; Lindroth, A.M.; Bogatyrova, O.; Claus, R.; Lichter, P. Mutations in regulators of the epigenome and their connections to global chromatin patterns in cancer. *Nat. Rev. Genet.* **2013**, 765–780. [CrossRef] [PubMed]
14. Shen, H.; Laird, P.W. Interplay between the cancer genome and epigenome. *Cell* **2013**, 38–55. [CrossRef] [PubMed]
15. Yan, X.J.; Xu, J.; Gu, Z.H.; Pan, C.M.; Lu, G.; Shen, Y.; Shi, J.Y.; Zhu, Y.M.; Tang, L.; Zhang, X.W.; et al. Exome sequencing identifies somatic mutations of DNA methyltransferase gene DNMT3A in acute monocytic leukemia. *Nat. Genet.* **2011**, *43*, 309–315. [CrossRef]
16. Creighton, C.; Morgan, M.; Gunaratne, P.; Wheeler, D.; Gibbs, R.; Robertson, R.; Chu, A.; Beroukhim, R.; Cibulskis, K.; Signoretti, S.; et al. Comprehensive molecular characterization of clear cell renal cell carcinoma. *Nature* **2013**, *499*, 43–49. [CrossRef]
17. Carvalho, S.; Vítor, A.C.; Sridhara, S.C.; Martins, F.B.; Raposo, A.C.; Desterro, J.M.; Ferreira, J.; de Almeida, S.F. SETD2 is required for DNA double-strand break repair and activation of the p53-mediated checkpoint. *Elife* **2014**, *3*, 1–19. [CrossRef]
18. Carvalho, S.; Raposo, A.C.; Martins, F.B.; Grosso, A.R.; Sridhara, S.C.; Rino, J.; Carmo-Fonseca, M.; de Almeida, S.F. Histone methyltransferase SETD2 coordinates FACT recruitment with nucleosome dynamics during transcription. *Nucleic Acids Res.* **2013**, *41*, 2881–2893. [CrossRef] [PubMed]
19. Grosso, A.R.; Leite, A.P.; Carvalho, S.; Matos, M.R.; Martins, F.B.; Vítor, A.C.; Desterro, J.M.; Carmo-Fonseca, M.; de Almeida, S.F. Pervasive transcription read-through promotes aberrant expression of oncogenes and RNA chimeras in renal carcinoma. *Elife* **2015**, *4*. [CrossRef]
20. Dhayalan, A.; Rajavelu, A.; Rathert, P.; Tamas, R.; Jurkowska, R.Z.; Ragozin, S.; Jeltsch, A. The Dnmt3a PWWP domain reads histone 3 lysine 36 trimethylation and guides DNA methylation. *J. Biol. Chem.* **2010**, *285*, 26114–26120. [CrossRef]
21. Timp, W.; Feinberg, A.P. Cancer as a dysregulated epigenome allowing cellular growth advantage at the expense of the host. *Nat. Rev. Cancer.* **2013**, 497–510. [CrossRef] [PubMed]
22. Hao, J.J.; Lin, D.C.; Dinh, H.Q.; Mayakonda, A.; Jiang, Y.Y.; Chang, C.; Jiang, Y.; Lu, C.C.; Shi, Z.Z.; Xu, X.; et al. Spatial intratumoral heterogeneity and temporal clonal evolution in esophageal squamous cell carcinoma. *Nat. Genet.* **2016**, *48*, 1500–1507. [CrossRef]
23. Mazor, T.; Pankov, A.; Johnson, B.E.; Hong, C.; Hamilton, E.G.; Bell, R.J.; Smirnov, I.V.; Reis, G.F.; Phillips, J.J.; Barnes, M.J.; et al. DNA Methylation and Somatic Mutations Converge on the Cell Cycle and Define Similar Evolutionary Histories in Brain Tumors. *Cancer Cell* **2015**, *28*, 307–317. [CrossRef] [PubMed]
24. Mroz, E.A.; Rocco, J.W. MATH, a novel measure of intratumor genetic heterogeneity, is high in poor-outcome classes of head and neck squamous cell carcinoma. *Oral Oncol.* **2013**, *49*, 211–215. [CrossRef] [PubMed]
25. Kandoth, C.; McLellan, M.D.; Vandin, F.; Ye, K.; Niu, B.; Lu, C.; Xie, M.; Zhang, Q.; McMichael, J.F.; Wyczalkowski, M.A.; et al. Mutational landscape and significance across 12 major cancer types. *Nature* **2013**, *502*, 333–339. [CrossRef] [PubMed]
26. Gerstung, M.; Pellagatti, A.; Malcovati, L.; Giagounidis, A.; Della Porta, M.G.; Jädersten, M.; Dolatshad, H.; Verma, A.; Cross, N.C.; Vyas, P.; et al. Combining gene mutation with gene expression data improves outcome prediction in myelodysplastic syndromes. *Nat. Commun.* **2015**, *6*, 5901. [CrossRef]
27. Yang, L.; Fang, J.; Chen, J. Tumor cell senescence response produces aggressive variants. *Cell Death Discov.* **2017**, *3*, 17049. [CrossRef]
28. Coppé, J.-P.; Desprez, P.-Y.; Krtolica, A.; Campisi, J. The Senescence-Associated Secretory Phenotype: The Dark Side of Tumor Suppression. *Annu. Rev. Pathol. Mech. Dis.* **2010**, *5*, 99–118. [CrossRef] [PubMed]
29. Castro-Vega, L.J.; Jouravleva, K.; Ortiz-Montero, P.; Liu, W.Y.; Galeano, J.L.; Romero, M.; Popova, T.; Bacchetti, S.; Vernot, J.P.; Londoño-Vallejo, A. The senescent microenvironment promotes the emergence of heterogeneous cancer stem-like cells. *Carcinogenesis* **2015**, *36*, 1180–1192. [CrossRef] [PubMed]
30. Roth, A.; Khattra, J.; Yap, D.; Wan, A.; Laks, E.; Biele, J.; Ha, G.; Aparicio, S.; Bouchard-Côté, A.; Shah, S.P. PyClone: Statistical inference of clonal population structure in cancer. *Nat. Methods* **2014**, *11*, 396–398. [CrossRef] [PubMed]
31. Porporato, P.E.; Filigheddu, N.; Pedro, J.M.B.-S.; Kroemer, G.; Galluzzi, L. Mitochondrial metabolism and cancer. *Cell Res.* **2017**. [CrossRef] [PubMed]
32. Tan, A.S.; Baty, J.W.; Berridge, M.V. The role of mitochondrial electron transport in tumorigenesis and metastasis. *Biochim. Biophys. Acta* **2014**, *1840*, 1454–1463. [CrossRef] [PubMed]

33. Alam, M.M.; Lal, S.; FitzGerald, K.E.; Zhang, L. A holistic view of cancer bioenergetics: Mitochondrial function and respiration play fundamental roles in the development and progression of diverse tumors. *Clin. Transl. Med.* **2016**, *5*, 3. [CrossRef]
34. Cherry, C.; Thompson, B.; Saptarshi, N.; Wu, J.; Hoh, J. A "Mitochondria" Odyssey. *Trends Mol. Med.* **2016**, 391–403. [CrossRef]
35. Raynaud, F.; Mina, M.; Tavernari, D.; Ciriello, G. Pan-cancer inference of intra-tumor heterogeneity reveals associations with different forms of genomic instability. *PLoS Genet.* **2018**. [CrossRef]
36. De, S.; Michor, F. DNA secondary structures and epigenetic determinants of cancer genome evolution. *Nat. Struct. Mol. Biol.* **2011**, *18*, 950–955. [CrossRef] [PubMed]
37. Schuster-Böckler, B.; Lehner, B. Chromatin organization is a major influence on regional mutation rates in human cancer cells. *Nature* **2012**, *488*, 504–507. [CrossRef] [PubMed]
38. Pfister, S.X.; Ahrabi, S.; Zalmas, L.P.; Sarkar, S.; Aymard, F.; Bachrati, C.Z.; Helleday, T.; Legube, G.; La Thangue, N.B.; Porter, A.C.; et al. SETD2-Dependent Histone H3K36 Trimethylation Is Required for Homologous Recombination Repair and Genome Stability. *Cell Rep.* **2014**, *7*, 2006–2018. [CrossRef]
39. Aymard, F.; Bugler, B.; Schmidt, C.K.; Guillou, E.; Caron, P.; Briois, S.; Iacovoni, J.S.; Daburon, V.; Miller, K.M.; Jackson, S.P.; et al. Transcriptionally active chromatin recruits homologous recombination at DNA double-strand breaks. *Nat. Struct. Mol. Biol.* **2014**, *21*, 366–374. [CrossRef]
40. Gerlinger, M.; Rowan, A.J.; Horswell, S.; Larkin, J.; Endesfelder, D.; Gronroos, E.; Martinez, P.; Matthews, N.; Stewart, A.; Tarpey, P.; et al. Intratumor Heterogeneity and Branched Evolution Revealed by Multiregion Sequencing. *N. Engl. J. Med.* **2012**, *366*, 883–892. [CrossRef] [PubMed]
41. Kanu, N.; Grönroos, E.; Martinez, P.; Burrell, R.A.; Goh, X.Y.; Bartkova, J.; Maya-Mendoza, A.; Mistrík, M.; Rowan, A.J.; Patel, H.; et al. SETD2 loss-of-function promotes renal cancer branched evolution through replication stress and impaired DNA repair. *Oncogene* **2015**, *34*, 5699–5708. [CrossRef] [PubMed]
42. Cerami, E.; Gao, J.; Dogrusoz, U.; Gross, B.E.; Sumer, S.O.; Aksoy, B.A.; Jacobsen, A.; Byrne, C.J.; Heuer, M.L.; Larsson, E.; et al. The cBio Cancer Genomics Portal: An open platform for exploring multidimensional cancer genomics data. *Cancer Discov.* **2012**, *2*, 401–404. [CrossRef] [PubMed]
43. R Core Team. *R: A Language and Environment for Statistical Computing*; R Foundation for Statistical Computing: Vienna, Austria, 2018; Available online: https://www.R-project.org/ (accessed on 19 March 2019).
44. Friedman, J.; Hastie, T.; Tibshirani, R. Regularization Paths for Generalized Linear Models via Coordinate Descent. *J. Stat. Softw.* **2010**, *33*. [CrossRef]
45. Rubio-Camarillo, M.; Gómez-López, G.; Fernández, J.M.; Valencia, A.; Pisano, D.G. RUbioSeq: A suite of parallelized pipelines to automate exome variation and bisulfite-seq analyses. *Bioinformatics* **2013**, *29*, 1687–1689. [CrossRef] [PubMed]
46. Li, H.; Durbin, R. Fast and accurate short read alignment with Burrows-Wheeler transform. *Bioinformatics* **2009**, *25*, 1754–1760. [CrossRef] [PubMed]
47. Homer, N.; Merriman, B.; Nelson, S.F. BFAST: An alignment tool for large scale genome resequencing. *PLoS ONE* **2009**, *4*. [CrossRef] [PubMed]
48. DePristo, M.A.; Banks, E.; Poplin, R.; Garimella, K.V.; Maguire, J.R.; Hartl, C.; Philippakis, A.A.; Del Angel, G.; Rivas, M.A.; Hanna, M.; et al. A framework for variation discovery and genotyping using next-generation DNA sequencing data. *Nat. Genet.* **2011**, *43*, 491–501. [CrossRef] [PubMed]
49. Forbes, S.A.; Beare, D.; Boutselakis, H.; Bamford, S.; Bindal, N.; Tate, J.; Cole, C.G.; Ward, S.; Dawson, E.; Ponting, L.; et al. COSMIC: Somatic cancer genetics at high-resolution. *Nucleic Acids Res.* **2017**, *45*, D777–D783. [CrossRef]
50. Cingolani, P.; Platts, A.; Wang, L.L.; Coon, M.; Nguyen, T.; Wang, L.; Land, S.J.; Lu, X.; Ruden, D.M. A program for annotating and predicting the effects of single nucleotide polymorphisms, SnpEff: SNPs in the genome of Drosophila melanogaster strain w1118; iso-2; iso-3. *Fly* **2012**, *6*, 80–92. [CrossRef] [PubMed]
51. Kuilman, T.; Velds, A.; Kemper, K.; Ranzani, M.; Bombardelli, L.; Hoogstraat, M.; Nevedomskaya, E.; Xu, G.; de Ruiter, J.; Lolkema, M.P.; et al. CopywriteR: DNA copy number detection from off-target sequence data. *Genome Biol.* **2015**, *16*. [CrossRef]
52. Wickham, H. ggplot2: Elegant Graphics for Data Analysis. In *eBook*; Springer: New York, NY, USA, 2016. [CrossRef]
53. Therneau, T.; Grambsch, P. Modeling Survival Data: Extending the Cox Model. *Technometrics* **2002**, *44*, 85–86. [CrossRef]

54. Govindan, R.; Ding, L.; Griffith, M.; Subramanian, J.; Dees, N.D.; Kanchi, K.L.; Maher, C.A.; Fulton, R.; Fulton, L.; Wallis, J.; et al. Genomic landscape of non-small cell lung cancer in smokers and never-smokers. *Cell* **2012**, *150*, 1121–1134. [CrossRef] [PubMed]
55. Fontebasso, A.M.; Schwartzentruber, J.; Khuong-Quang, D.A.; Liu, X.Y.; Sturm, D.; Korshunov, A.; Jones, D.T.; Witt, H.; Kool, M.; Albrecht, S.; et al. Mutations in SETD2 and genes affecting histone H3K36 methylation target hemispheric high-grade gliomas. *Acta Neuropathol.* **2013**, *125*, 659–669. [CrossRef] [PubMed]

7

Identification of Novel MicroRNAs and their Diagnostic and Prognostic Significance in Oral Cancer

Luca Falzone [1,†], Gabriella Lupo [1,2,†], Giusy Rita Maria La Rosa [3], Salvatore Crimi [4], Carmelina Daniela Anfuso [1,2], Rossella Salemi [1], Ernesto Rapisarda [3], Massimo Libra [1,2,*] and Saverio Candido [1,2]

1 Department of Biomedical and Biotechnological Sciences, Oncologic, Clinic and General Pathology Section, University of Catania, 95123 Catania, Italy; luca.falzone@unict.it (L.F.); lupogab@unict.it (G.L.); anfudan@unict.it (C.D.A.); rossellasalemi@alice.it (R.S.); scandido@unict.it (S.C.)
2 Research Center for Prevention, Diagnosis and Treatment of Cancer, University of Catania, 95123 Catania, Italy
3 Department of General Surgery and Surgical-Medical Specialties, University of Catania, 95125 Catania, Italy; g_larosa92@live.it (G.R.M.L.R.); errapis@tin.it (E.R.)
4 Department of Surgical and Biomedical Sciences, University of Catania, 95123 Catania, Italy; torecrimi@gmail.com
* Correspondence: mlibra@unict.it;
† The authors contribute equally to this work.

Abstract: *Background*: Oral cancer is one of the most prevalent cancers worldwide. Despite that the oral cavity is easily accessible for clinical examinations, oral cancers are often not promptly diagnosed. Furthermore, to date no effective biomarkers are available for oral cancer. Therefore, there is an urgent need to identify novel biomarkers able to improve both diagnostic and prognostic strategies. In this context, the development of innovative high-throughput technologies for molecular and epigenetics analyses has generated a huge amount of data that may be used for the identification of new cancer biomarkers. *Methods*: In the present study, GEO DataSets and TCGA miRNA profiling datasets were analyzed in order to identify miRNAs with diagnostic and prognostic significance. Furthermore, several computational approaches were adopted to establish the functional roles of these miRNAs. *Results*: The analysis of datasets allowed for the identification of 11 miRNAs with a potential diagnostic role for oral cancer. Additionally, eight miRNAs associated with patients' prognosis were also identified; six miRNAs predictive of patients' overall survival (OS) and one, hsa-miR-let.7i-3p, associated with tumor recurrence. *Conclusions*: The integrated analysis of different miRNA expression datasets allows for the identification of a set of miRNAs that, after validation, may be used for the early detection of oral cancers.

Keywords: oral cancer; miRNA; bioinformatics; datasets; biomarkers; TCGA; GEO DataSets

---

1. Introduction

Oral cancer is one of the most prevalent cancers worldwide, accounting for about 354,864 new diagnoses and approximately 177,384 new deaths annually [1]. Generally, the term oral cancer identifies a subset of head and neck cancers arising in the lips, hard palate, upper and lower alveolar ridges, anterior two-thirds of the tongue, sublingual region, buccal mucosa, retro-molar trigone and floor of the mouth [2]. Among these cancers, the most frequent histotype is oral squamous cell carcinoma (OSCC) representing about 95% of all oral cancers [3]. Recent epidemiological data demonstrated that despite the development of novel screening strategies together with the advancement of pharmacological treatments, the incidence and mortality rates of head and neck cancer, and in particular that of oral cancer, are almost stable or increased during the last years [4,5].

Behind the increase of both oral cancer incidence and mortality rates, there are several modifiable factors, including dietary and lifestyles habits, together contributing to cancer development. Among these factors, alcohol consumption and smoking represent the most recognized factors predisposing to OSCC [6,7]. Additionally, viruses and other microbes have been intensively associated with a higher increase of OSCC development, such as infections sustained by human papilloma viruses (HPVs), Epstein-Barr virus (EBV) or Candida albicans [8–10]. Although the majority of the studies are focused on the investigation of microbial factors as cancer risk factors, recently several studies were pursued with the aim of establishing a potential role of the human microbiota in protecting the host from several tumors, including those of the oral cavity [11–13].

Along with these well-recognized risk factors, oral cancer development is also associated with several molecular alterations affecting key genes involved in the regulation of pivotal cellular processes, such as cell cycle, cell proliferation and apoptosis. The most frequent gene alterations found linked with OSCC affect *TP53*, *NOTCH1*, *CDKN2A*, *SYNE1*, *PIK3CA*, as well as the EGFR pathway-related genes (including *TGF-β*, fibroblastic growth factor-BP (*FGF-BP*) and *MMK6*) [14,15]. Recently, epigenetic modifications, including promoter/intragenic methylation and microRNAs (miRNAs) de-regulation, have been linked to the development of oral cancers by mediating the alteration of cellular homeostasis and physiological processes [16–18].

Despite that the oral cavity is readily explorable, most oral tumors are diagnosed at an advanced stage reducing the survival rate of patients [19,20]. Currently, there are no effective biomarkers for the early diagnosis of oral cancer. Several studies have proposed the evaluation of the salivary and serum levels of IL-6 and/or IL-8 as promising biomarkers for oral cancer lesions, however, the sensitivity and specificity of these markers were low because they increase also in presence of various oral cavity inflammatory conditions [21,22]. Other studies focused the attention on tumor markers already used for the diagnosis of other solid tumors, such as the salivary levels of the carcino-embryonic antigen (CEA; 68.9% sensitivity, 73.3% specificity) [23], carcinoantigen 19-9 (CA19-9; no diagnostic value) [24] and CA125 (80.0% sensitivity, 66.0% specificity) [25]. However, the sensitivity and specificity of these markers were not high enough to diagnose effectively all oral tumors.

Therefore, there is an urgent need to identify novel biomarkers for the early diagnosis of oral cancer. In this context, the role of non-coding RNAs, of which miRNAs are the most studied, has been recently acquiring remarkable importance in the development of several pathologies, including cancer [26–28]. In particular, several studies demonstrated that miRNAs, a class of small non-coding RNAs with a length of 20–22 nucleotides, are involved in cancer, including that of oral cavity cancer, inducing epigenetic modifications altering key cellular processes, such as cell differentiation, growth, apoptosis and drug resistance [29,30]. Notably, miRNAs are able to regulate gene expression by controlling mRNA translation, either by translational repression of the targeted mRNA or by enhancing its degradation through an RNA interference mechanism [31]. Furthermore, a growing body of evidence demonstrated that dysregulated miRNAs may be used for diagnostic and prognostic purposes. In fact, it is well established that certain miRNAs are specifically associated with the presence of tumors, even in the early stages, or associated with a worse prognosis [32,33].

Therefore, miRNAs may represent good candidate biomarkers also for oral cancer. On this matter, during the last decade, a huge amount of molecular and bioinformatics data has been generated, with the final goal of characterizing miRNAs' expression profile in several cancers. These databases were therefore used to identify new effective biomarkers identified through computational approaches [34]. Several studies analyzed the data deriving from miRNAs microarray or sequencing profiling in oral cancer samples. However, the lack of integration between the different data matrix generated has generated confusing data on this matter. For instance, Manikandan M and colleagues (2016) have performed a miRNA microarray analysis in a discovery cohort ($n = 29$) and validation cohort ($n = 61$) of primary OSCC tissue specimens identifying a set of miRNAs (let-7a, let-7d, let-7f, miR-16, miR-29b, miR-142-3p, miR-144, miR-203, miR-223 and miR-1275) potentially involved in oral cancer development and progression [35]. Other microarray studies have identified miRNAs different from those identified by Manikandan et al. In particular, Chamorro Petronacci and colleagues (2019) have recently identified two potential miRNAs, miR-497-5p and miR-4417 associated with the presence of OSCC [36]. Yan ZY and co-workers (2017) have identified seven key miRNAs (miR-21, miR-31, miR-338, miR-125b, hsa-miR-133a, miR-133b and miR-139) associated with the tumor [37]. Therefore, it is evident that there are no concordant data generated by the single and independent analysis of different miRNA microarray datasets for oral cancer.

To our best knowledge, no previous studies have analyzed simultaneously different oral cancer tissue miRNAs profiling datasets. In the present study, miRNA expression datasets, contained in both the Gene Expression Omnibus DataSets (GEO DataSets) and The Cancer Genome Atlas (TCGA) Head and Neck Cancer (HNSC), were analyzed to identify a panel of miRNAs used as potential diagnostic and/or prognostic biomarkers for oral cancer.

2. Results

2.1. *Identification of Oral Cancer-Associated miRNAs*

The differential analysis performed by GEO2R on the two datasets of the GEO DataSets database allowed the identification of two lists of de-regulated miRNAs in oral tumors compared to non-tumor controls. By comparing these two lists of miRNAs, it was possible to identify 28 miRNAs differentially expressed in the tumor tissue, 12 of which were up-regulated and 16 were down-regulated (Table 1).

Table 1. Up-regulated and down-regulated miRNAs in tumor samples compared to the healthy controls.

miRNA ID	GSE45238		GSE31277	
	Fold Change	*p*-Value *	Fold Change	*p*-Value *
Up-regulated miRNAs				
hsa-miR-196a-5p	8.096	9.45×10^{-12}	8.132	1.42×10^{-6}
hsa-miR-503-5p	5.010	4.83×10^{-21}	2.622	4.69×10^{-4}
hsa-miR-7-5p	3.505	9.41×10^{-20}	2.297	5.00×10^{-4}
hsa-miR-542-5p	3.348	9.21×10^{-12}	2.700	1.10×10^{-4}
hsa-miR-142-5p	3.323	3.98×10^{-8}	2.633	2.12×10^{-3}
hsa-miR-19a-3p	3.068	3.81×10^{-7}	2.910	4.75×10^{-4}
hsa-miR-18a-5p	2.646	2.34×10^{-10}	1.554	2.66×10^{-3}
hsa-miR-19b-3p	2.179	1.28×10^{-5}	2.415	7.73×10^{-4}
hsa-miR-32-5p	1.997	1.76×10^{-5}	3.874	3.28×10^{-5}
hsa-miR-196b-5p	1.791	2.05×10^{-8}	1.874	2.00×10^{-4}
hsa-miR-33b-5p	1.581	9.26×10^{-4}	2.541	2.00×10^{-3}
hsa-miR-34b-3p	1.558	1.95×10^{-4}	2.079	1.13×10^{-3}
Down-Regulated miRNAs				
hsa-miR-195-5p	−1.778	1.25×10^{-12}	−1.620	1.71×10^{-6}
hsa-miR-378a-5p	−1.799	9.47×10^{-12}	−2.194	4.45×10^{-3}
hsa-miR-363-3p	−1.869	1.56×10^{-5}	−1.951	4.16×10^{-5}
hsa-miR-100-5p	−1.883	8.04×10^{-14}	−2.199	1.19×10^{-4}
hsa-miR-328-5p	−2.471	1.18×10^{-8}	−1.599	2.32×10^{-3}
hsa-miR-99a-5p	−2.732	4.83×10^{-16}	−2.441	7.82×10^{-5}
hsa-miR-218-5p	−3.021	1.08×10^{-10}	−1.853	1.72×10^{-4}
hsa-miR-432-5p	−3.155	1.55×10^{-13}	−1.718	3.14×10^{-3}
hsa-miR-379-5p	−3.513	1.83×10^{-11}	−2.345	9.63×10^{-4}
hsa-miR-154-5p	−4.021	4.01×10^{-13}	−1.826	2.00×10^{-3}
hsa-miR-133a-3p	−4.202	6.37×10^{-9}	−3.446	8.47×10^{-3}
hsa-miR-487b-5p	−4.366	6.96×10^{-15}	−1.899	9.71×10^{-3}
hsa-miR-135a-5p	−4.910	1.11×10^{-14}	−3.324	1.90×10^{-3}
hsa-miR-411-5p	−5.574	3.25×10^{-16}	−2.542	6.18×10^{-3}
hsa-miR-1-3p	−9.783	3.47×10^{-9}	−5.786	2.16×10^{-3}
hsa-miR-375	−16.589	1.95×10^{-17}	−3.198	5.12×10^{-4}

* *p*-values were automatically obtained by using the GEO2R software by performing Student's *t*-test.

The analysis of the expression data of miRNAs contained in the TCGA HNSC dataset allowed us to obtain a list of 514 de-regulated miRNAs associated with the presence of a tumor ($p < 0.01$;

Table S1). Furthermore, 21 of the 28 miRNAs identified with the GEO DataSets analysis were contained in this list of 514 miRNAs (Table S1), thus confirming that the results obtained from the two analyses were overlapping.

To further narrow the search towards miRNAs showing a strong diagnostic significance, the 25 most up-regulated and the 25 most down-regulated miRNAs were selected from the list of 514 miRNAs. The analysis of the TCGA HNSC dataset showed a list of 50 miRNAs that were strongly associated with the presence of the tumor (Table 2).

Table 2. TCGA analysis of up-regulated and down-regulated miRNAs in the tumor compared to the normal samples.

miRNA ID	miRNA Name	FC Cancer vs Normal	*p*-Value *
Up-regulated			
MIMAT0000226	**hsa-miR-196a-5p**	**12.145**	**3.12×10^{-19}**
MIMAT0001080	**hsa-miR-196b-5p**	**11.639**	**5.43×10^{-20}**
MIMAT0000267	hsa-miR-210-3p	9.733	1.18×10^{-9}
MIMAT0000089	hsa-miR-31-5p	7.684	8.42×10^{-12}
MIMAT0004784	hsa-miR-455-3p	7.165	9.21×10^{-18}
MIMAT0005923	hsa-miR-1269a	5.899	1.99×10^{-11}
MIMAT0000102	hsa-miR-105-5p	5.510	9.64×10^{-13}
MIMAT0004504	hsa-miR-31-3p	5.298	1.59×10^{-9}
MIMAT0003882	hsa-miR-767-5p	5.294	5.40×10^{-13}
MIMAT0000281	hsa-miR-224-5p	4.789	5.39×10^{-11}
MIMAT0002874	**hsa-miR-503-5p**	**4.044**	**3.86×10^{-19}**
MIMAT0002819	hsa-miR-193b-3p	3.407	8.17×10^{-15}
MIMAT0005951	hsa-miR-1307-3p	3.395	1.14×10^{-11}
MIMAT0000076	hsa-miR-21-5p	3.209	3.05×10^{-10}
MIMAT0000266	hsa-miR-205-5p	3.040	1.64×10^{-5}
MIMAT0016895	hsa-miR-2355-5p	3.023	6.22×10^{-14}
MIMAT0004987	hsa-miR-944	3.020	7.56×10^{-7}
MIMAT0005797	hsa-miR-1301-3p	2.902	6.39×10^{-17}
MIMAT0000761	hsa-miR-324-5p	2.878	7.41×10^{-12}
MIMAT0000758	hsa-miR-135b-5p	2.859	4.08×10^{-8}
MIMAT0001341	hsa-miR-424-5p	2.856	4.57×10^{-13}
MIMAT0000072	**hsa-miR-18a-5p**	**2.829**	**8.10×10^{-10}**
MIMAT0001545	hsa-miR-450a-5p	2.828	1.20×10^{-15}
MIMAT0000688	hsa-miR-301a-3p	2.807	5.32×10^{-13}
MIMAT0003150	hsa-miR-455-5p	2.799	3.50×10^{-12}
Down-regulated			
MIMAT0002870	hsa-miR-499a-5p	−3.296	3.76×10^{-5}
MIMAT0000733	**hsa-miR-379-5p**	**−3.298**	**1.29×10^{-10}**
MIMAT0002890	hsa-miR-299-5p	−3.504	8.97×10^{-7}
MIMAT0000461	**hsa-miR-195-5p**	**−3.510**	**7.79×10^{-14}**
MIMAT0022721	hsa-miR-1247-3p	−3.553	3.40×10^{-7}
MIMAT0016847	hsa-miR-378c	−3.670	4.61×10^{-8}
MIMAT0002171	hsa-miR-410-3p	−3.684	9.33×10^{-12}
MIMAT0004603	hsa-miR-125b-2-3p	−3.694	1.52×10^{-18}
MIMAT0004606	hsa-miR-136-3p	−3.797	1.08×10^{-12}
MIMAT0004550	hsa-miR-30c-2-3p	−3.881	1.03×10^{-12}
MIMAT0004552	hsa-miR-139-3p	−3.937	3.02×10^{-14}
MIMAT0000099	hsa-miR-101-3p	−4.017	3.64×10^{-23}
MIMAT0000087	hsa-miR-30a-5p	−4.132	6.93×10^{-14}
MIMAT0003329	**hsa-miR-411-5p**	**−4.160**	**2.03×10^{-10}**
MIMAT0000265	hsa-miR-204-5p	−4.519	1.28×10^{-17}
MIMAT0000681	hsa-miR-29c-3p	−4.539	5.24×10^{-17}
MIMAT0000064	hsa-let-7c-5p	−4.674	3.68×10^{-22}
MIMAT0000462	hsa-miR-206	−5.228	4.62×10^{-3}
MIMAT0000736	hsa-miR-381-3p	−5.293	5.06×10^{-8}
MIMAT0000770	hsa-miR-133b	−5.580	3.66×10^{-4}
MIMAT0000088	hsa-miR-30a-3p	−5.696	2.66×10^{-13}
MIMAT0000097	**hsa-miR-99a-5p**	**−5.746**	**1.85×10^{-27}**
MIMAT0000427	**hsa-miR-133a-3p**	**−7.055**	**2.93×10^{-4}**
MIMAT0000416	**hsa-miR-1-3p**	**−10.663**	**8.80×10^{-6}**
MIMAT0000728	**hsa-miR-375-3p**	**−18.183**	**1.33×10^{-11}**

In bold the miRNAs in common with the results of the GEO DataSets analysis; * *p*-values were calculated by Student's *t*-test.

In Table 2, in bold, are reported the miRNAs matching between the analyses of GEO DataSets and TCGA datasets. These common-shared miRNAs are presumably more involved in neoplastic transformation mechanisms underlying the development of oral cancers. As shown in Table 2, most of these miRNAs presented the highest levels of up-regulation (miR-196a-5p and miR-196b-5p) and down-regulation (miR-99a-5p, miR-133a-3p, miR-1-3p and miR-375-3p).

In summary, the two differential analyses between tumor samples and normal samples performed on GEO DataSets and TCGA datasets, showed that 11 miRNAs, of which four up-regulated and seven down-regulated, were strictly related to the presence of a tumor (Table 3).

Table 3. Summary table of GEO DataSets and TCGA HNSC datasets "Cancer vs Normal" differential analyses.

miRNA Name	GEO DataSets				TCGA HNSC Datasets	
	GSE45238		GSE31277			
	FC Cancer vs Normal	*p*-Value *	FC Cancer vs Normal	*p*-Value *	FC Cancer vs Normal	*p*-Value **
Up-regulated						
hsa-miR-196a-5p	8.096	9.45×10^{-12}	8.132	1.42×10^{-6}	12.145	3.12×10^{-19}
hsa-miR-196b-5p	1.791	2.05×10^{-8}	1.874	2.00×10^{-4}	11.639	5.43×10^{-20}
hsa-miR-503-5p	5.010	4.83×10^{-21}	2.622	4.69×10^{-4}	4.044	3.86×10^{-19}
hsa-miR-18a-5p	2.646	2.34×10^{-10}	1.554	2.66×10^{-3}	2.829	8.10×10^{-10}
Down-regulated						
hsa-miR-379-5p	−3.513	1.83×10^{-11}	−2.345	9.63×10^{-4}	−3.298	1.29×10^{-10}
hsa-miR-195-5p	−1.778	1.25×10^{-12}	−1.620	1.71×10^{-6}	−3.510	7.79×10^{-14}
hsa-miR-411-5p	−5.574	3.25×10^{-16}	−2.542	6.18×10^{-3}	−4.160	2.03×10^{-10}
hsa-miR-99a-5p	−2.732	4.83×10^{-16}	−2.441	7.82×10^{-5}	−5.746	1.85×10^{-27}
hsa-miR-133a-3p	−4.202	6.37×10^{-9}	−3.446	8.47×10^{-3}	−7.055	2.93×10^{-4}
hsa-miR-1-3p	−9.783	3.47×10^{-9}	−5.786	2.16×10^{-3}	−10.663	8.80×10^{-6}
hsa-miR-375-3p	−16.589	1.95×10^{-17}	−3.198	5.12×10^{-4}	−18.183	1.33×10^{-11}

* *p*-values were already calculated by GEO2R software; ** *p*-values were calculated by applying Student's *t*-test.

As shown in Table 3, the miRNA miR-196a-5p and the two miRNAs miR-1-3p and miR-375-3p, respectively up-regulated and down-regulated, presented the higher levels of over-expression or down-regulation in all three datasets (two GEO DataSets and one TCGA).

For the further prediction analyses of target genes and altered molecular pathways, the 11 miRNAs reported in Table 3 were considered: hsa-miR-196a-5p, hsa-miR-196b-5p, hsa-miR-503-5p, hsa-miR-18a-5p, hsa-miR-379-5p, hsa-miR-195-5p, hsa-miR-411-5p, hsa-miR-99a-5p, hsa-miR-133a-3p, hsa-miR- 1-3p and hsa-miR-375-3p.

2.2. Levels of Interaction Between the 11 Selected miRNAs and Oral Cancer Altered Genes

Through the use of COSMIC and mirDIP, the majority of mutated and altered genes in oral cavity tumors were identified and miRNA-gene interaction specificity was determined, respectively. First, by using COSMIC the 10 most frequent mutations and gene alteration found in oral cancers were identified. These altered genes were the *TP53* genes (43%), *FAT1* (28%), *CASP8* (23%), *TERT* (22%), *NOTCH1* (20%), *CDKN2A* (16%), *HRAS* (10%), *KMT2D* (10%), *FGFR3* (8%) and *PIK3CA* (8%).

Then, through mirDIP it was possible to establish the interaction levels with the selected 11 oral cancer-associated miRNAs and the genes identified by using COSMIC (Table S2). For the 10 interacting genes, also gene expression levels were analyzed using the TCGA HNSC IlluminaHiSeq pancan normalized dataset (Table S3). This analysis revealed that all the identified miRNAs were able to target the commonly mutated genes in oral cancers. In fact, the majority of the interactions occurred with medium-high specificity underlining the strong correlation between deregulated miRNAs in cancer patients and the aforementioned genes involved in fundamental cellular and cancer pathways (Figure 1). However, the analysis of the TCGA HNSC IlluminaHiSeq pancan normalized dataset showed that only six out of the 10 (*TP53, FAT1, CASP8, TERT, CDKN2A* and *PIK3CA*) genes were significantly de-regulated in oral cancers (Table S3).

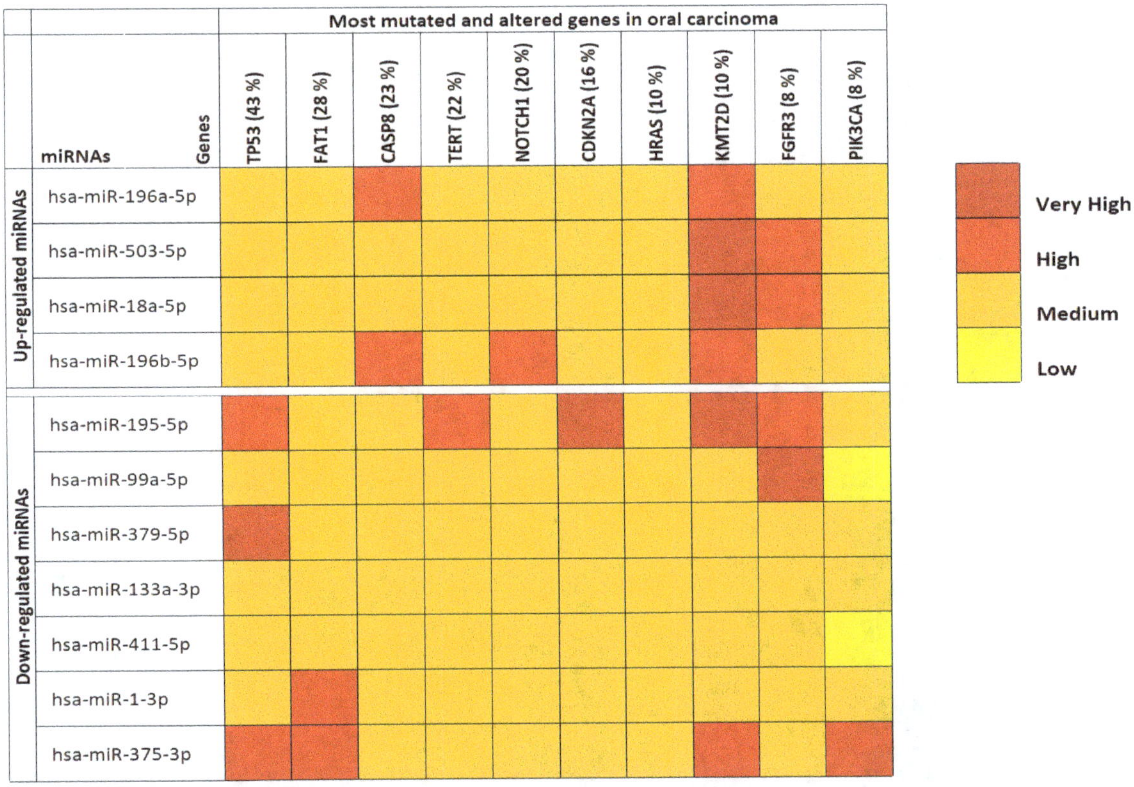

Figure 1. mirDIP analysis of interaction levels between selected miRNAs and the main mutated and altered genes in oral cavity tumors.

The most interesting data showed in Figure 1 were relative to the *KMT2D* gene where it is possible to note how all up-regulated miRNAs were able to target this gene by reducing its expression levels. This is important if we consider that KMT2D is a tumor suppressor gene, therefore its down-regulation due to the suppressive action of up-regulated miRNAs triggers cellular neoplastic transformation. Taking into account the miRNAs, it can instead be noted that, generally, the 11 selected miRNAs have medium levels of interaction with the target genes (medium interaction orange). However, the down-regulated hsa-miR-195-5p and hsa-miR-375-3p miRNAs showed the highest interaction levels with the analyzed genes (Figure 1). The expression levels of the 10 targeted genes showed that the *FAT1, CASP8, TERT, CDKN2A* and *PIK3CA* genes were significantly up-regulated in tumor samples, while *TP53* was significantly down-regulated.

2.3. Correlation Analysis Between the 11 Selected Tumor-Associated miRNAs and Ene Expression

The correlation value of each miRNA with different genes was obtained by using the bioinformatics tool miRCancerdb. This tool is a free easy-to-use database of microRNA-gene/protein expression and correlation in cancer where the correlation levels are calculated using the Pearson correlation coefficient (ρ). Therefore, the correlation levels are denoted by "*r*" [38].

In particular, for each miRNA a list of miRNAs-correlated genes, ranging from 4493 to 9042, was obtained through miRCancerdb analysis. Subsequently, these lists of genes were compared showing a total of 121 genes in common and altered by the 11 selected miRNAs. However, only the genes shared by the 11 miRNAs and belonging to the first quartile of the genes most positively and negatively correlated to each miRNA were considered (Figure 2). This selection unveiled the correlation levels of 105 different genes (Figure 2A).

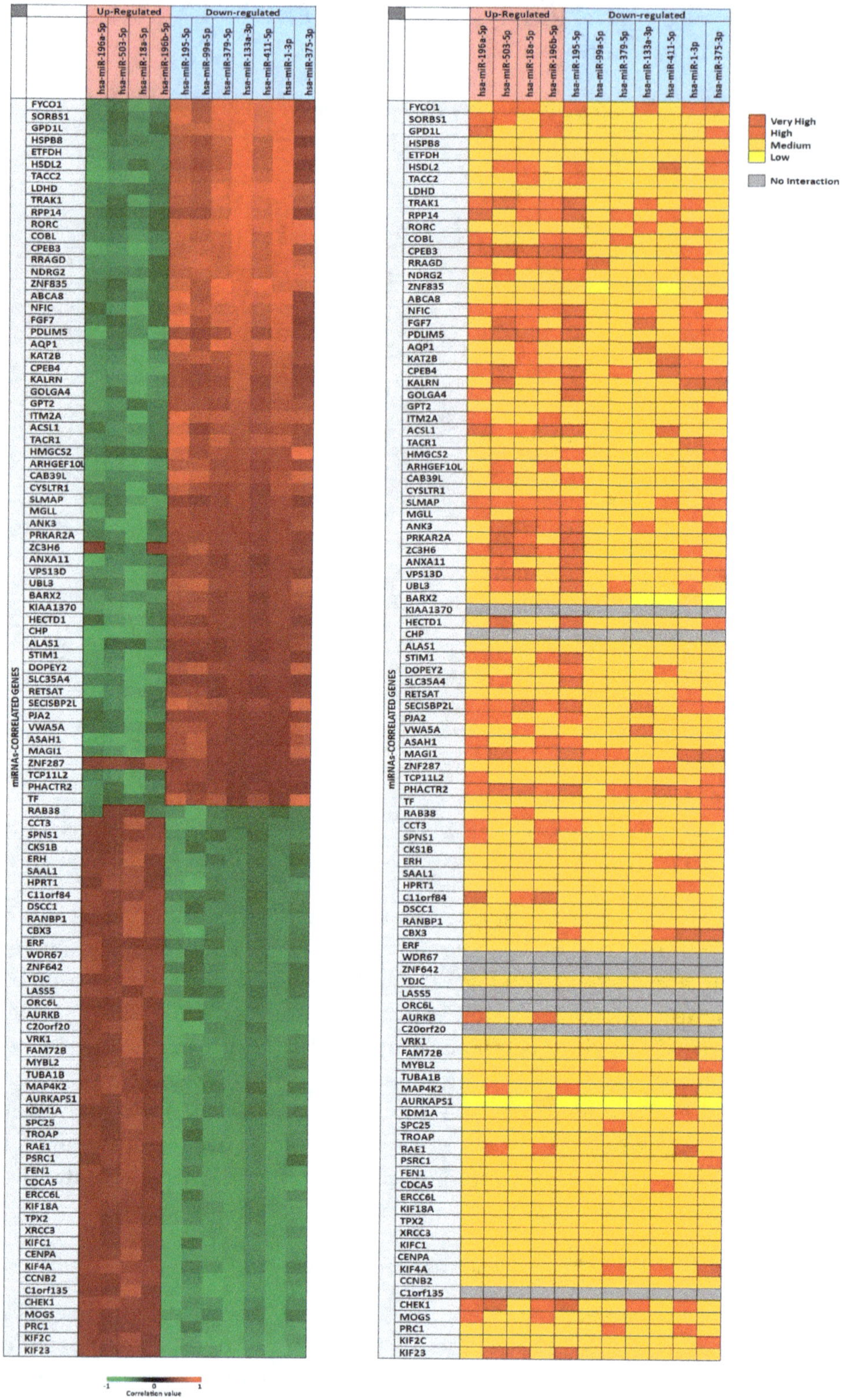

Figure 2. Panel (**A**) miRCancerdb analysis of genes whose expression is positively and negatively related to the 11 selected miRNAs; panel (**B**) mirDIP analysis of interaction levels between miRNAs and related genes.

In Figure 2A, the heat map showed that the down-regulated miRNAs miR-133a-3p and miR-1-3p were those with the highest positive correlation levels; instead, the miRNA with lower negative correlation levels was the up-regulated miRNA miR-18a-5p. Moreover, it can be observed that *FYCO1*,

SORBS1 and *GPD1L* genes were strongly positively correlated with the selected miRNAs; on the other hand, *ASA1*, *NFIC* and *SECISBP2L* genes were the least correlated with the analyzed miRNAs.

To further confirm the correlation levels existing among miRNAs and genes, the mirDIP tool was used. In Figure 2B, the interaction levels between the 11 selected miRNAs and the positively and negatively correlated genes are showed (Figure 2B). The figure shows that for eight genes there were no interactions with the selected miRNAs (*KIAA1370, CHP, WDR67, ZNF642, LASS5, ORC6L, C20orf20, C1orf135*). Overall, such analysis revealed that miR-195-5p, miR-503-5p, miR-18a-5p (up-regulated) and miR-375-3p (down-regulated) showed highest interaction levels with the 105 genes. On the other hand, the genes *CPEB3, CPEB4, MAGI1, PHACTR2, PDLIM5, NFIC, SLMAP* and *SECISBP2L* were strongly targeted by the 11 selected miRNAs (Figure 2B).

2.4. Determination of the Functional Roles of Tumor-Associated MiRNAs Through Pathway and GO Enrichment Analyses

For the pathway prediction analysis, all the 11 tumor-associated miRNAs were inputted into the bioinformatics prediction tool DIANA-mirPath. The analysis revealed that for the miRNAs miR-503-5p, miR-133a-3p and miR-1-3p there were not modulated pathways and targeted genes according to the TarBase Version 7.0 database of DIANA-mirPath. For the remaining miRNAs the cumulative pathway analysis showed that, overall, the miRNAs were able to alter 48 different pathways and over 2100 genes. However, the pathways involved in the tumor processes were 22 and the modulated genes amounted to 345 univocal genes (Table 4).

Table 4. Pathways involved in neoplastic transformation and modulated by the 11 computationally selected miRNAs.

No.	KEGG Pathway	Up-Regulated miRNAs			Down-Regulated miRNAs		
		p-Value *	#Genes	#miRNAs	*p*-Value *	#Genes	#miRNAs
1	Bladder cancer (hsa05219)	2.25×10^{-3}	14	3	2.78×10^{-3}	19	5
2	Cell cycle (hsa04110)	1.11×10^{-2}	27	3	5.48×10^{-3}	43	6
3	Central carbon metabolism in cancer (hsa05230)	/	/	/	4.59×10^{-2}	20	5
4	Chronic myeloid leukemia (hsa05220)	3.61×10^{-4}	22	3	1.99×10^{-2}	25	5
5	Colorectal cancer (hsa05210)	7.53×10^{-5}	18	3	/	/	/
6	FoxO signaling pathway (hsa04068)	7.64×10^{-3}	28	3	4.50×10^{-3}	44	6
7	Glioma (hsa05214)	2.56×10^{-3}	16	3	3.70×10^{-3}	23	5
8	Hippo signaling pathway (hsa04390)	1.74×10^{-11}	41	3	4.22×10^{-8}	51	6
9	Melanoma (hsa05218)	1.48×10^{-2}	15	3	/	/	/
10	mTOR signaling pathway (hsa04150)	/	/	/	1.82×10^{-2}	22	5
11	Non-small cell lung cancer (hsa05223)	2.54×10^{-2}	14	3	/	/	/
12	p53 signaling pathway (hsa04115)	1.84×10^{-3}	19	3	6.53×10^{-4}	28	6
13	Pancreatic cancer (hsa05212)	2.90×10^{-2}	17	3	4.79×10^{-2}	23	5
14	Pathways in cancer (hsa05200)	1.33×10^{-3}	62	3	1.68×10^{-4}	111	6
15	Prostate cancer (hsa05215)	3.73×10^{-2}	19	3	3.83×10^{-3}	33	6
16	Proteoglycans in cancer (hsa05205)	2.13×10^{-4}	35	3	1.11×10^{-12}	73	6
17	Renal cell carcinoma (hsa05211)	/	/	/	1.65×10^{-2}	23	6
18	Small cell lung cancer (hsa05222)	2.34×10^{-2}	19	3	1.65×10^{-2}	29	5
19	TGF-beta signaling pathway (hsa04350)	8.01×10^{-6}	19	3	6.45×10^{-3}	26	6
20	Thyroid cancer (hsa05216)	3.68×10^{-2}	7	3	/	/	/
21	TNF signaling pathway (hsa04668)	/	/	/	1.88×10^{-2}	36	6
22	Viral carcinogenesis (hsa05203)	1.53×10^{-2}	35	3	3.77×10^{-6}	65	6

* *p*-values were already calculated by the DIANA-mirPath by automatically applying the Fisher's Exact Test.

As shown in Table 4, the identified miRNAs play a key role in the modulation of different pathways involved in neoplastic development and in different types of tumors, highlighting their potential pro-oncogenic role when de-regulated (Table 4). The pathways found highly modulated were: "Pathways in cancer (hsa05200)", "Cell cycle (hsa04110)", various signal transduction pathways, including "FoxO signaling pathway (hsa04068)", "p53 signaling pathway (hsa04115)" and "Hippo signaling pathways (hsa04390)".

Within these pathways, *MAPK1* (18 counts), *CCND1* (17 counts), *AKT3* and *PIK3CA* (15 counts), *PIK3CB* (14 counts), *NRAS* (13 counts), *BRAF* (12 counts), *CDK4* and *CDKN1A* (11 counts) and *E2F2* (10 counts) genes were found commonly altered by the selected miRNAs. All these genes, when de-regulated, were notoriously involved in cancer development and progression.

To further confirm the functional roles of miRNAs and their modulated genes, gene enrichment analyses were performed on both miRCancerdb and DIANA-mirPath lists of genes by using both GO PANTHER and STRING software.

Both enrichment analyses were performed on the list of the 105 miRCancerdb genes correlated to the 11 cancer-associated miRNAs giving back similar results regarding the three ontological categories "biological process", "molecular function" and "cellular component". Figure 3 shows the results of the GO PANTHER and STRING analyses (Figure 3).

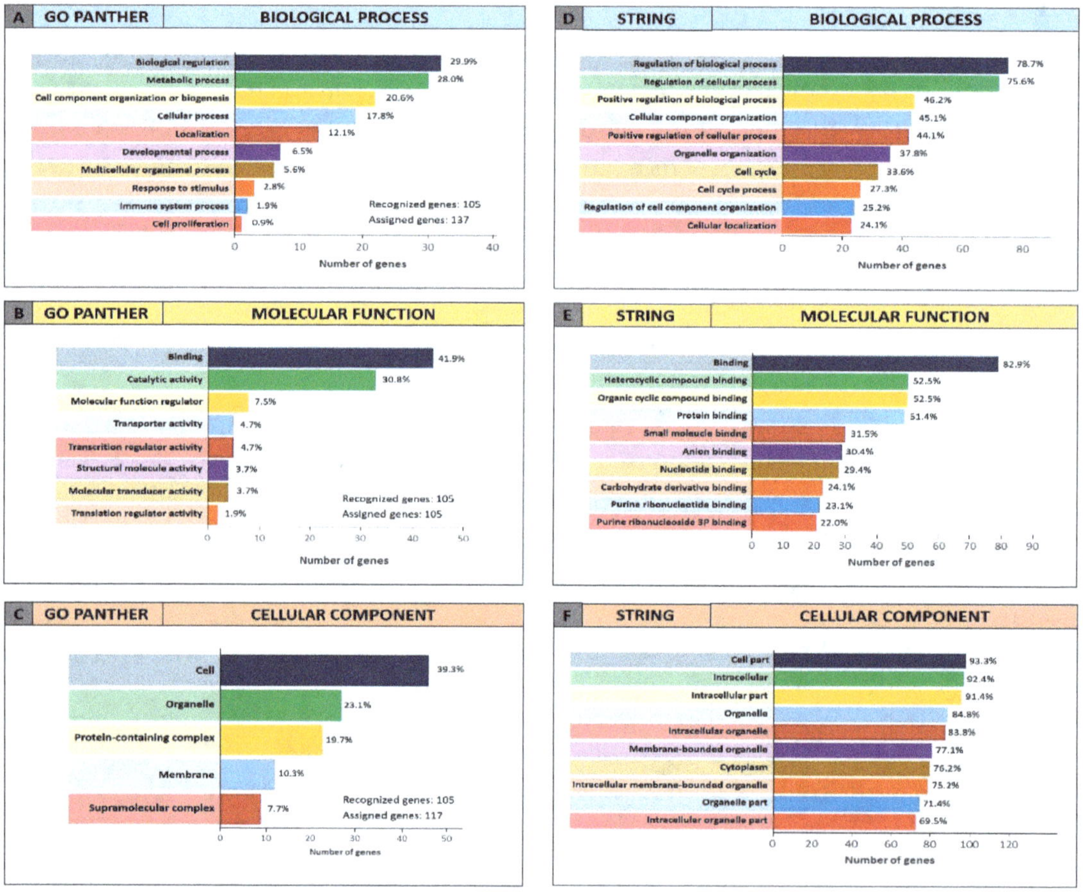

Figure 3. Gene Ontology enrichment of the 105 genes identified through miRCancerdb. Panel (**A**,**D**) GO PANTHER and STRING analyses of the "biological process" category; panel (**B**,**E**) GO PANTHER and STRING analyses of the "molecular function" category; panel (**C**,**F**) GO PANTHER and STRING analyses of the "cellular component" category.

Regarding the "biological process" category, it was demonstrated that most of the miRNAs-modulated genes are involved in the regulation of biological (29.9% and 78.7%, GO PANTHER and STRING, respectively) and cellular (17.8% and 75.6%, GO PANTHER and STRING, respectively) processes (Figure 3A,D). In Figure 3B,E, the genes were clustered according to their "molecular function" and the results showed that the genes were all involved in protein binding, cyclic compounds and nucleotides binding (STRING analysis Figure 3E). While the GO PANTHER analysis for the same category (molecular function) showed that the genes were mainly involved in the binding and, to a lesser extent, in the catalytic, molecular and transport activities (Figure 3B). Finally, with regard to the "cellular component" category, the majority of the genes were components of the cell (39.3% and

93.3, GO PANTHER and STRING, respectively) and organelles (23.1% and 84.8%, GO PANTHER and STRING, respectively; Figure 3C,F).

The same GO enrichment analyses were performed on the 345 genes identified by DIANA-mirPath showing similar results to those described above (Figure 4).

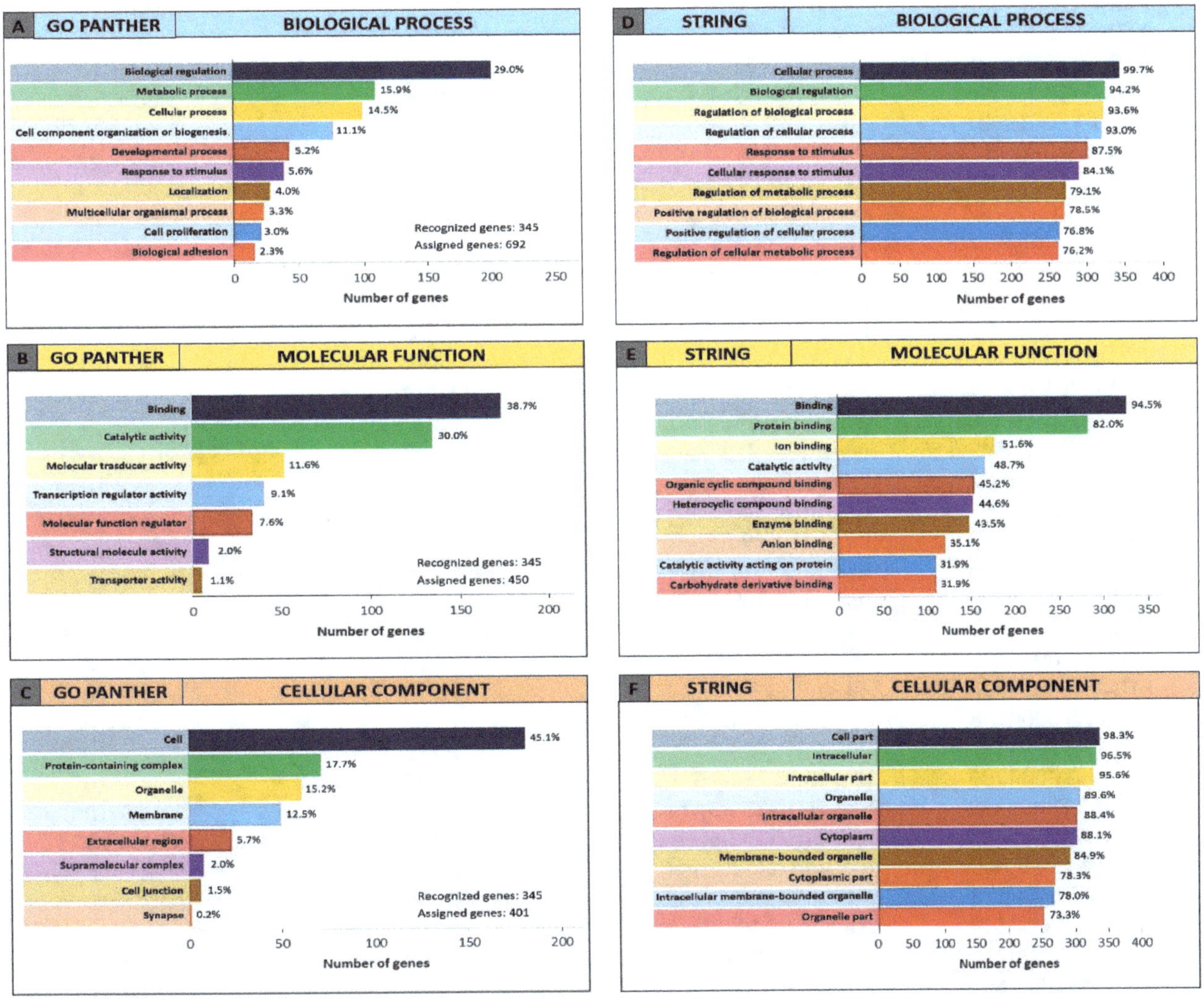

Figure 4. Gene Ontology enrichment of the 345 genes identified through DIANA-mirPath. Panel (**A**,**D**) GO PANTHER and STRING analyses of the "biological process" category; panel (**B**,**E**) GO PANTHER and STRING analyses of the "molecular function" category; panel (**C**,**F**) GO PANTHER and STRING analyses of the "cellular component" category.

Figure 4 (Panel A and D) shows that, in the "biological process" category, the genes identified by DIANA-mirPath were involved in the regulation of the biological and cellular processes as observed in Figure 3. Similarly, in the "molecular function" and "cellular component" categories, the 345 genes were involved, respectively, in molecular binding and catalytic activities (Figure 4B,E), and were components of the cell and intracellular organelles (Figure 4C,F).

2.5. *Identification of Oral Cancer Stage-Related miRNAs*

The same differential analysis performed to find the oral cancer-associated miRNAs was also performed between high-grade tumor samples (254 stage III and IV samples—high-grade) and low-grade tumor samples (94 Stage I and II samples—low-grade) in order to find oral cancer stage-related miRNAs with a prognostic significance. This second differential analysis showed that 36 miRNAs were de-regulated in high-grade samples compared to low-grade ($p < 0.01$; Table 5).

Table 5. TCGA analysis of up-regulated and down-regulated miRNAs in high-grade compared with low-grade tumors.

miRNA ID	miRNA Name	FC High-Grade vs Low-Grade	*p*-Value **
Up-regulated			
MIMAT0001536	hsa-miR-429	1.279	3.20×10^{-3}
MIMAT0003233	hsa-miR-551b-3p	1.205	1.31×10^{-3}
MIMAT0004697	hsa-miR-151a-5p	1.172	3.78×10^{-3}
MIMAT0003246	hsa-miR-581	1.078	3.88×10^{-3}
MIMAT0019931	hsa-miR-4775	1.064	1.31×10^{-3}
Down-regulated			
MIMAT0004594	hsa-miR-132-5p	−1.141	4.88×10^{-3}
MIMAT0000727	hsa-miR-374a-5p	−1.148	7.65×10^{-3}
MIMAT0022272	hsa-miR-664b-3p	−1.159	9.42×10^{-4}
MIMAT0000415	hsa-let-7i-5p	−1.180	2.57×10^{-3}
MIMAT0003338	hsa-miR-660-5p	−1.202	5.19×10^{-3}
MIMAT0004775	hsa-miR-502-3p	−1.206	4.61×10^{-3}
MIMAT0000082	hsa-miR-26a-5p	−1.209	4.96×10^{-3}
MIMAT0004694	hsa-miR-342-5p	−1.213	4.45×10^{-3}
MIMAT0004766	hsa-miR-146b-3p	−1.222	7.84×10^{-3}
MIMAT0025849	hsa-miR-6718-5p	−1.223	3.61×10^{-4}
MIMAT0004682	hsa-miR-361-3p	−1.224	8.00×10^{-4}
MIMAT0004597	hsa-miR-140-3p	−1.232	5.38×10^{-5}
MIMAT0004673	hsa-miR-29c-5p	−1.234	1.88×10^{-3}
MIMAT0002808	hsa-miR-511-5p	−1.246	9.53×10^{-3}
MIMAT0000250	hsa-miR-139-5p	−1.248	2.75×10^{-3}
MIMAT0004585	hsa-let-7i-3p	−1.251	7.09×10^{-3}
MIMAT0019071	hsa-miR-4532	−1.256	3.56×10^{-3}
MIMAT0019927	hsa-miR-4772-3p	−1.258	6.01×10^{-3}
MIMAT0000258	hsa-miR-181c-5p	−1.267	1.17×10^{-3}
MIMAT0004570	hsa-miR-223-5p	−1.285	7.97×10^{-3}
MIMAT0000086	hsa-miR-29a-3p	−1.290	1.94×10^{-3}
MIMAT0004552	**hsa-miR-139-3p**	**−1.314**	$\mathbf{2.04 \times 10^{-3}}$
MIMAT0000433	**hsa-miR-142-5p**	**−1.329**	$\mathbf{3.76 \times 10^{-3}}$
MIMAT0000646	hsa-miR-155-5p	−1.349	5.08×10^{-3}
MIMAT0000274	hsa-miR-217-5p	−1.354	6.83×10^{-3}
MIMAT0000449	hsa-miR-146a-5p	−1.375	1.56×10^{-3}
MIMAT0000280	hsa-miR-223-3p	−1.397	1.40×10^{-3}
MIMAT0000681	**hsa-miR-29c-3p**	**−1.430**	$\mathbf{1.90 \times 10^{-3}}$
MIMAT0000451	hsa-miR-150-5p	−1.644	3.98×10^{-4}
* **MIMAT0000427**	**hsa-miR-133a-3p**	**−2.168**	$\mathbf{6.39 \times 10^{-3}}$
MIMAT0000462	hsa-miR-206	−3.070	1.29×10^{-3}

In bold, miRNAs detected in the differential analysis "Cancer vs Normal" performed in both the TCGA and GEO Datasets; * miRNA included in the list of 11 selected miRNAs; ** *p*-values were calculated by Student's *t*-test.

As shown in Table 5, among the 36 identified miRNAs, 31 were down-regulated and five were up-regulated. Furthermore, among the 31 down-regulated miRNAs, three were in common with those obtained by the lists of differentially expressed miRNAs in tumor samples compared to the normal one, i.e. miRNAs miR-139-3p, miR-142-5p and miR-29c-3p, which therefore may have both diagnostic and prognostic significance in oral cancers. Furthermore, the down-regulated miRNA miR-133a-3p was in common with the list of 11 miRNAs obtained from the comparison between GEO DataSets and TCGA analyses (Table 3) suggesting that these miRNAs may have both a diagnostic and prognostic role for oral cancer.

2.6. *Prognostic Value of Oral Cancer Stage-Related miRNAs*

The OncoLnc analysis performed on the 36 differently expressed miRNAs in high-grade oral cancers revealed the real prognostic significance of each miRNA in terms of patients' overall survival (OS). As shown in Figure 5, of 36 miRNAs analyzed only nine were statistically associated with patients' OS (log-rank test, $p < 0.05$). These prognostic miRNAs were all down-regulated miRNAs, i.e., miR-181c-5p, miR-342-5p, miR-361-3p, miR-29c-5p, miR-142-5p, miR-146a-5p, miR-150-5p, miR-146b-3p and miR-206 (Figure 5).

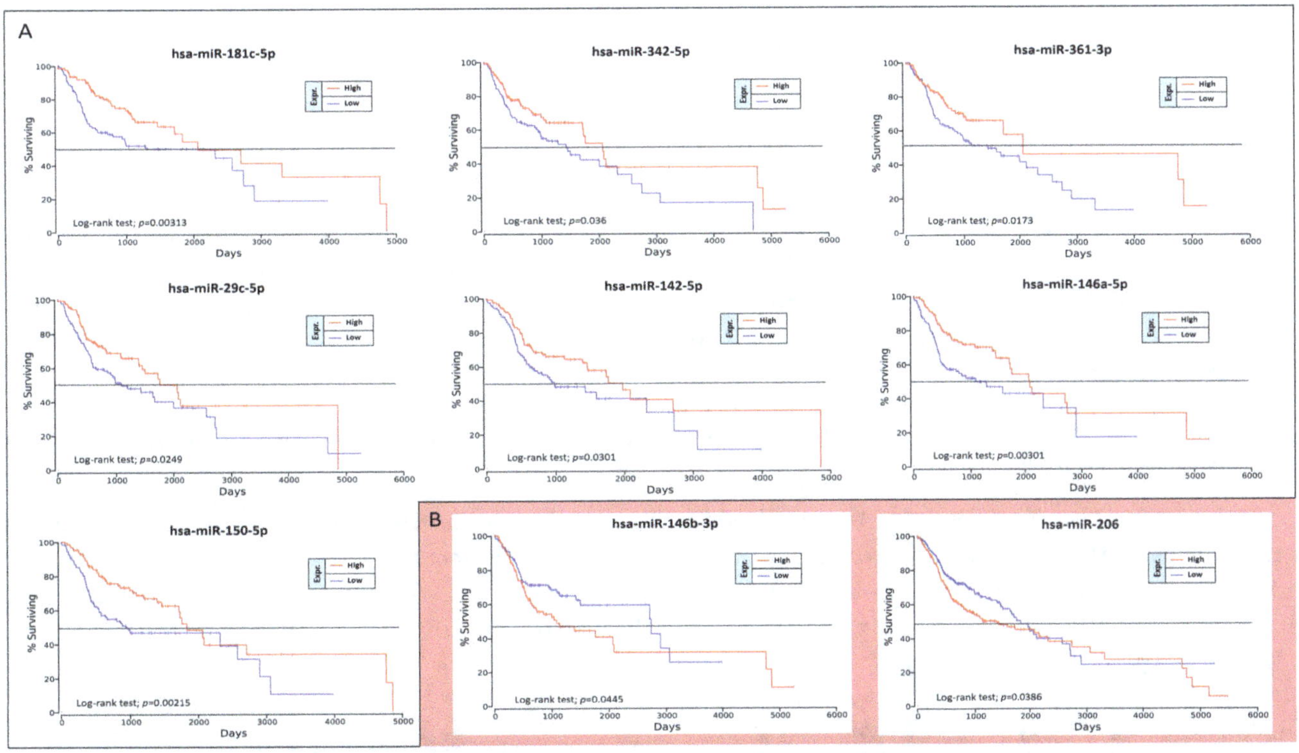

Figure 5. Survival analysis performed by OncoLnc. Panel (**A**) down-regulated miRNAs statistically associated with patients' overall survival (OS) whose expression is concordant with survival curves; panel (**B**) miRNAs statistically associated with patients' OS whose expression levels are not concordant with the survival curves.

However, two of these miRNAs, miR-146b-3p and miR-206, have shown results of dubious interpretation. In fact, despite these miRNAs are down-regulated in high-grade tumors, their down-regulation is not associated with a worse OS, but with a better prognosis (Figure 5B).

To confirm the Kaplan-Meier results obtained by using OncoLnc, the OS curves were also calculated by using GraphPad v.6 and analyzing the TGCA HNSC survival data previously downloaded from the UCSC Xena Browser. Overall, this analysis revealed the same results previously obtained.

The TCGA HNSC data were also used for the identification of miRNAs able to predict the risk of oral cancer recurrence. For this purpose, GraphPad Kaplan-Meier curves showed that two out of 36 tumor stage-related miRNAs were statistically linked to the patients' recurrence-free survival (RFS). Of these miRNAs, miR-581 was up-regulated and miR-let-7i-3p was down-regulated. Unexpectedly the over-expression of the up-regulated miR-581 was not associated with a worse prognosis, but with a minor RFS (Figure 6).

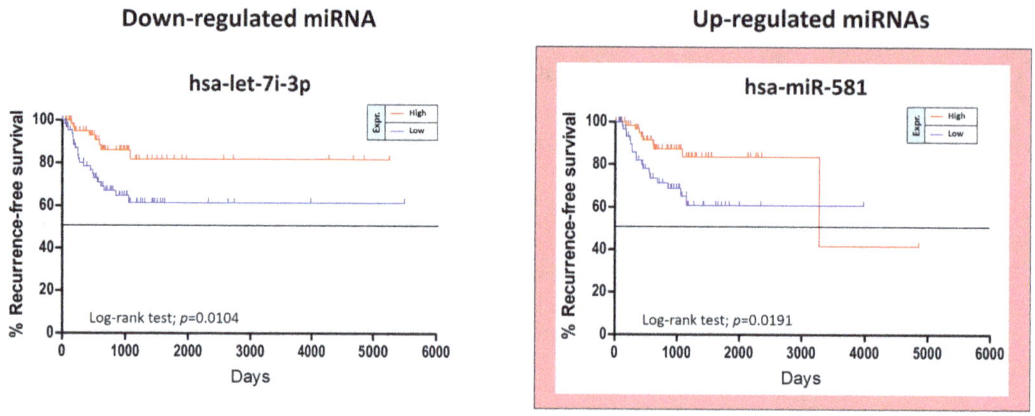

Figure 6. Recurrence-free survival analysis performed on the TCGA HNSC data.

Other five miRNAs, miR-151a-5p, miR-6718-5p, miR-660-5p, miR-4772-3p and miR-217-5p, showed a weak correlation with RFS when de-regulated, however no statistical significance was reached.

These analyses allowed us to identify 11 miRNAs significantly associated to both tumor grade and patients' OS and RFS, of these only eight were related to patients' OS (seven miRNAs) and RFS (one miRNA), respectively.

2.7. Determination of the Functional Roles of the 11 Tumor-Grade Associated miRNAs Through Pathway and GO Enrichment Analyses

As previously described for the analysis of the 11 selected miRNAs associate to the presence of tumor, the miRCancerdb and mirDIP analyses were performed for the 11 miRNAs associated to patients' prognosis in order to identify the miRNAs-correlated and -targeted genes. The miRCancerdb analysis showed that 19 different genes were positively and negatively correlated to the 11 selected miRNAs (Figure 7A).

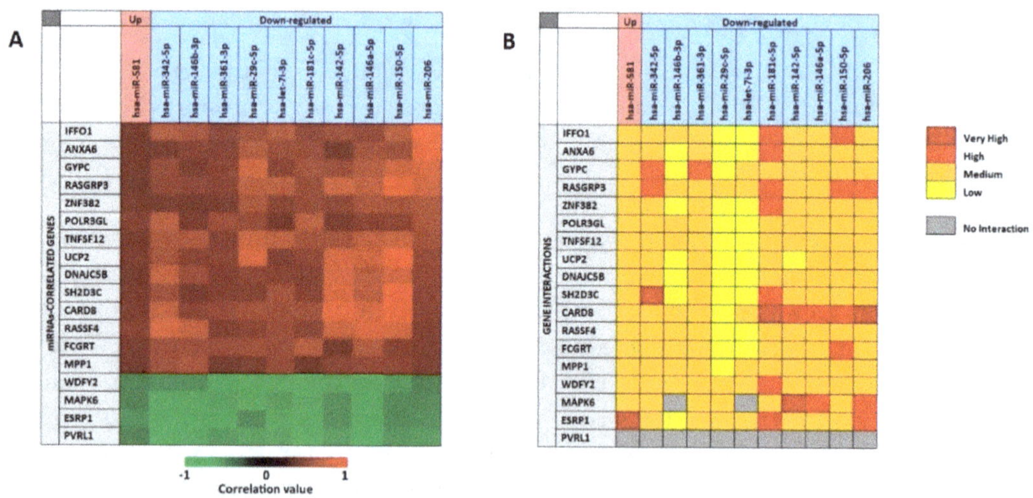

Figure 7. Panel (**A**) miRCancerdb analysis of genes whose expression is positively and negatively related to the 11 selected miRNAs; panel (**B**) mirDIP analysis of interaction levels between miRNAs and related genes.

The heat map showed that the down-regulated miRNAs miR-150-5p and miR-206 are those with the highest positive correlation levels. Of note, these two miRNAs were also those with the higher levels of down-regulation among the 36 differentially expressed miRNAs showed in Table 5. Figure 7 also shows that the miRNAs miR-181c-5p and miR-146a-5p were those more negatively correlated with the identified genes. By considering the genes, it was observed that *CARD8* and *RASGAP3* genes were those that were more positively correlated with the selected miRNAs, while the four genes *WDFY2, MAPK6, ESRP1* and *PVRL1* were all negatively correlated with the 11 miRNAs with similar correlation levels.

The mirDIP analysis performed on the 19 genes and the 11 miRNAs showed that for the *PVRL1* gene no interaction levels were available. Overall, the analysis revealed the existence of medium interaction levels between miRNAs and genes. However, the down-regulated miR-29c-5p and let-7i-3p showed lower interaction levels with most of the 19 genes, while the miR-181c-5p was the miRNA with the higher interaction levels. On the other hand, the *CARD8* gene was the most targeted by the 11 selected miRNAs, while the *UCP2* was the less targeted (Figure 7B).

After the gene targets analysis, the DIANA-mirPath analysis of the 11 prognostic miRNAs revealed that for the miRNA miR-581 there were not modulated pathways and targeted genes according to the TarBase Version 7.0 database of the mirPath tool. For the other 10 miRNAs the cumulative pathway analysis showed that, the miRNAs were able to modulate 44 different pathways and over than 1300 genes. The selection of the 21 pathways involved in the tumor processes showed that the selected miRNAs were able to modulate 292 univocal genes (Table 6).

Table 6. Tumor pathways modulated by the 11 computationally selected miRNAs associated to patients' prognosis.

N.	KEGG Pathway	*p*-Value *	#Genes	#miRNAs
1	PI3K-Akt signaling pathway (hsa04151)	8.22×10^{-3}	82	10
2	Cell cycle (hsa04110)	1.91×10^{-5}	45	10
3	Proteoglycans in cancer (hsa05205)	6.81×10^{-5}	48	9
4	Transcriptional misregulation in cancer (hsa05202)	2.00×10^{-2}	46	9
5	FoxO signaling pathway (hsa04068)	2.66×10^{-3}	43	9
6	Hippo signaling pathway (hsa04390)	9.14×10^{-4}	39	9
7	Melanoma (hsa05218)	7.56×10^{-3}	22	9
8	Viral carcinogenesis (hsa05203)	1.08×10^{-6}	62	8
9	Prostate cancer (hsa05215)	6.33×10^{-3}	29	8
10	Small cell lung cancer (hsa05222)	2.63×10^{-3}	29	8
11	Renal cell carcinoma (hsa05211)	6.92×10^{-6}	27	8
12	Chronic myeloid leukemia (hsa05220)	7.67×10^{-4}	26	8
13	Glioma (hsa05214)	1.74×10^{-4}	23	8
14	TGF-beta signaling pathway (hsa04350)	7.03×10^{-4}	23	8
15	Pancreatic cancer (hsa05212)	3.18×10^{-2}	21	8
16	Non-small cell lung cancer (hsa05223)	8.22×10^{-3}	18	8
17	p53 signaling pathway (hsa04115)	2.00×10^{-3}	26	7
18	Central carbon metabolism in cancer (hsa05230)	1.96×10^{-5}	24	7
19	Colorectal cancer (hsa05210)	4.50×10^{-2}	19	6
20	Acute myeloid leukemia (hsa05221)	3.52×10^{-2}	17	6
21	Endometrial cancer (hsa05213)	4.46×10^{-2}	16	6

* *p*-values were already calculated by the DIANA-mirPath by automatically applying the Fisher's Exact Test.

The DIANA-mirPath analysis showed that all the selected miRNAs were involved in the modulation of the "PI3K-Akt signaling pathway (hsa04151)" and the "Cell cycle (hsa04110)", both involved in various neoplastic processes when altered (Table 6). Of note, "Cell cycle (hsa04110)" pathways were also strongly altered by the 11 cancer-associated miRNAs previously analyzed (Table 4). The genes altered by these miRNAs were all involved in neoplastic processes, such as *CCND1* (18 counts), *MAPK1* (16 counts), *MAP2K1* (14 counts), *PIK3CB* and *PIK3R3* (16 counts), *AKT2* and *AKT3* (15 counts), *CDK4* and *CDK6* (11 counts), etc.

The genes identified through miRCancerdb and DIANA-mirPath analyses were finally analyzed with GO PANTHER and STRING to establish for which molecular processes and functions these miRNAs were enriched.

For the 19 genes identified by miRCancerdb analysis only the GO PANTHER evaluation was performed because the gene ontology enrichment performed by STRING requires a wide number of analyzed genes. The GO PANTHER analysis showed that most of selected genes were involved in the cellular processes (23.3% of genes) and in biological regulation (20.0% of genes) for the "biological process" category (Figure 8A). Regarding the "molecular function" category, the analysis demonstrated that the 43.5% and 17.4% of genes were involved in binding and molecular regulatory functions, respectively (Figure 8B); while for the "cellular component" category, the results showed that the 19 genes constitute mainly part of the cell, of the organelles and of the cell junctions (37.5%, 25.0% and 18.8% respectively; Figure 8C).

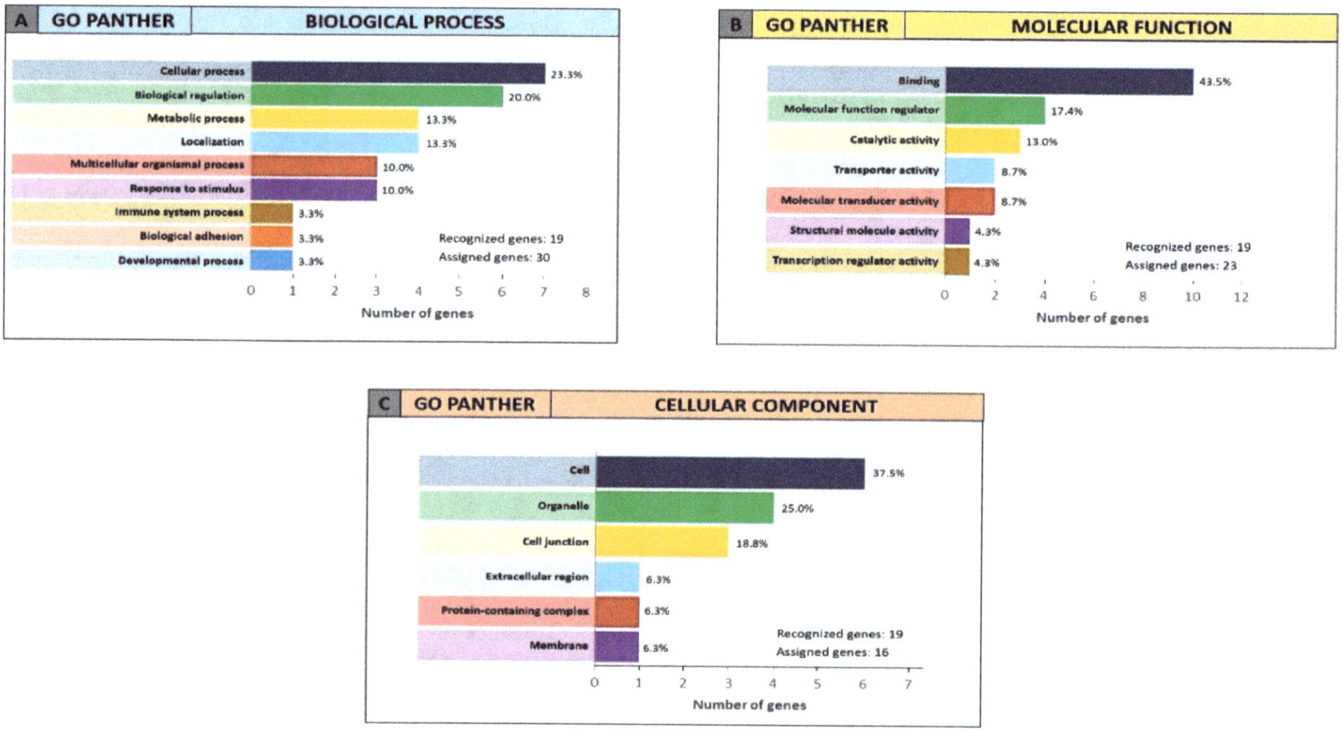

Figure 8. Gene Ontology enrichment of the 19 genes identified through miRCancerdb. Panel (**A**) GO PANTHER analysis of the "biological process" category; panel (**B**) GO PANTHER analysis of the "molecular function" category; panel (**C**) GO PANTHER analysis of the "cellular component" category.

The same enrichment analysis was performed on the 292 genes identified by DIANA-mirPath carrying out both GO PANTHER and STRING analyses.

The results obtained for the "biological process" category showed that the identified genes were mainly involved in the cellular processes (23.3% of genes) and in biological regulation (20.0% of genes) as observed for the 19 genes identified by miRCancerdb (Figure 9A,D). Furthermore, both the analyses (GO PANTHER and STRING) showed that the 292 genes were involved in molecular binding and catalytic activities (Figure 9B,E), as observed in the previous evaluations. Regarding the "cellular component" category, it was finally demonstrated that the genes were part of the cell and of the intracellular organelles (Figure 9C,F).

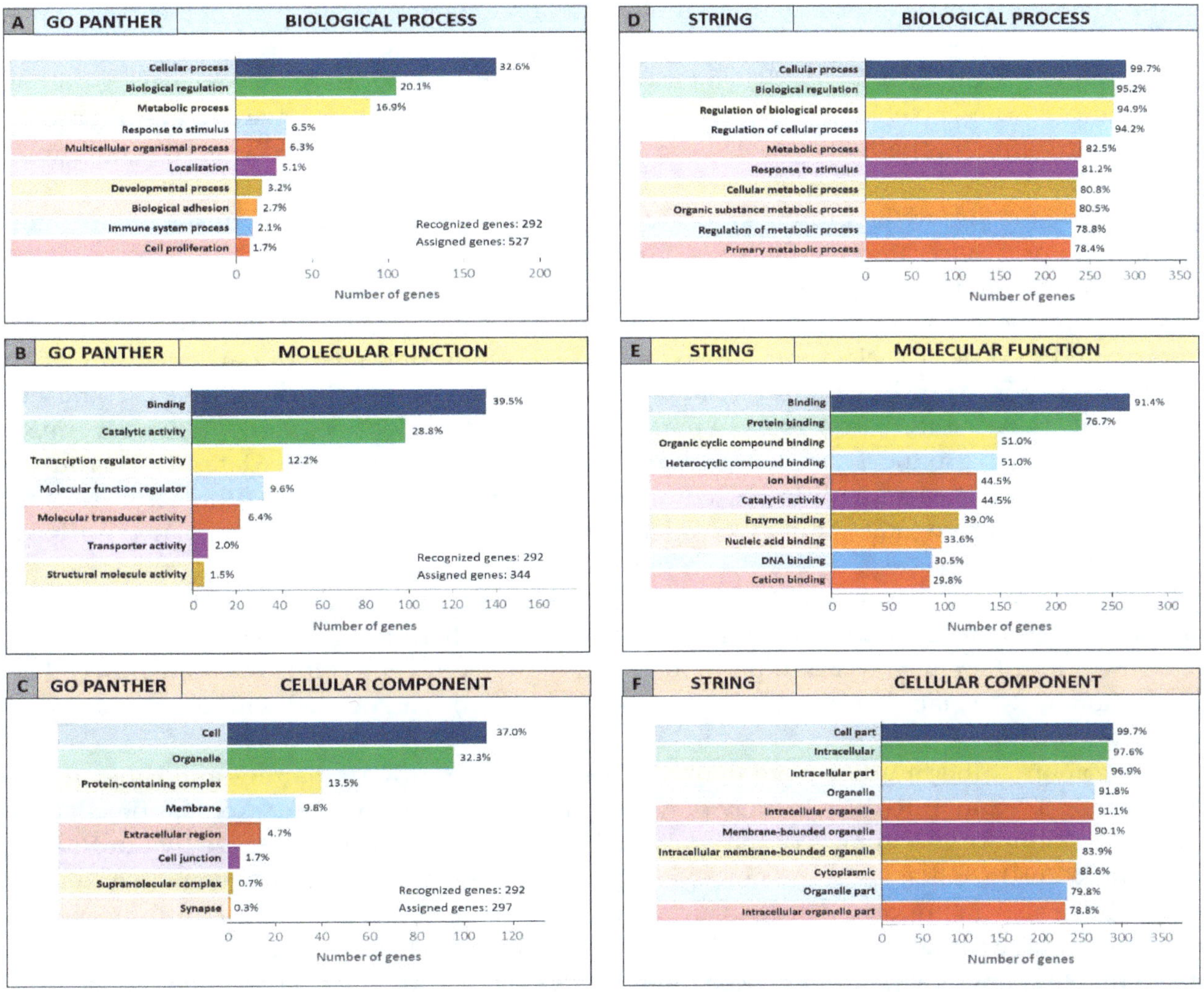

Figure 9. Gene Ontology enrichment of the 345 genes identified through DIANA-mirPath. Panel (**A,D**) GO PANTHER and STRING analyses of the "biological process" category; panel (**B,E**) GO PANTHER and STRING analyses of the "molecular function" category; panel (**C,F**) GO PANTHER and STRING analyses of the "cellular component" category.

3. Discussion

During the last decade, the advancement of bioinformatics and high-throughput technologies led to the development of omics sciences, as well as to the collection of thousands of petabytes of molecular data related to various human diseases, including tumors [39].

The increase in the number of available bioinformatics data allowing the understanding of various physio-pathological aspects of tumors. However, the huge amount of data, either deriving from individual basic science experiments, or collected by large international consortia, such as TCGA and ENCODE, are often incorrectly analyzed, thus generating conflicting results [40–42].

In order to best analyze the so-called "Big Data", in recent years different researchers have created several bioinformatics software useful for a fast and efficient analysis of a large number of data thus interpretation through a process named "data mining" [43,44].

Thanks to the availability of new software for the computational analysis of Big Data, numerous studies tried to establish the molecular mechanisms responsible for neoplastic transformation, as well as to identify novel molecular targets or biomarkers useful for the management of tumors [45].

In recent years, several genetic, epigenetic and proteomic data were also generated for oral cancer. These data allowed the researchers to obtain important information regarding the main molecular and clinical-pathological characteristics of this kind of tumor. However, the analysis of the data contained in the various oral cancer datasets generated conflicting data difficult to interpret due to the lack of data integration among the different data matrices [46]. Furthermore, despite the increasing number of bioinformatics studies, no effective diagnostic and prognostic biomarkers have been yet identified for oral cancers, making this pathology one of the most aggressive, since in most cases it is not promptly diagnosed [47].

Therefore, the aim of the present study was to identify new specific diagnostic and prognostic biomarkers for oral cancer through the analysis and integration of different miRNAs profiling datasets, using several computational approaches.

For this purpose, two of the biggest worldwide genomics databases, TCGA and GEO DataSets were analyzed in order to select miRNA expression profiling datasets. In particular, the analysis of the TCGA HNSC "miRNA mature strand expression RNAseq by Illumina Hiseq" dataset and of two GEO DataSets miRNA microarray matrices allowed the identification of a panel of miRNAs with diagnostic and prognostic value for oral cancer patients. From these datasets, a group of 11 de-regulated miRNAs was identified by comparing cancer patients with healthy controls. Among these miRNAs, the up-regulated miR-196a-5p and miR-196b-5p and the down-regulated miR-99a-5p, miR-133a-3p, miR-1-3p and miR-375-3p were the most de-regulated and therefore these miRNAs may be used to improve the actual diagnostic strategies for oral cancers. Indeed, different research groups are currently investigating all these miRNAs because their deregulation is associated with the development of different cancers. In particular, Sutliff and colleagues (2019) demonstrated that the de-regulation miR-196 family (miR-196a-5p and miR-196b-5p) is associated with the development of lung cancer [48].

Furthermore, other studies have demonstrated that the miR-196 family and other miRNAs, including miR-375 and miR-133a-3p, may play a key role as diagnostic biomarkers for head and neck cancers, especially for the tumors of the oral cavity [49–51]. In addition to these five miRNAs, the miRNAs miR-139-3p, miR-142-5p and miR-29c-3p are also noteworthy because beyond their diagnostic role, they have also an important prognostic role. On this regard, the analysis of miRNA expression levels in high-grade tumors compared to the low-grade tumors contained in the TCGA HNSC dataset revealed that the down-regulation of these three miRNAs, together with the aforementioned miRNA miR-133a-3p, was associated with a more aggressive and infiltrating phenotype. Accordingly, these results are supported by several studies performed on different tumors where it has been shown that the de-regulation of these miRNAs is associated with a more aggressive tumor phenotype [32,52–54].

Furthermore, the OncoLnc analysis revealed that among the 36 tumor-stage associated miRNAs only eight were related to patients' OS and RFS (seven and one, respectively). Of note, all these miRNAs were found all down-regulated in high-grade tumors compared to low-grade. In particular, the most statistically significant miRNAs associated with OS, and therefore to a worse prognosis, were the miRNAs miR-150-5p, miR-181c-5p and miR-146a-5p. Regarding the RFS, only the miRNA miR-let-7i-3p was a good indicator of disease recurrence. These data are also supported by several studies since the miR-7i (both 3p and 5p strands) is associated with a poorer prognosis when down-regulated [55]. Furthermore, other studies showed that the down-regulation of other miRNAs, such as miR-375 and miR-181c, is associated with a cancer aggressive phenotype [56,57].

Therefore, these first computational data demonstrated that by using an integrated computational approach for the analysis of miRNAs datasets it is possible to identify a set of miRNAs potentially used as specific biomarkers for oral cancers. As described above, the validity of the obtained results is further strengthened by the results obtained by other research groups in independent experimental studies.

Once identified which miRNAs bear a diagnostic and/or prognostic significance, it was also established which genes and pathways they were able to modulate to uncover their functional roles. As described in previous studies, the DIANA-mirPath analysis showed that the computationally selected miRNAs were strictly related to cancer development since they were able to alter key oncogenic pathways [32–34,58]. On this regard, the oral cancer-associated miRNAs identified in the present study were able to alter several intracellular signal transduction pathways, including mTOR, p53 and TGF-β pathways, whose implication in the development of oral carcinoma has been widely demonstrated [59–61]. Similarly, the selected miRNAs were also able to target genes frequently down-regulated or over-expressed in oral cancers. Some of these genes, including *AKT*, *BRAF*, *PIK3CA*, *NRAS*, *GSK3*, *CNND1*, etc., are involved not only in oral cancers but, generally, in several solid tumors [62–65]. The subsequent gene ontology enrichment analyses further demonstrated that the miRNAs' targeted genes were involved in the biological process linked to the cell proliferation, biological regulation, protein binding, catalytic activities and metabolic processes.

Similarly, the prediction and GO enrichment analyses performed on the 11 miRNAs associated to the patients' OS and RFS revealed that all the miRNAs with a significant diagnostic and/or prognostic role were able to modulate several cancer pathways by modulating numerous genes known to be involved in neoplastic transformation.

Overall, the computational approaches adopted in the present studies allowed us to identify a set of specific miRNAs for the diagnosis of oral cancer and the definition of patients' prognosis through the integrated analysis of different bioinformatics datasets that allowed us to understand the functional role of each miRNA. However, the results obtained from this study represent only the starting point for identifying effective markers for oral carcinoma. Therefore, further experimental and functional studies will have to be performed on a large number of samples in order to evaluate the expression levels of these putative miRNAs biomarkers and to validate their predictive role for oral cancer. With the advancement of both bioinformatics and high-throughput and high-sensitive molecular technologies this future goal can be easily achieved thanks to the detection of even small variations in the expression levels of selected miRNAs indicative of the presence of a possible pathological state [66–68].

4. Materials and Methods

4.1. Oral Cancer MicroRNA Datasets Selection

In order to identify miRNAs potentially involved in the development and progression of oral cancer, several oral cancer miRNAs datasets were taken into account. Firstly, the oral cancer datasets of microRNA profiling by array were selected by checking within the datasets registered in the GEO DataSets portal publicly available on NCBI (www.ncbi.nlm.nih.gov/geo/) [69]. In particular, for the selection of the suitable datasets an advanced search was carried out by inserting the search terms "(("non coding RNA profiling by array"[DataSet Type]) and oral carcinoma) and "Homo sapiens"[porgn:__txid9606]". With this first approach, a list of all oral cancer datasets containing miRNA expression levels was obtained. Of these datasets, only those that respect the following inclusion and exclusion criteria were selected for the subsequent evaluations:

Inclusion criteria, i) datasets containing miRNA expression levels of oral cancer tissues, excluding tumor arising in the hypopharynx, larynx, esophagus and tonsil; ii) datasets reporting miRNAs expression levels of both tumor and normal tissue samples; iii) datasets containing the miRNA expression data of at least 30 samples (tumor + normal).

Exclusion criteria, i) datasets constructed only with tumor samples; ii) datasets containing information about miRNAs of oral cancer or normal cell lines; iii) datasets containing information on miRNAs expression levels of serum samples.

The search criteria for the selection of the datasets contained in the GEO DataSets database allowed us to preliminarily identify 37 different datasets of oral carcinoma microRNA profiling by array (published up to December 2018). However, most of these datasets did not respect the exclusion and inclusion criteria because they were datasets reporting the miRNA expression data relative to tumor cell lines and not from oral cancer patients. Hence, after the application of the abovementioned criteria only two datasets were selected for performing the differential analyses (Table 7).

Table 7. Features of the two selected datasets from GEO DataSets.

Series Accession	n. Normal	n. Cancer	Samples	Platform	Author Ref	Total Number
GSE45238	40	40	Fresh Frozen Tissues	GPL8179 Illumina Human v2 MicroRNA expression beadchip	Shiah SG et al, Cancer Res 2014	80
GSE31277	15	15	Fresh Frozen Tissues	GPL9770 Illumina miR arrays version 1.0	Severino P et al, BMC Cancer 2013	30

In addition to the datasets contained in the GEO DataSets database, also the TCGA Head and Neck Cancer (HNSC) database was selected. Among the 25 datasets available in the TCGA HNSC database, the "Phenotype" and "miRNA mature strand expression RNAseq by Illumina Hiseq" HNSC datasets were downloaded for the analyses by using the UCSC Xena Browser (https://xenabrowser.net/) portal where all the HNSC molecular profiling data, generated by the TCGA consortium, were deposited, including those of oral cancer. In particular, the first dataset contained the clinical-pathological data of 604 samples (530 cancer patients and 74 normal individuals) while the second one contained the miRNAs expression profile of 529 samples. Since the TCGA HNSC database also contains tumor samples obtained not only from the oral cavity but also from other sites (oropharynx, hypopharynx, larynx and tonsil), for the purposes of this study only the data of samples derived from alveolar ridge, base of tongue, buccal mucosa, floor of mouth, hard palate, lip, oral cavity and oral tongue were analyzed. In this way, the number of analyzed samples was reduced to 399. By selecting only samples of the oral cavity also the number of samples with available miRNAs expression profile it was reduced passing from 529 to 351 samples.

4.2. Differential Analysis of miRNAs Expression Between Groups

Two distinct differential analyses were performed by using the datasets selected from the GEO DataSets and TCGA databases. A first differential analysis was performed to both GEO DataSets and TCGA data matrices by integrating the different GEO DataSets platform and by comparing the miRNAs expression levels of tumor samples with a normal one in order to identify new diagnostic biomarkers.

The second differential analysis was conducted only for the TCGA dataset comparing the expression levels of miRNAs of advanced tumors with that of low-grade tumors to identify miRNAs able to define the prognosis of patients.

In particular, the data matrices of each dataset selected from GEO DataSets were downloaded to identify the down-regulated or up-regulated miRNAs in oral cancer. The differential analysis between cancer and normal samples was performed by using the GEO2R tool [69]. The fold change value (FC) obtained for each miRNA was indicated as base-2 logarithm of FC (logFC) in order to normalize the data derived from different microarray platforms. Then, for each dataset only the differentially expressed miRNAs with a statistical significance $p < 0.01$ were taken into account. The lists of the de-regulated miRNAs of the two selected GEO DataSets platforms were subsequently compared in order to select only the miRNAs shared by the two datasets and with a logFC value greater than ±1.5.

In parallel, other differential analyses of miRNAs expression levels between tumor vs normal samples and between high-grade vs low-grade tumors of TCGA HNSC dataset were performed.

For the differential analyses, the samples were clustered according to the presence or absence of tumor (Tumor (348 samples) vs Normal (51 samples)) and according to the tumor stage (T3–T4 (319 samples) vs. T1–T2 (32 samples)). After patients' stratification, the down-regulated and up-regulated miRNAs were identified by calculating the fold change value obtained through the differential analysis between the different clusters of samples. Of note, for some of the oral cancer patients the miRNA expression levels were missing (NA value). Therefore, in order to avoid the identification of non-representative miRNAs, for further analysis only the differentially expressed miRNAs with reported expression data for at least 50% of the patients and with p-value of $p < 0.01$ were selected.

Moreover, with reference to the differential analysis between tumor and normal samples, only the 25 most up-regulated and down-regulated miRNAs were considered to obtain more significant data; while for the differential analysis between high-grade and low-grade tumors all the differentially expressed miRNAs were considered.

Finally, the annotation of the TCGA HNSC miRNAs was performed using miRBase V.22 (http://www.mirbase.org/) by converting the miRNA IDs 'MIMAT00' in 'hsa-miR-'.

4.3. *Analysis of the Interaction Levels Between the Selected miRNAs and Oral Cancer-Altered Genes*

After the identification of the most de-regulated miRNAs in tumor samples compared to normal samples, their functional roles were studied using different bioinformatics approaches. At first, using the data reported in the Catalogue of Somatic Mutations in Cancer (COSMIC) (http://cancer.sanger.ac.uk/cosmic), the most mutated and altered genes of oral cavity tumors were identified. Subsequently, for each of the COSMIC genes, the specificity of miRNA-gene interaction was highlighted by using the bioinformatics prediction software miRNA Data Integration Portal (mirDIP; (http://ophid.utoronto.ca/mirDIP). In particular, this software is able to integrate the data related to 26 different databases for miRNAs (including miRBase, microrna.org and DIANA microT-CDS v5) allowing the users to centralize the data related to the miRNAs-target genes interactions obtaining more robust data. The levels of interaction between the miRNAs and the targeted gene are expressed as very high, high, medium and low according to the integrated score calculated by the mirDIP algorithm that combines the confidence scores from all available predictions data of the 26 different databases [70,71]. Furthermore, the expression levels of the 10 interacting genes identified with COSMIC were analyzed by performing the differential analysis of the gene expression data contained in the TCGA HNSC IlluminaHiSeq pancan normalized dataset.

4.4. *Analysis of TCGA HNSC Genes Positively and Negatively Correlated with the Selected Tumor-Associated/Grade-Associated miRNAs*

In addition to the COSMIC analysis, a global correlation analysis was also performed on the genes contained in the TCGA HNSC dataset whose expression is modulated, positively or negatively, by the selected tumor-associated miRNAs. In particular, for this analysis the bioinformatics tool miRCancerdb (https://mahshaaban.shinyapps.io/miRCancerdb/) was used. miRCancerdb is a free R software for the correlation analysis between gene expression and miRNAs levels with a web interface based on data contained in the TCGA and TargetScan databases [38]. In particular, through miRCancerdb, for each selected miRNA was obtained the correlation value (ρ) with different genes. The lists of genes generated for each miRNA were subsequently combined using the tool Draw Venn Diagrams of the Bioinformatics & Evolutionary Genomics (BEG) (http://bioinformatics.psb.ugent.be/webtools/Venn/) to identify the genes correlated and shared among all miRNAs.

However, since miRCancerdb uses interaction data between miRNAs and genes derived exclusively from the TargetScan database, the previously described mirDIP tool, that uses 26 different miRNA databases, was also used to establish the levels of miRNAs-genes interaction. These analyses were performed for the 11 miRNAs associated to the presence of oral cancer and for the 11 miRNAs that after OncoLnc analysis were associated to both tumor grade and patients' OS and RFS.

4.5. *Prediction Pathway Analysis, Gene Ontology (GO) and Functional Roles of Tumor-Associated Selected miRNAs*

To better understand the functional role of the tumor-associated selected miRNAs, a pathway prediction analysis was performed. For this purpose, the bioinformatics tool DIANA-mirPath v.3 was used [72]. With this computational approach it was possible to identify the main molecular pathways altered by selected miRNAs, especially those related to tumor development and hence to oral carcinoma.

Finally, the functional role of the selected miRNAs was determined by performing the pathways enrichment analysis of the lists of genes obtained from the miRCancerdb and DIANA-mirPath v.3 analyses. For this purpose, both GO PANTHER version 14.0 (http://pantherdb.org/) and STRING version 11.0 (https://string-db.org/) software were used [73,74]. The two software were used to perform a more robust analysis. In fact, STRING database uses a number of functional classification systems including GO, Pfam and KEGG and therefore provide more comprehensive results than those obtained with the GO PANTHER analysis. Furthermore, the data derived from the biological functional prediction analyses performed with DIANA-mirPath, GO PANTHER and STRING tools are already normalized with data used as reference or negative control, therefore, no additional datasets were used for the normalization of the data.

The DIANA-mirPath, GO PANTHER and STRING analyses were performed for the 11 selected miRNAs associated to the presence of oral cancer and for the 11 miRNAs that after OncoLnc analysis were associated to both tumor grade and patients' OS and RFS.

4.6. Kaplan-Meier Estimate of Overall Survival (OS) and Recurrence-Free Survival (RFS) in Patients with Down-regulated and Up-regulated Tumor Stage-Related miRNAs

In order to establish the prognostic significance of the tumor stage-related miRNAs identified, the bioinformatics tool OncoLnc (http://www.oncolnc.org/) was used [75]. OncoLnc is a tool able to derive the mortality data from the TCGA datasets, including that of HNSC, allowing the user to obtain the Kaplan-Meier survival curves for each miRNA. The software identifies which of the selected tumor stage-related miRNAs were correlated to a patients' overall survival (OS). The OncoLnc analysis was performed according to the instruction given by the software developers that suggest to perform the analysis between the expression levels of bottom quartile samples and top quartile samples.

To further confirm the OS Kaplan-Meier results obtained by OncoLnc, the survival curves were also calculated by using the TGCA survival data downloaded only for the oral cancer (excluding tumor arising in hypopharynx, oropharynx, larynx and tonsil) analyzed with GraphPad v.6.

Furthermore, to our best knowledge no bioinformatics tools are available for the analysis of TCGA recurrence-free survival data; therefore, the RFS curves were calculated by using the TGCA HNSC progression data analyzed with a GraphPad survival curve sheet. In particular, RFS was calculated from the date of diagnosis to patient progression, or to the end of follow-up, whichever occurred first. The times of follow-up were different from patient to patient up to a maximum follow-up time of 5480 days, however, for some patients RFS data were not available.

4.7. Statistical Analyses

The miRNAs expression data derived from the GEO DataSets were already normalized by the GEO2R software, while the fold change values of TCGA HNSC miRNA expression levels were calculated through differential analysis. Student's t-test was performed to select the differentially expressed miRNAs of the TCGA dataset with a statistical significance. The GEO2R software already calculated the p-values of the GEO DataSets data. For the Kaplan-Meier analyses, GraphPad survival sheet and log-rank non-parametric test were used. Data with a p-value of ≤ 0.05 and ≤ 0.01 were considered statistically significant.

5. Conclusions

In conclusion, in the present study the integrated analysis of different miRNA expression datasets and the use of several tools for the interpretation of bioinformatics data allowed us to identify a set of miRNAs that, after in vitro and in vivo validations, may be used in clinical practice for the early detection of pre-cancerous and cancerous oral lesions.

Author Contributions: Conceptualization, L.F., M.L. and S.C.; Formal analysis, G.R.M.L.R.; Investigation, L.F. and G.R.M.L.R.; Supervision, E.R. and M.L.; Writing – original draft, L.F.; Writing—review & editing, G.L., S.C., C.D.A., R.S., E.R. and M.L. All authors have approved the final version of the manuscript.

Acknowledgments: The authors would like to thank the support kindly provided by the researcher of the Research Center for Prevention, Diagnosis and Treatment of Cancer, University of Catania, Catania.

References

1. Bray, F.; Ferlay, J.; Soerjomataram, I.; Siegel, R.L.; Torre, L.A.; Jemal, A. Global cancer statistics 2018: GLOBOCAN estimates of incidence and mortality worldwide for 36 cancers in 185 countries. *CA Cancer J. Clin.* **2018**, *68*, 394–424. [CrossRef]
2. Dhanuthai, K.; Rojanawatsirivej, S.; Thosaporn, W.; Kintarak, S.; Subarnbhesaj, A.; Darling, M.; Kryshtalskyj, E.; Chiang, C.P.; Shin, H.I.; Choi, S.Y.; et al. Oral cancer: A multicenter study. *Med. Oral Patol. Oral Cir. Bucal* **2018**, *23*, e23–e29. [CrossRef]
3. Rivera, C.; Venegas, B. Histological and molecular aspects of oral squamous cell carcinoma (Review). *Oncol. Lett.* **2014**, *8*, 7–11. [CrossRef] [PubMed]
4. Falzone, L.; Salomone, S.; Libra, M. Evolution of Cancer Pharmacological Treatments at the Turn of the Third Millennium. *Front. Pharmacol.* **2018**, *9*, 1300. [CrossRef] [PubMed]
5. Gupta, N.; Gupta, R.; Acharya, A.K.; Patthi, B.; Goud, V.; Reddy, S.; Garg, A.; Singla, A. Changing Trends in oral cancer—A global scenario. *Nepal. J. Epidemiol.* **2016**, *6*, 613–619.
6. Santos, H.B.; dos Santos, T.K.; Paz, A.R.; Cavalcanti, Y.W.; Nonaka, C.F.; Godoy, G.P.; Alves, P.M. Clinical findings and risk factors to oral squamous cell carcinoma in young patients: A 12-year retrospective analysis. *Med. Oral Patol. Oral Cir. Bucal* **2016**, *21*, e151–e156. [CrossRef] [PubMed]
7. Polesel, J.; Franceschi, S.; Talamini, R.; Negri, E.; Barzan, L.; Montella, M.; Libra, M.; Vaccher, E.; Franchin, G.; La Vecchia, C.; et al. Tobacco smoking, alcohol drinking, and the risk of different histological types of nasopharyngeal cancer in a low-risk population. *Oral. Oncol.* **2011**, *47*, 541–545. [CrossRef] [PubMed]
8. Yete, S.; D'Souza, W.; Saranath, D. High-Risk Human Papillomavirus in Oral Cancer: Clinical Implications. *Oncology.* **2018**, *94*, 133–141. [CrossRef] [PubMed]
9. She, Y.; Nong, X.; Zhang, M.; Wang, M. Epstein-Barr virus infection and oral squamous cell carcinoma risk: A meta-analysis. *PLoS ONE* **2017**, e0186860. [CrossRef]
10. Mohd Bakri, M.; Mohd Hussaini, H.; Rachel Holmes, A.; David Cannon, R.; Mary Rich, A. Revisiting the association between candidal infection and carcinoma, particularly oral squamous cell carcinoma. *J. Oral Microbiol.* **2010**, *2*. [CrossRef] [PubMed]
11. Vivarelli, S.; Salemi, R.; Candido, S.; Falzone, L.; Santagati, M.; Stefani, S.; Torino, F.; Banna, G.L.; Tonini, G.; Libra, M. Gut Microbiota and Cancer: From Pathogenesis to Therapy. *Cancers (Basel)* **2019**, *11*, 38. [CrossRef]
12. Karpiński, T.M. Role of Oral Microbiota in Cancer Development. *Microorganisms.* **2019**, *7*, 20. [CrossRef] [PubMed]
13. Banna, G.L.; Torino, F.; Marletta, F.; Santagati, M.; Salemi, R.; Cannarozzo, E.; Falzone, L.; Ferraù, F.; Libra, M. Lactobacillus rhamnosus GG: An Overview to Explore the Rationale of Its Use in Cancer. *Front. Pharmacol.* **2017**, *8*, 603. [CrossRef]
14. Nakagaki, T.; Tamura, M.; Kobashi, K.; Koyama, R.; Fukushima, H.; Ohashi, T.; Idogawa, M.; Ogi, K.; Hiratsuka, H.; Tokino, T.; et al. Profiling cancer-related gene mutations in oral squamous cell carcinoma from Japanese patients by targeted amplicon sequencing. *Oncotarget* **2017**, *8*, 59113–59122. [CrossRef] [PubMed]
15. Bavle, R.M.; Venugopal, R.; Konda, P.; Muniswamappa, S.; Makarla, S. Molecular Classification of Oral Squamous Cell Carcinoma. *J. Clin. Diagn. Res.* **2016**, *10*, ZE18–ZE21. [CrossRef]
16. Irimie, A.I.; Ciocan, C.; Gulei, D.; Mehterov, N.; Atanasov, A.G.; Dudea, D.; Berindan-Neagoe, I. Current Insights into Oral Cancer Epigenetics. *Int. J. Mol. Sci.* **2018**, *19*, 670. [CrossRef] [PubMed]
17. Hema, K.N.; Smitha, T.; Sheethal, H.S.; Mirnalini, S.A. Epigenetics in oral squamous cell carcinoma. *J. Oral Maxillofac. Pathol.* **2017**, *21*, 252–259. [CrossRef] [PubMed]
18. Falzone, L.; Salemi, R.; Travali, S.; Scalisi, A.; McCubrey, J.A.; Candido, S.; Libra, M. MMP-9 overexpression is associated with intragenic hypermethylation of MMP9 gene in melanoma. *Aging (Albany NY)* **2016**, *8*, 933–944. [CrossRef] [PubMed]

19. Grafton-Clarke, C.; Chen, K.W.; Wilcock, J. Diagnosis and referral delays in primary care for oral squamous cell cancer: a systematic review. *Br. J. Gen. Pract.* **2019**, *69*, e112–e126. [CrossRef] [PubMed]
20. Akbulut, N.; Oztas, B.; Kursun, S.; Evirgen, S. Delayed diagnosis of oral squamous cell carcinoma: A case series. *J. Med. Case. Rep.* **2011**, *5*, 291. [CrossRef]
21. Sahibzada, H.A.; Khurshid, Z.; Khan, R.S.; Naseem, M.; Siddique, K.M.; Mali, M.; Zafar, M.S. Salivary IL-8, IL-6 and TNF-α as Potential Diagnostic Biomarkers for Oral Cancer. *Diagnostics (Basel)* **2017**, *7*, 21. [CrossRef] [PubMed]
22. St John, M.A.; Li, Y.; Zhou, X.; Denny, P.; Ho, C.M.; Montemagno, C.; Shi, W.; Qi, F.; Wu, B.; Sinha, U.; et al. Interleukin 6 and interleukin 8 as potential biomarkers for oral cavity and oropharyngeal squamous cell carcinoma. *Arch. Otolaryngol. Head Neck Surg.* **2004**, *130*, 929–935. [CrossRef] [PubMed]
23. Zheng, J.; Sun, L.; Yuan, W.; Xu, J.; Yu, X.; Wang, F.; Sun, L.; Zeng, Y. Clinical value of Naa10p and CEA levels in saliva and serum for diagnosis of oral squamous cell carcinoma. *J. Oral Pathol. Med.* **2018**, *47*, 830–835. [CrossRef]
24. Yuan, C.; Yang, K.; Tang, H.; Chen, D. Diagnostic values of serum tumor markers Cyfra21-1, SCCAg, ferritin, CEA, CA19-9, and AFP in oral/oropharyngeal squamous cell carcinoma. *Onco. Targets Ther.* **2016**, *9*, 3381–3386.
25. Geng, X.F.; Du, M.; Han, J.X.; Zhang, M.; Tang, X.F.; Xing, R.D. Saliva CA125 and TPS levels in patients with oral squamous cell carcinoma. *Int. J. Biol. Markers.* **2013**, *28*, 216–220. [CrossRef] [PubMed]
26. Yang, C.X.; Sedhom, W.; Song, J.; Lu, S.L. The Role of MicroRNAs in Recurrence and Metastasis of Head and Neck Squamous Cell Carcinoma. *Cancers (Basel)* **2019**, *11*, 395. [CrossRef]
27. Dias, F.; Morais, M.; Teixeira, A.L.; Medeiros, R. Involving the microRNA Targetome in Esophageal-Cancer Development and Behavior. *Cancers (Basel)* **2018**, *10*, 381. [CrossRef]
28. Wang, M.; Yu, F.; Li, P. Circular RNAs: Characteristics; Function and Clinical Significance in Hepatocellular Carcinoma. *Cancers (Basel)* **2018**, *10*, 258. [CrossRef]
29. Russo, D.; Merolla, F.; Varricchio, S.; Salzano, G.; Zarrilli, G.; Mascolo, M.; Strazzullo, V.; Di Crescenzo, R.M.; Celetti, A.; Ilardi, G. Epigenetics of oral and oropharyngeal cancers. *Biomed. Rep.* **2018**, *9*, 275–283.
30. Castilho, R.M.; Squarize, C.H.; Almeida, L.O. Epigenetic Modifications and Head and Neck Cancer: Implications for Tumor Progression and Resistance to Therapy. *Int. J. Mol. Sci.* **2017**, *18*, 1506. [CrossRef] [PubMed]
31. Duchaine, T.F.; Fabian, M.R. Mechanistic Insights into MicroRNA-Mediated Gene Silencing. *Cold Spring Harb. Perspect. Biol.* **2019**, *11*. [CrossRef]
32. Falzone, L.; Romano, G.L.; Salemi, R.; Bucolo, C.; Tomasello, B.; Lupo, G.; Anfuso, C.D.; Spandidos, D.A.; Libra, M.; Candido, S. Prognostic significance of deregulated microRNAs in uveal melanomas. *Mol. Med. Rep.* **2019**, *19*, 2599–2610. [CrossRef]
33. Hafsi, S.; Candido, S.; Maestro, R.; Falzone, L.; Soua, Z.; Bonavida, B.; Spandidos, D.A.; Libra, M. Correlation between the overexpression of Yin Yang 1 and the expression levels of miRNAs in Burkitt's lymphoma: A computational study. *Oncol. Lett.* **2016**, *11*, 1021–1025. [CrossRef]
34. Falzone, L.; Scola, L.; Zanghì, A.; Biondi, A.; Di Cataldo, A.; Libra, M.; Candido, S. Integrated analysis of colorectal cancer microRNA datasets: identification of microRNAs associated with tumor development. *Aging (Albany NY)* **2018**, *10*, 1000–1014. [CrossRef]
35. Manikandan, M.; Deva Magendhra Rao, A.K.; Arunkumar, G.; Manickavasagam, M.; Rajkumar, K.S.; Rajaraman, R.; Munirajan, A.K. Oral squamous cell carcinoma: microRNA expression profiling and integrative analyses for elucidation of tumourigenesis mechanism. *Mol. Cancer* **2016**, *15*, 28. [CrossRef]
36. Chamorro Petronacci, C.M.; Pérez-Sayáns, M.; Padín Iruegas, M.E.; Suárez Peñaranda, J.M.; Lorenzo Pouso, A.I.; Blanco Carrión, A.; García García, A. miRNAs expression of oral squamous cell carcinoma patients: Validation of two putative biomarkers. *Medicine (Baltimore)* **2019**, *98*, e14922. [CrossRef]
37. Yan, Z.Y.; Luo, Z.Q.; Zhang, L.J.; Li, J.; Liu, J.Q. Integrated Analysis and MicroRNA Expression Profiling Identified Seven miRNAs Associated With Progression of Oral Squamous Cell Carcinoma. *J. Cell Physiol.* **2017**, *232*, 2178–2185. [CrossRef]
38. Ahmed, M.; Nguyen, H.; Lai, T.; Kim, D.R. miRCancerdb: A database for correlation analysis between microRNA and gene expression in cancer. *BMC Res. Notes* **2018**, *11*, 103. [CrossRef]

39. Greene, C.S.; Tan, J.; Ung, M.; Moore, J.H.; Cheng, C. Big data bioinformatics. *J. Cell Physiol.* **2014**, *22*, 1896–1900. [CrossRef]
40. Cheng, P.F.; Dummer, R.; Levesque, M.P. Data mining The Cancer Genome Atlas in the era of precision cancer medicine. *Swiss Med. Wkly.* **2015**, *145*, w14183. [CrossRef]
41. Cancer Genome Atlas Research Network; Weinstein, J.N.; Collisson, E.A.; Mills, G.B.; Shaw, K.R.; Ozenberger, B.A.; Ellrott, K.; Shmulevich, I.; Sander, C.; Stuart, J.M. The Cancer Genome Atlas Pan-Cancer analysis project. *Nat. Genet.* **2013**, *45*, 1113–1120. [CrossRef]
42. ENCODE Project Consortium. An integrated encyclopedia of DNA elements in the human genome. *Nature* **2012**, *489*, 57–74. [CrossRef]
43. Gauthier, J.; Vincent, A.T.; Charette, S.J.; Derome, N. A brief history of bioinformatics. *Brief. Bioinform.* **2018**, *3*. [CrossRef]
44. Gill, S.K.; Christopher, A.F.; Gupta, V.; Bansal, P. Emerging role of bioinformatics tools and software in evolution of clinical research. *Perspect. Clin. Res.* **2016**, *7*, 115–122.
45. Shukla, H.D. Comprehensive Analysis of Cancer-Proteogenome to Identify Biomarkers for the Early Diagnosis and Prognosis of Cancer. *Proteomes.* **2017**, *5*, 28. [CrossRef]
46. Giacomelli, L.; Covani, U. Bioinformatics and data mining studies in oral genomics and proteomics: new trends and challenges. *Open. Dent. J.* **2010**, *4*, 67–71. [CrossRef] [PubMed]
47. Santosh, A.B.; Jones, T.; Harvey, J. A review on oral cancer biomarkers: Understanding the past and learning from the present. *J. Cancer Res. Ther.* **2016**, *12*, 486–492. [CrossRef] [PubMed]
48. Sutliff, A.K.; Watson, C.J.W.; Chen, G.; Lazarus, P. Regulation of UGT2A1 by miR-196a-5p and miR-196b-5p and its implications for lung cancer risk. *J. Pharmacol. Exp. Ther.* **2019**. [CrossRef] [PubMed]
49. Mazumder, S.; Datta, S.; Ray, J.G.; Chaudhuri, K.; Chatterjee, R. Liquid biopsy: miRNA as a potential biomarker in oral cancer. *Cancer Epidemiol.* **2019**, *58*, 137–145. [CrossRef]
50. Gissi, D.B.; Morandi, L.; Gabusi, A.; Tarsitano, A.; Marchetti, C.; Cura, F.; Palmieri, A.; Montebugnoli, L.; Asioli, S.; Foschini, M.P.; et al. A Noninvasive Test for MicroRNA Expression in Oral Squamous Cell Carcinoma. *Int. J. Mol. Sci.* **2018**, *19*, 1789. [CrossRef]
51. He, B.; Lin, X.; Tian, F.; Yu, W.; Qiao, B. MiR-133a-3p Inhibits Oral Squamous Cell Carcinoma (OSCC) Proliferation and Invasion by Suppressing COL1A1. *J. Cell. Biochem.* **2018**, *119*, 338–346. [CrossRef]
52. Mizuno, K.; Mataki, H.; Seki, N.; Kumamoto, T.; Kamikawaji, K.; Inoue, H. MicroRNAs in non-small cell lung cancer and idiopathic pulmonary fibrosis. *J. Hum. Genet.* **2017**, *62*, 57–65. [CrossRef]
53. Li, Z.; Yu, X.; Shen, J.; Law, P.T.; Chan, M.T.; Wu, W.K. MicroRNA expression and its implications for diagnosis and therapy of gallbladder cancer. *Oncotarget* **2015**, *6*, 13914–13921.
54. Srivastava, S.K.; Arora, S.; Singh, S.; Bhardwaj, A.; Averett, C.; Singh, A.P. MicroRNAs in pancreatic malignancy: Progress and promises. *Cancer Lett.* **2014**, *347*, 167–174. [CrossRef]
55. Du, M.; Giridhar, K.V.; Tian, Y.; Tschannen, M.R.; Zhu, J.; Huang, C.C.; Kilari, D.; Kohli, M.; Wang, L. Plasma exosomal miRNAs-based prognosis in metastatic kidney cancer. *Oncotarget* **2017**, *8*, 63703–63714. [CrossRef]
56. Yamazaki, N.; Koga, Y.; Taniguchi, H.; Kojima, M.; Kanemitsu, Y.; Saito, N.; Matsumura, Y. High expression of miR-181c as a predictive marker of recurrence in stage II colorectal cancer. *Oncotarget.* **2017**, *8*, 6970–6983. [CrossRef]
57. Feng, X.; Matsuo, K.; Zhang, T.; Hu, Y.; Mays, A.C.; Browne, J.D.; Zhou, X.; Sullivan, C.A. MicroRNA Profiling and Target Genes Related to Metastasis of Salivary Adenoid Cystic Carcinoma. *Anticancer Res.* **2017**, *37*, 3473–3481.
58. Falzone, L.; Candido, S.; Salemi, R.; Basile, M.S.; Scalisi, A.; McCubrey, J.A.; Torino, F.; Signorelli, S.S.; Montella, M.; Libra, M. Computational identification of microRNAs associated to both epithelial to mesenchymal transition and NGAL/MMP-9 pathways in bladder cancer. *Oncotarget* **2016**, *7*, 72758–72766. [CrossRef]
59. Lakshminarayana, S.; Augustine, D.; Rao, R.S.; Patil, S.; Awan, K.H.; Venkatesiah, S.S.; Haragannavar, V.C.; Nambiar, S.; Prasad, K. Molecular pathways of oral cancer that predict prognosis and survival: A systematic review. *J. Carcinog.* **2018**, *17*, 7. [CrossRef]
60. Ji, L.; Xu, J.; Liu, J.; Amjad, A.; Zhang, K.; Liu, Q.; Zhou, L.; Xiao, J.; Li, X. Mutant p53 promotes tumor cell malignancy by both positive and negative regulation of the transforming growth factor β (TGF-β) pathway. *J. Biol. Chem.* **2015**, *290*, 11729–11740. [CrossRef]

61. Vander Broek, R.; Mohan, S.; Eytan, D.F.; Chen, Z.; Van Waes, C. The PI3K/Akt/mTOR axis in head and neck cancer: functions; aberrations; cross-talk; and therapies. *Oral Dis.* **2015**, *21*, 815–825. [CrossRef]
62. Salemi, R.; Falzone, L.; Madonna, G.; Polesel, J.; Cinà, D.; Mallardo, D.; Ascierto, P.A.; Libra, M.; Candido, S. MMP-9 as a Candidate Marker of Response to BRAF Inhibitors in Melanoma Patients with BRAFV600E Mutation Detected in Circulating-Free DNA. *Front. Pharmacol.* **2018**, *9*, 856. [CrossRef]
63. Leonardi, G.C.; Falzone, L.; Salemi, R.; Zanghì, A.; Spandidos, D.A.; Mccubrey, J.A.; Candido, S.; Libra, M. Cutaneous melanoma: From pathogenesis to therapy (Review). *Int. J. Oncol.* **2018**, *52*, 1071–1080. [CrossRef]
64. McCubrey, J.A.; Fitzgerald, T.L.; Yang, L.V.; Lertpiriyapong, K.; Steelman, L.S.; Abrams, S.L.; Montalto, G.; Cervello, M.; Neri, L.M.; Cocco, L.; et al. Roles of GSK-3 and microRNAs on epithelial mesenchymal transition and cancer stem cells. *Oncotarget* **2017**, *8*, 14221–14250. [CrossRef] [PubMed]
65. Vogelstein, B.; Papadopoulos, N.; Velculescu, V.E.; Zhou, S.; Diaz, L.A. Jr.; Kinzler, K.W. Cancer genome landscapes. *Science* **2013**, *339*, 1546–1558. [CrossRef]
66. Battaglia, R.; Palini, S.; Vento, M.E.; La Ferlita, A.; Lo Faro, M.J.; Caroppo, E.; Borzì, P.; Falzone, L.; Barbagallo, D.; Ragusa, M.; et al. Identification of extracellular vesicles and characterization of miRNA expression profiles in human blastocoel fluid. *Sci. Rep.* **2019**, *9*, 84. [CrossRef] [PubMed]
67. Hasin, Y.; Seldin, M.; Lusis, A. Multi-omics approaches to disease. *Genome Biol.* **2017**, *18*, 83. [CrossRef]
68. Casamassimi, A.; Federico, A.; Rienzo, M.; Esposito, S.; Ciccodicola, A. Transcriptome Profiling in Human Diseases: New Advances and Perspectives. *Int. J. Mol. Sci.* **2017**, *18*, 1652. [CrossRef] [PubMed]
69. Barrett, T.; Wilhite, S.E.; Ledoux, P.; Evangelista, C.; Kim, I.F.; Tomashevsky, M.; Marshall, K.A.; Phillippy, K.H.; Sherman, P.M.; Holko, M.; et al. NCBI GEO: Archive for functional genomics data sets—Update. *Nucleic Acids Res.* **2013**, *41*, D991–D995. [CrossRef]
70. Tokar, T.; Pastrello, C.; Rossos, A.E.M.; Abovsky, M.; Hauschild, A.C.; Tsay, M.; Lu, R.; Jurisica, I. mirDIP 4.1-integrative database of human microRNA target predictions. *Nucleic Acids Res.* **2018**, *46*, D360–D370. [CrossRef] [PubMed]
71. Shirdel, E.A.; Xie, W.; Mak, T.W.; Jurisica, I. NAViGaTing the Micronome. Using Multiple MicroRNA Prediction Databases to Identify Signalling Pathway-Associated MicroRNAs. *PLoS ONE* **2011**, *6*, e17429. [CrossRef]
72. Vlachos, I.S.; Zagganas, K.; Paraskevopoulou, M.D.; Georgakilas, G.; Karagkouni, D.; Vergoulis, T.; Dalamagas, T.; Hatzigeorgiou, A.G. DIANA-miRPath v3.0: Deciphering microRNA function with experimental support. *Nucleic Acids Res.* **2015**, *43*, W460–W466. [CrossRef]
73. Mi, H.; Muruganujan, A.; Ebert, D.; Huang, X.; Thomas, P.D. PANTHER version 14: More genomes, a new PANTHER GO-slim and improvements in enrichment analysis tools. *Nucleic Acids Res.* **2019**, *47*, D419–D426. [CrossRef]
74. Szklarczyk, D.; Gable, A.L.; Lyon, D.; Junge, A.; Wyder, S.; Huerta-Cepas, J.; Simonovic, M.; Doncheva, N.T.; Morris, J.H.; Bork, P.; et al. STRING v11: Protein-protein association networks with increased coverage, supporting functional discovery in genome-wide experimental datasets. *Nucleic Acids Res.* **2019**, *47*, D607–D613. [CrossRef] [PubMed]
75. Anaya, J. OncoLnc: Linking TCGA survival data to mRNAs, miRNAs, and lncRNAs. *PeerJ. Comput. Sci.* **2016**, *2*, e67. [CrossRef]

8

Breast Cancer Prognosis Using a Machine Learning Approach

Patrizia Ferroni [1,2,*], Fabio M. Zanzotto [3], Silvia Riondino [1,4], Noemi Scarpato [2], Fiorella Guadagni [1,2] and Mario Roselli [4]

1 BioBIM (InterInstitutional Multidisciplinary Biobank), IRCCS San Raffaele Pisana, Via di Val Cannuta 247, 00166 Rome, Italy; silvia.riondino@sanraffaele.it (S.R.); fiorella.guadagni@sanraffaele.it (F.G.)
2 Department of Human Sciences & Quality of Life Promotion, San Raffaele Roma Open University, Via di Val Cannuta 247, 00166 Rome, Italy; noemi.scarpato@unisanraffaele.gov.it
3 Department of Enterprise Engineering, University of Rome "Tor Vergata", Viale Oxford 81, 00133 Rome, Italy; fabio.massimo.zanzotto@uniroma2.it
4 Department of Systems Medicine, Medical Oncology, Tor Vergata Clinical Center, University of Rome "Tor Vergata", Viale Oxford 81, 00133 Rome, Italy; mario.roselli@uniroma2.it
* Correspondence: patrizia.ferroni@sanraffaele.it or ferronipatrizia@gmail.com;

Abstract: Machine learning (ML) has been recently introduced to develop prognostic classification models that can be used to predict outcomes in individual cancer patients. Here, we report the significance of an ML-based decision support system (DSS), combined with random optimization (RO), to extract prognostic information from routinely collected demographic, clinical and biochemical data of breast cancer (BC) patients. A DSS model was developed in a training set (n = 318), whose performance analysis in the testing set (n = 136) resulted in a C-index for progression-free survival of 0.84, with an accuracy of 86%. Furthermore, the model was capable of stratifying the testing set into two groups of patients with low- or high-risk of progression with a hazard ratio (HR) of 10.9 ($p < 0.0001$). Validation in multicenter prospective studies and appropriate management of privacy issues in relation to digital electronic health records (EHR) data are presently needed. Nonetheless, we may conclude that the implementation of ML algorithms and RO models into EHR data might help to achieve prognostic information, and has the potential to revolutionize the practice of personalized medicine.

Keywords: breast cancer prognosis; artificial intelligence; machine learning; decision support systems

---

1. Introduction

The breast cancer (BC) death rate has declined steadily over the past two decades, progress that can be attributed to the deployment of innovative management pathways, from early detection to treatment. Nevertheless, BC still represents the leading cause of cancer death among females worldwide [1]. Accordingly, BC survivability prediction represents a challenging task that could strongly benefit from the development of personalized predictive models. In this context, contemporary oncology has witnessed a growing interest in digital technologies, whose integration with big healthcare data has raised new hopes for personalized medicine.

Artificial intelligence (AI) and machine learning (ML) have been used to diagnose and classify cancer for nearly 20 years, but only a few studies have investigated their relevance in cancer prognosis [2]. In particular, ML or semi-supervised learning techniques have been recently applied to develop models for BC progression and survivability. Most of them, however, were built on datasets from the SEER (Surveillance Program, Epidemiology, and End Results), not including important prognostic parameters such as the St. Gallen criteria (hormones receptor status, HER2/Neu expression or Ki67 proliferation index) [3–5], while other studies were performed on hybrid models containing microarray data [6] or on mammographic images [7,8]. Lately, an unsupervised ML approach that can admit any number of prognostic factors, was used to build prognostic systems for cancer patients [9]. Also, in this case, the SEER dataset used did not include information on HER2/Neu expression, whose prognostic significance has been emphasized in the 8th edition TNM staging system for BC [10]. Thus, the unmet need to develop prognostic classification models that embody the newest AI technologies and can be used to predict outcomes in individual cancer patients for personalized patient care has been highlighted [11].

In this context, we have recently demonstrated the potential of a semi-explainable decision support system (DSS), based on multiple kernel learning (MKL) [12], that can be adapted to different medical problems [13,14] and gives the possibility to inspect the learned model. The model combines a support vector machine (SVM) [15] algorithm and random optimization (RO) [16]. Hence, it can offer an explanation on how routinely collected demographic, clinical and biochemical data are important in predictions. This MKL model, originally developed for cancer-associated thrombosis risk assessment [13], has been here adapted to estimate the risk of disease progression in an oncology setting of BC patients. To achieve this objective, a proof-of-concept study was specifically designed to assess whether a customized MKL-based DSS could be a useful prognostic tool in the clinical management of BC patients.

2. Results

A set of predictors (named ML-RO) was identified using a 3-fold cross-validation technique on a training set (n = 318). A testing set (n = 136) was used to compute the final performance of risk predictors. To devise the DSS, we selected ML-RO-4 as the best performing out of a range of ten runs, in terms of the area under the curve (AUC), on the training set (Table 1).

Table 1. Analytical performance of machine learning with random optimization in the training set.

ML Predictor	AUC (SE)	95% CI	Sensitivity (95% CI)	Specificity (95% CI)	+LR	−LR
ML-RO-4	0.778 (0.0290)	0.728–0.822	67.1 (55.4–77.5)	88.4 (83.7–92.2)	5.80	0.37
ML-RO-1	0.769 (0.0293)	0.719–0.814	65.8 (54.0–76.3)	88.0 (83.2–91.8)	5.49	0.39
ML-RO-7	0.767 (0.0293)	0.717–0.813	67.1 (55.4–77.5)	86.4 (81.4–90.4)	4.92	0.38
ML-RO-3	0.759 (0.0296)	0.708–0.805	65.8 (54.0–76.3)	86.0 (80.9–90.1)	4.68	0.40
ML-RO-6	0.759 (0.0296)	0.708–0.805	65.8 (54.0–76.3)	86.0 (80.9–90.1)	4.68	0.40
ML-RO-8	0.755 (0.0297)	0.703–0.801	65.8 (54.0–76.3)	85.1 (80.0–89.4)	4.42	0.40
ML-RO-0	0.753 (0.0297)	0.701–0.799	65.8 (54.0–76.3)	84.7 (79.5–89.0)	4.30	0.40
ML-RO-2	0.748 (0.0299)	0.697–0.795	64.5 (52.7–75.1)	85.1 (80.0–89.4)	4.33	0.42
ML-RO-9	0.739 (0.0302)	0.687–0.786	61.8 (50.0–72.8)	86.0 (80.9–90.1)	4.40	0.44
ML-RO-5	0.722 (0.0306)	0.669–0.770	59.2 (47.3–70.4)	85.1 (80.0–89.4)	3.98	0.48

AUC: Area under the curve; CI: Confidence interval; LR: Likelihood ratio; ML: Machine learning; RO: Random optimization.

As shown in Table 1, most predictors had a receiver operating characteristic (ROC) curve with an AUC $\geq$0.75 (the threshold generally accepted as clinically useful) [17]. Among these, ML-RO-0 was further selected as it provided a major relative importance to the group of features linked to glucose metabolism (Group 5) (Table 2), which is currently considered an important contributor to BC progression [18,19], at the point that metformin—an anti-diabetic drug with insulin-lowering effects—has been proposed in combination with chemotherapy [20,21] and is currently being considered vs. placebo in a phase-III randomized trial in early stage BC (ClinicalTrials.gov Identifier: NCT01101438).

Table 2. Weights of attribute groups in the training set.

Method	Group					Sum of the Weights	Normalized Group Weights				
	1	2	3	4	5		1	2	3	4	5
ML+RO-4	0.41890	1.04551	0.60311	0.33909	0.58969	2.996321	0.13980	0.34893	0.20128	0.11316	0.19680
ML+RO-0	0.77299	1.86062	1.39445	0.90456	1.00740	5.940053	0.13013	0.31323	0.23475	0.15228	0.16959
ML+RO-6	0.42756	0.91373	1.16514	0.39297	0.58755	3.486968	0.12261	0.26204	0.33414	0.11269	0.16849
ML+RO-8	0.44878	1.28224	0.63075	0.44350	0.53398	3.339267	0.13439	0.38399	0.18888	0.13281	0.15991
ML+RO-1	0.46149	1.17742	0.55782	0.34141	0.47660	3.014770	0.15307	0.39055	0.18503	0.11324	0.15809
ML+RO-7	0.54682	1.40025	0.79264	0.59119	0.61023	3.941154	0.13874	0.35529	0.20112	0.15000	0.15483
ML+RO-3	0.64274	1.13249	0.36078	0.39482	0.45241	2.983255	0.21545	0.37961	0.12093	0.13234	0.15165

Data are absolute numbers for group weights. ML: Machine Learning; RO: Random Optimization.

When both predictors were incorporated into a DSS model for BC progression, their combined use (both positive, either positive, both negative) in the testing set translated in a c-statistic = 0.84 (95% CI: 0.76–0.90). The level with the best Youden index at ROC analysis (>1, i.e., risk estimate achieved by both predictors, according to voting on the positive class) was then selected as the cutoff value for further evaluation of the combined DSS. A comparison of the analytical performance of the trained models and derived DSS on the testing set is reported in Table 3.

Table 3. Analytical performance of machine learning with random optimization in the testing set.

Performance Parameter	ML-RO-0	ML-RO-4	DSS Model [a]
F-measure [b]	0.696	0.677	0.698
Accuracy	0.853	0.838	0.860
Area under the curve (AUC)	0.822	0.813	0.815
(+)LR (95% CI)	9.1 (4.3–20.8)	8.5 (3.9–19.6)	8.6 (4.2–18.0)
(−)LR (95% CI)	0.4 (0.3–0.6)	0.4 (0.3–0.6)	0.4 (0.2–0.5)
HR (95% CI)	10.7 (4.6–24.8)	10.3 (4.5–23.7)	10.9 (4.5–26.6)

LR: Likelihood ratio; C.I.: Confidence interval; HR: Hazard ratio; [a] Analytical performance was evaluated after categorization 0/1 based on risk estimate achieved by both predictors; [b] F-measure represents a harmonic mean of precision [(P) positive predictive value in machine learning] and recall [(R) sensitivity in machine learning] and is calculated as: 2PR/(P+R).

At a criterion >1, the DSS model was capable of stratifying primary BC patients into two groups with a low- or high-risk of progression, either in the training (n = 279; log-rank = 3.23, p = 0.001) or in the testing set (n = 118; log-rank = 3.42, p < 0.001). Figure 1 reports the Kaplan–Meier curves of progression-free survival (PFS) in the 136 BC women included in the testing set and followed-up for a mean time of 3.5 years (ranging from 0.3–9.7 years). As shown, patients estimated at high risk (>1) of progression by the combined DSS model had a 5-year progression-free survival probability significantly lower than that observed in BC patients estimated at low-risk ($\leq$1) (26% vs. 85%, respectively; log-rank = 6.82, p < 0.0001).

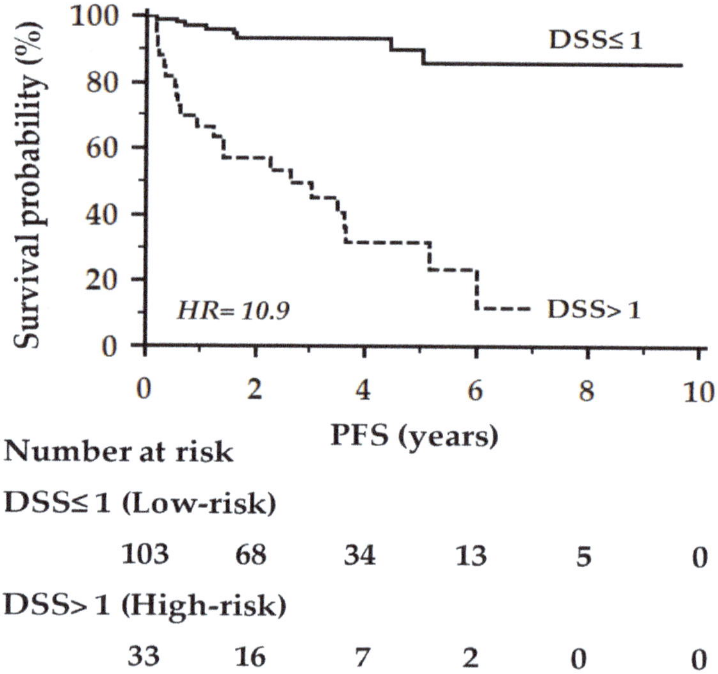

Figure 1. Kaplan–Meier curves of progression-free survival (PFS) of the 136 BC women included in the testing set. Comparison between patients at high (>1) or low-risk (≤1) of progression by the combined decision support system (DSS) model.

3. Discussion

Treatment decisions are particularly challenging in early-stage BC patients with conflicting prognostic features, especially node-negative ones, in which the question of whether to pursue an adjuvant treatment with chemotherapy or endocrine therapies is still unclear. Putative biomarkers, so far, have not demonstrated sufficient predictive ability to be clinically useful. Ki67 itself lacks reproducibility and its use, if not part of an AI model, has been largely re-dimensioned [22].

Identification of predictive tools of tumor responsiveness, risk of recurrence, and mortality, providing the possibility to avoid unnecessary toxicities are thus very appealing. As reported above, ML has started to take hold across the oncology community to develop prognostic classifications models of BC progression and survivability [9]. In this regard, the possibility to perform an automated survival prediction in metastatic cancer patients using high-dimensional electronic health records (EHR) data has been recently highlighted [23]. By using an ML approach on EHR-derived predictor variables (clustered into categories), Gensheimer et al., in fact, devised an AI system, with a better c-statistic than previously reported prognostic models, which could be deployed in a DSS to help improve quality of care in the metastatic setting [23]. More recently, four major nonlinear ML methods (integrating multiple clinicopathological features and genomic data) were used to compare survival predictions in a large cohort of BC patients [24]. Although no model significantly outperformed others, the Nottingham Prognostic Index, age, tumor stage and size, ER/PR/HER2 and breast surgery status strongly influenced survival across repeated runs and models, while the gene expression cluster was a moderately influential factor [24].

The results here reported confirm and extend the findings by Zhao et al., as the use of an SVM has proven effective in devising an AI-based DSS for the prognostic assessment of non-metastatic BC patients. In particular, the combined use of ML and RO techniques, allowed the construction of a set of prognostic discriminators from routinely collected clinicopathological features and biochemical data of BC patients, which showed a better performance than the predictors developed by Zhao et al. (c-statistic 0.82 vs. 0.66 and an accuracy of 86% vs. 73%, respectively) [24]. In our opinion, this combined approach might hold potential for improving model precision through weighting the relative importance of attributes. Moreover, with respect to models based on neural networks [7], the combination of ML and RO techniques offers a model that can be learned with small datasets and that is more interpretable, as were Bayesian networks applied to BC [25]. Furthermore, the devised DSS included a number of prognostic and metabolic parameters, not previously analyzed, that could be easily extracted by EHR, meaning that ML may add significant and sustained benefits to personalized medicine at no additional cost to the health system.

Of course, there are limitations to acknowledge. First, the study was mono-institutional. Second, the sample size was relatively small, which may have lowered the power of ML. Nonetheless, we believe that implementation of ML algorithms and RO models into high-dimensional EHR data might help to achieve prognostic information, and has the potential to revolutionize the practice of personalized medicine.

4. Patients and Methods

Starting from January 2007, the PTV Bio.Ca.Re. (Policlinico Tor Vergata Biospecimen Cancer Repository) and the SR-BioBIM (Interinstitutional Multidisciplinary Biobank, IRCCS San Raffaele Pisana, Rome, Italy) are actively involved in the recruitment of ambulatory patients with primary or metastatic cancer, who are prospectively followed under the appropriate institutional ethics approval, as part of a Clinical Database and Biobank project. Among these, a cohort of 454 consecutive BC patients in whom prognostic and pre-treatment biochemical factors were available, were selected for the present analysis. The study was performed in accordance with the principles embodied in the Declaration of Helsinki. All patients gave written informed consent, previously approved by our Institutional Ethics Committee (ISR/DMLBA/405, 15 November 2006). BC was pathologically staged according to the latest prognostic TNM staging system [8]. Three hundred and ninety-seven women (87%) had primary BC and underwent radical surgery followed by radiation and/or adjuvant treatment as per current guidelines. The remaining 57 (13%) patients presented with metastatic disease. Prognostic routinely-collected factors such as BC stage, menopausal status, pathological grading as well as the St. Gallen criteria (e.g., estrogen and progesterone receptors, HER2/neu expression and the proliferation index Ki67) were available for each patient. In particular, grading was assessed according to the Nottingham grading system (Elston–Ellis modification of the Scarff–Bloom–Richardson grading system) for BC [8]. The immunohistochemical analyses were performed on formalin-fixed, paraffin-embedded tumor sections for hormone receptor presence [26], HER2/neu expression [27] and proliferation index (Ki67) [28]. HER2/neu positivity was defined according to the American Society of Clinical Oncology-College of American Pathologists (ASCO-CAP) guidelines as an immunohistochemical staining of 3+ or 2+ with evidence of gene amplification by fluorescence in situ hybridization (FISH) [27]. The Ki67 proliferative index in surgical specimens was assigned by the pathologist based on the percentage of positivity on at least 500 neoplastic cells counted in the peripheral area of the nodule. A cut–off value of $\geq$20% was used in all association analyses, according to the recommendations of the St. Gallen International Expert Consensus on the primary therapy of early BC 2013 [28].

Furthermore, given the increasing awareness that metabolic features might represent an important contributor to BC progression, Type 2 diabetes, glycemic parameters and the body mass index (BMI) were introduced in the model [18,19]. Routine biochemical analyses were performed on fresh blood samples taken in the morning after an overnight fast at the time of enrolment and prior to any treatment (surgery, adjuvant, either chemotherapy or endocrine, or metastatic). The demographic and clinical characteristics of the recruited population are summarized in Table 4.

Table 4. Clinical-pathological characteristics of breast cancer (BC) patients. Comparison between training and testing set.

Clinical-Pathological Characteristics	Training Set (n = 318)	Testing Set (n = 136)
Age (years), Mean ± SD	56 ± 13	57 ± 12
Menopausal status, N (%)		
Pre	141 (44)	51 (38)
Post	177 (56)	85 (63)
Body Mass Index, Mean ± SD	25.2 ± 4.5	25.7 ± 5.2
Histological diagnosis, N (%)		
Ductal	263 (83)	121 (89)
Lobular	37 (12)	9 (7)
Others	18 (5)	6 (4)
Molecular Type [a], N (%)		
Triple-negative	39 (12)	17 (12)
Luminal-like A	97 (31)	37 (27)
Luminal-like B	172 (54)	77 (57)
HER2 pos	10 (3)	5 (4)
Grading, N (%) [b]		
1	20 (7)	15 (13)
2	108 (39)	45 (38)
3	151 (54)	58 (49)
Tumor, N (%) [b]		
T1	141 (50)	59 (50)
T2	91 (33)	42 (36)
T3	28 (10)	5 (4)
T4	19 (7)	12 (10)
Node, N (%) [b]		
N0	134 (48)	54 (46)
N+	145 (52)	64 (54)
Prognostic stage, N (%)		
I	177 (56)	70 (50)
II	53 (17)	20 (15)
III	45 (14)	26 (19)
IV	4 (1)	2 (1)
Metastatic	39 (12)	18 (13)
Receptor status, N (%) [c]		
ER+/PR+	235 (74)	94 (69)
ER+/PR−	29 (9)	19 (14)
ER-/PR+	5 (2)	1 (1)
ER-/PR−	49 (15)	22 (16)
HER2/neu+, N (%) [c]	66 (21)	34 (25)
Ki67 proliferation index ≥20%, N (%) [c]	204 (67)	93 (71)
Type 2 Diabetes, N (%)	39 (12)	11 (8%)
Glucose metabolic asset [d]		
Fasting blood glucose (mg/dl), Mean ± SD	105 ± 31	102 ± 32
Fasting insulin (μIU/ml), Median (IQR)	11.9 (6.4–27.0)	10.6 (5.6–19.6)
HbA_{1c} (%), Mean ± SD	5.8 ± 0.8	5.8 ± 0.7
HOMA Index, Mean ± SD	3.0 (1.4–8.3)	2.9 (1.2–6.3)
Follow-up (years)		
Mean (range)	3.4 (0.29–10.5)	3.5 (0.26–9.65)

[a] According to St. Gallen Consensus Conference. [b] Evaluated at time of diagnosis. [c] Evaluated in a population of 397 primary breast cancer patients. [d] Evaluated at time of enrollment and prior to any treatment. ER/PR: estrogen/progesterone receptors; HER2: Human epidermal growth factor receptor 2; IQR: Interquartile range; HbA_{1c}: Glycosylated hemoglobin; HOMA Index: Homeostasis model assessment index.

The machine learning used for the primary analysis was run using the kernel-based learning platform (KeLP) [29], as previously reported [13]. Multiple kernel learning (MKL), based on support vector machines (SVM) and random optimization (RO) models, were used to produce prognostic discriminators (referred as machine-learning (ML)-RO) yielding the best classification performance over a training (3-fold cross-validation) and testing set. The training set consisted of 318 BC patients (70% of the dataset); the remaining 136 patients were allocated to the testing set (30% of the cases). No significant difference was observed for demographic, clinical and biochemical characteristics between the training and testing set (Table 4). The numerical attributes were analyzed as continuous values. Missing clinical attribute values were treated according to the predictive value imputation (PVI) method by replacing missing values with the average of the attribute observed in the training set. The variables were clustered into five groups according to clinical significance. A detailed list of all the features applied to construct the predictor is reported in Table 5. RO was used to devise their relative weights in the final prediction. In RO, relative weights are initialized with a random number and estimated by maximizing performance in the 3-fold cross-validation. These weights can be used to interpret the importance of the groups of features within the model. Thus, the final DSS is interpretable.

Table 5. Features included in the model.

Patient-Related	Tumor-Related	Biochemical
Group 1: Age Menopausal status Body Mass Index	**Group 2:** Molecular type Histological diagnosis Grading TNM stage **Group 3:** Estrogen receptors Progesterone receptors HER2/NEU Ki67 proliferation index	**Group 4:** Total BilirubinCreatinine **Group 5:** Fasting glycemia Fasting insulinemia Glycosylated hemoglobin HOMA index (insulin resistance) Type 2 diabetes

Statistical analysis

The receiver operating characteristic (ROC) curve and univariate Cox proportional hazards analyses were performed by MedCalc Statistical Software version 13.1.2 (MedCalc Software bvba, Ostend, Belgium). The area under the curve (AUC) was calculated on a three-level risk: 2 (if both predictors estimated the risk), 1 (if only one predictor estimated the risk) or 0 (if both predictors did not estimate the risk) to investigate whether the combined DSS could distinguish between recurrent and non-recurrent patients. The level with the best Youden index (>1, i.e., risk estimate achieved by both predictors) was selected as the cutoff value for the combined DSS. Bayesian analysis was performed, and positive (+LR) and negative (−LR) likelihood ratios were used to estimate the probability of BC progression. The survival curves were calculated by the Kaplan–Meier and log-rank methods using computer software packages (MedCalc Software bvba, Ostend, Belgium and Statistica 8.0, StatSoft Inc., Tulsa, OK, USA). The PFS represented the study endpoint and was calculated from the date of enrollment until disease progression. The patients who had no disease progression were censored at the time of the last follow-up. For administrative censoring, the follow-up ended on 31 December, 2017. All tests were two-tailed and only p-values lower than 0.05 were regarded as statistically significant.

5. Conclusions

ML has recently started to take hold across the oncology community to develop prognostic classifications models of cancer progression and survivability. In our opinion, a combined approach of ML algorithms and RO models might hold potential for improving model precision through weighting the relative importance of attributes. In line with the actual trend, in fact, the proposed model seeks not only decision, but also interpretability of the model itself, which, together with the use of a real-world BC dataset, represents the novel aspect of our research. Validation in multicenter prospective studies and appropriate management of privacy issues in relation to digital EHR data are required before making any ML approach into the clinical practice available.

Author Contributions: P.F. and M.R. designed the study, analyzed and interpreted the clinical data, and wrote the manuscript; F.M.Z. and N.S. designed the algorithm, performed the machine learning experiments, and wrote the manuscript; S.R. collected clinical and laboratory data, interpreted the data and wrote the manuscript; F.G. designed the study, analyzed and interpreted the data, and critically revised the manuscript. All authors revised and approved the final version of the manuscript.

References

1. Torre, L.A.; Bray, F.; Siegel, R.L.; Ferlay, J.; Lortet-Tieulent, J.; Jemal, A. Global cancer statistics, 2012. *CA Cancer J. Clin.* **2015**, *65*, 87–108. [CrossRef] [PubMed]
2. Kourou, K.; Exarchos, T.P.; Exarchos, K.P.; Karamouzis, M.V.; Fotiadis, D.I. Machine learning applications in cancer prognosis and prediction. *Comput. Struct. Biotechnol. J.* **2014**, *13*, 8–17. [CrossRef] [PubMed]
3. Delen, D.; Walker, G.; Kadam, A. Predicting breast cancer survivability: A comparison of three data mining methods. *Artif. Intell. Med.* **2005**, *34*, 113–127. [CrossRef] [PubMed]
4. Kim, J.; Shin, H. Breast cancer survivability prediction using labeled, unlabeled, and pseudo-labeled patient data. *J. Am. Med. Inform. Assoc.* **2013**, *20*, 613–618. [CrossRef] [PubMed]
5. Park, K.; Ali, A.; Kim, D.; An, Y.; Kim, M.; Shin, H. Robust predictive model for evaluating breast cancer survivability. *Eng. Appl. Artif. Intell.* **2013**, *26*, 2194–2205. [CrossRef]
6. Sun, Y.; Goodison, S.; Li, J.; Liu, L.; Farmerie, W. Improved breast cancer prognosis through the combination of clinical and genetic markers. *Bioinformatics* **2007**, *23*, 30–37. [CrossRef] [PubMed]
7. Burt, J.R.; Torosdagli, N.; Khosravan, N.; RaviPrakash, H.; Mortazi, A.; Tissavirasingham, F.; Hussein, S.; Bagci, U. Deep learning beyond cats and dogs: Recent advances in diagnosing breast cancer with deep neural networks. *Br. J. Radiol.* **2018**, *91*, 20170545. [CrossRef] [PubMed]
8. Yousefi, B.; Ting, H.N.; Mirhassani, S.M.; Hosseini, M. Development of computer-aided detection of breast lesion using gabor-wavelet BASED features in mammographic images. In Proceedings of the 2013 IEEE International Conference on Control System, Computing and Engineering (ICCSCE), Penang, Malaysia, 29 November–1 December 2013; pp. 127–131.
9. Hueman, M.T.; Wang, H.; Yang, C.Q.; Sheng, L.; Henson, D.E.; Schwartz, A.M.; Chen, D. Creating prognostic systems for cancer patients: A demonstration using breast cancer. *Cancer Med.* **2018**, *7*, 3611–3621. [CrossRef] [PubMed]
10. Amin, M.B.; Edge, S.; Greene, F.; Byrd, D.R.; Brookland, R.K.; Washington, M.K.; Gershenwald, J.E.; Compton, C.C.; Hess, K.R.; Sullivan, D.C.; et al. (Eds.) *AJCC Cancer Staging Manual*, 8th ed.; Springer: New York, NY, USA, 2017.
11. O'Sullivan, B.; Brierley, J.; Byrd, D.; Bosman, F.; Kehoe, S.; Kossary, C.; Piñeros, M.; Van Eycken, E.; Weir, H.K.; Gospodarowicz, M. The TNM classification of malignant tumours-towards common understanding and reasonable expectations. *Lancet Oncol.* **2017**, *18*, 849–851. [CrossRef]
12. Gönen, M.; Alpaydın, E. Multiple kernel learning algorithms. *J. Mach. Learn. Res.* **2011**, *12*, 2211–2268.
13. Ferroni, P.; Zanzotto, F.M.; Scarpato, N.; Riondino, S.; Nanni, U.; Roselli, M.; Guadagni, F. Risk assessment for venous thromboembolism in chemotherapy treated ambulatory cancer patients: A precision medicine approach. *Med. Dec. Mak.* **2017**, *37*, 234–242. [CrossRef] [PubMed]
14. Ferroni, P.; Roselli, M.; Zanzotto, F.M.; Guadagni, F. Artificial Intelligence for cancer-associated thrombosis risk assessment. *Lancet Haematol.* **2018**, *5*, e391. [CrossRef]
15. Cristianini, N.; Shawe-Taylor, J. An Introduction to Support Vector Machines and other kernel based learning methods. *Ai Magazine* **2000**, *22*, 190.
16. Matyas, J. Random optimization. *Automat. Rem. Control* **1965**, *26*, 246–253.
17. Fan, J.; Upadhye, S.; Worster, A. Understanding receiver operating characteristic (ROC) curves. *Can. J. Emerg. Med.* **2006**, *8*, 19–20. [CrossRef]
18. Zhu, Q.L.; Xu, W.H.; Tao, M.H. Biomarkers of the Metabolic Syndrome and Breast Cancer Prognosis. *Cancers* **2010**, *2*, 721–739. [CrossRef] [PubMed]
19. Ferroni, P.; Riondino, S.; Laudisi, A.; Portarena, I.; Formica, V.; Alessandroni, J.; D'Alessandro, R.; Orlandi, A.; Costarelli, L.; Cavaliere, F.; et al. Pre-treatment insulin levels as a prognostic factor for breast cancer progression. *Oncologist* **2016**, *21*, 1041–1049. [CrossRef] [PubMed]

20. Yam, C.; Esteva, F.J.; Patel, M.M.; Raghavendra, A.S.; Ueno, N.T.; Moulder, S.L.; Hess, K.R.; Shroff, G.S.; Hodge, S.; Koenig, K.H.; et al. Efficacy and safety of the combination of metformin, everolimus and exemestane in overweight and obese postmenopausal patients with metastatic, hormone receptor-positive, HER2-negative breast cancer: A phase II study. *Investig. New Drugs* **2019**. [CrossRef] [PubMed]
21. Martin-Castillo, B.; Pernas, S.; Dorca, J.; Álvarez, I.; Martínez, S.; Pérez-Garcia, J.M.; Batista-López, N.; Rodríguez-Sánchez, C.A.; Amillano, K.; Domínguez, S.; et al. A phase 2 trial of neoadjuvant metformin in combination with trastuzumab and chemotherapy in women with early HER2-positive breast cancer: The METTEN study. *Oncotarget* **2018**, *9*, 35687–35704. [CrossRef] [PubMed]
22. Thakur, S.S.; Li, H.; Chan, A.M.Y.; Tudor, R.; Bigras, G.; Morris, D.; Enwere, E.K.; Yang, H. The use of automated Ki67 analysis to predict Oncotype DX risk-of-recurrence categories in early-stage breast cancer. *PLoS ONE* **2018**, *13*, e0188983. [CrossRef] [PubMed]
23. Gensheimer, M.F.; Henry, A.S.; Wood, D.J.; Hastie, T.J.; Aggarwal, S.; Dudley, S.A.; Pradhan, P.; Banerjee, I.; Cho, E.; Ramchandran, K.; et al. Automated survival prediction in metastatic cancer patients using high-dimensional electronic medical record data. *J. Natl. Cancer Inst.* **2019**, *111*, djy178. [CrossRef] [PubMed]
24. Zhao, M.; Tang, Y.; Kim, H.; Hasegawa, K. Machine learning with k-means dimensional reduction for predicting survival outcomes in patients with breast cancer. *Cancer Inf.* **2018**, *17*, 1–7. [CrossRef] [PubMed]
25. Cruz-Ramírez, N.; Acosta-Mesa, H.G.; Carrillo-Calvet, H.; Nava-Fernández, L.A.; Barrientos-Martínez, R.E. Diagnosis of breast cancer using Bayesian networks: A case study. *Comput. Biol. Med.* **2007**, *37*, 1553–1564. [CrossRef] [PubMed]
26. Hammond, M.E.; Hayes, D.F.; Dowsett, M.; Allred, D.C.; Hagerty, K.L.; Badve, S.; Fitzgibbons, P.L.; Francis, G.; Goldstein, N.S.; Hayes, M.; et al. American Society of Clinical Oncology/College of American Pathologists guideline recommendations for immunohistochemical testing of estrogen and progesterone receptors in breast cancer. *J. Clin. Oncol.* **2010**, *28*, 2784–2795. [CrossRef] [PubMed]
27. Wolff, A.C.; Hammond, M.E.; Schwartz, J.N.; Hagerty, K.L.; Allred, D.C.; Cote, R.J.; Dowsett, M.; Fitzgibbons, P.L.; Hanna, W.M.; Langer, A.; et al. American Society of Clinical Oncology/College of American Pathologists. American Society of Clinical Oncology/College of American Pathologists guideline recommendations for human epidermal growth factor receptor 2 testing in breast cancer. *Arch. Pathol. Lab. Med.* **2007**, *131*, 18–43. [PubMed]
28. Goldhirsch, A.; Winer, E.P.; Coates, A.S.; Gelber, R.D.; Piccart-Gebhart, M.; Thürlimann, B.; Senn, H.J.; Panel Members. Personalizing the treatment of women with early breast cancer: Highlights of the St Gallen International Expert Consensus on the Primary Therapy of Early Breast Cancer 2013. *Ann. Oncol.* **2013**, *24*, 2206–2223. [CrossRef] [PubMed]
29. Filice, S.; Castellucci, G.; Croce, D.; Basili, R. KeLP: A Kernel-based Learning Platform for Natural Language Processing. In Proceedings of the ACL-IJCNLP 2015 System Demonstrations, Beijing, China, 26–31 July 2015; pp. 19–24.

9

Nucleotide Weight Matrices Reveal Ubiquitous Mutational Footprints of AID/APOBEC Deaminases in Human Cancer Genomes

Igor B. Rogozin [1,*,†], Abiel Roche-Lima [2,†], Artem G. Lada [3,†], Frida Belinky [1], Ivan A. Sidorenko [4], Galina V. Glazko [5], Vladimir N. Babenko [4], David N. Cooper [6] and Youri I. Pavlov [7,8,*]

1 National Center for Biotechnology Information, National Library of Medicine, National Institutes of Health, Bethesda, MD 20894-6075, USA; frida.belinky@gmail.com

2 Center for Collaborative Research in Health Disparities–RCMI Program, Medical Sciences Campus, University of Puerto Rico, San Juan, PR 00936, USA; abiel.roche@upr.edu

3 Department Microbiology and Molecular Genetics, University of California, Davis, CA 95616, USA; alada@ucdavis.edu

4 Institute of Cytology and Genetics, Novosibirsk 630090, Russia; vanyasidorenko22@gmail.com (I.A.S.); babenko@yahoo.com (V.N.B.)

5 Department of Biomedical Informatics, University of Arkansas for Medical Sciences, Little Rock, AR 72205, USA; GVGlazko@uams.edu

6 Institute of Medical Genetics, Cardiff University, Cardiff CF14 4AY, UK; CooperDN@cardiff.ac.uk

7 Departments of Microbiology and Pathology; Biochemistry and Molecular Biology; Genetics, Cell Biology and Anatomy, University of Nebraska Medical Center, Omaha, NE 68198, USA

8 Eppley Institute for Research in Cancer and Allied Diseases, Omaha, NE 68198, USA

* Correspondence: rogozin@ncbi.nlm.nih.gov (I.B.R.); ypavlov@unmc.edu (Y.I.P.)

† These authors contributed equally.

Abstract: Cancer genomes accumulate nucleotide sequence variations that number in the tens of thousands per genome. A prominent fraction of these mutations is thought to arise as a consequence of the off-target activity of DNA/RNA editing cytosine deaminases. These enzymes, collectively called activation induced deaminase (AID)/APOBECs, deaminate cytosines located within defined DNA sequence contexts. The resulting changes of the original C:G pair in these contexts (mutational signatures) provide indirect evidence for the participation of specific cytosine deaminases in a given cancer type. The conventional method used for the analysis of mutable motifs is the consensus approach. Here, for the first time, we have adopted the frequently used weight matrix (sequence profile) approach for the analysis of mutagenesis and provide evidence for this method being a more precise descriptor of mutations than the sequence consensus approach. We confirm that while mutational footprints of APOBEC1, APOBEC3A, APOBEC3B, and APOBEC3G are prominent in many cancers, mutable motifs characteristic of the action of the humoral immune response somatic hypermutation enzyme, AID, are the most widespread feature of somatic mutation spectra attributable to deaminases in cancer genomes. Overall, the weight matrix approach reveals that somatic mutations are significantly associated with at least one AID/APOBEC mutable motif in all studied cancers.

Keywords: DNA sequence profile; Monte Carlo; mixture of normal distributions; somatic mutation; tumor; mutable motif; activation induced deaminase; AID/APOBEC

1. Introduction

The sequencing of genomes of solid tumors and liquid malignancies associated with different types and stages of cancer has revealed a plethora of genetic changes, from nucleotide substitutions and insertions/deletions to chromosomal rearrangements and chromosome copy number alterations [1–3]. As predicted decades ago by the mutator theory of cancer [4], the elevated mutability in tumors contributes both to their onset and to their further evolution. The underlying causes of this mutagenesis are diverse, from the appearance of mutator mutations to DNA damage by intrinsic or environmental mutagens (e.g., oxidative stress, tobacco smoke, UV light, etc.) [5]. Somatic genome instability leads to the activation of oncogenes and inactivation of tumor suppressors and helps tumor cells to emerge, proliferate, elude immune surveillance, and acquire resistance to anticancer drugs.

In some cancers, the number of single nucleotide variations (SNVs) is in the order of tens of thousands per genome. A few driver mutations [6,7] ultimately lead to cancer, while the role, if any, of the vast majority of mutations, termed "passengers", during tumor development is poorly understood [8,9]. One crucial principle stands out: mutations can be classified into 'families' based upon their flanking DNA sequences [10,11]. Different mutagenic processes generate mutations within different contexts of a neighboring nucleotide sequence (the bases upstream and/or downstream of the mutations, termed "mutation signatures"). Sophisticated approaches have been developed to extract the most prominent signatures from a complex mix of mutational targets resulting from the action of a variety of mutagens, both exogenous and endogenous, operating during tumor evolution [12,13]. Both driver and passenger mutations have been used in the analysis. One of the clearest mutational signatures, found in breast and other cancers [14,15], is characterized by C:G to T:A or C:G to G:C substitutions that are found predominantly in the 5′-TC sequence motif (signatures #2 and 13; listed in the COSMIC database). These signatures have been attributed to the action of nucleic acid-editing enzymes, cytosine deaminases. These enzymes, collectively called APOBECs, deaminate cytosine in single-stranded DNA, yielding uracil. DNA replication past the uracil leads to the insertion of A, thereby giving rise to the C-to-T transition. Also, abasic sites that are produced as intermediates of uracil repair are bypassed by the cytidine transferase activity of REV1 translesion DNA polymerase, leading to C:G to G:C transversions. Cytosine deaminases possess inherent sequence specificity. Thus, for example, activation induced deaminase (AID) prefers to deaminate within 5′-WRC motifs (W = A or T, R = A or G), whereas APOBEC3G acts preferentially on the last cytosine in the 5′-CCC motif, while two other APOBEC3 enzymes, APOBEC3A and APOBEC3B, exhibit a preference for 5′-TC sequences. Another prominent feature of APOBEC enzymes is their ability to act in a processive fashion, i.e., to catalyze multiple deamination events per substrate-binding event [16], thereby inducing kataegis (clustered mutations); however, it should be noted that APOBEC action is only one possible explanation for kataegis in cancer cells [17]. Mutational signatures of cytosine deaminases are detected in many cancers [15]. It is unlikely to be a mere coincidence that the APOBEC3 enzymes are frequently upregulated in tumors [18,19]. It should be noted that if deaminases act on 5-methylcytosine generating "T", a specialized G:T mismatch repair mechanism operates, and the genetic consequences could be different because of the disappearance of an epigenetic mark [20]. There is evidence for the contribution of this process to cancer [21].

Cancer genome studies necessitate working with huge datasets; the obvious problems posed by the analysis of such data are partially solved by the advent of the "mutational signature" technique [12,22,23]. It is not usually possible to define the DNA strand upon which the vast majority of mutations has occurred (but see [24,25]); for example, both a C>T change on one strand and a G>A change on the opposite strand lead to the same CG to TA transition. Therefore, in practice, the analysis may be reduced to the study of only six different types of substitution. Similarly, there are 96 context-dependent mutations (mutation types) that consider two nucleotides in the flanking 5′ and 3′ positions of the mutated nucleotide [23]. Analysis of the mutational spectra of context-dependent mutations in cancer genomes involves pooling all the mutations from cancer samples into a discrete distribution according to the mutation types, while further analysis involves the so-called non-negative matrix factorization (NMF) method [12,22,23]. There are some variations of this basic technique; indeed, Temiz et al. [26] presented a 32 × 12 mutation matrix, which captures the nucleotide pattern two nucleotides upstream and downstream of each mutation. In this study, a somatic autosomal mutation matrix (SAMM) representing tumor-specific mutations and mechanistic template mutation matrices (MTMMs) representing oxidative DNA damage, ultraviolet-induced DNA damage, (5m)CpG deamination, and APOBEC-mediated cytosine mutation were constructed. MTMMs were mapped to the individual tumor SAMMs to identify mutational mechanisms corresponding to each overall mutational pattern. The method appeared to be sensitive enough to retrospectively allocate the origins of tumors to specific tissues [26].

In an attempt to increase the specificity and sensitivity of the arsenal of techniques available for mutation analysis in whole genomes, we have employed mutable motifs of cytosine deaminases represented in the form of weight matrices (sequence profiles) [27–29]. This approach may be expected to be a more general descriptor of nucleotide sequences as compared to the sequence consensus approach, because it takes into account the variability in the information content ("conservation") across neighboring positions. Control experiments using various constrained samples of randomly selected sequences indicated that the level of false positives obtained using this approach is even lower than the expected false discovery rate (~0.05, see Sections 4.5–4.8 for details). These analyses suggest that the weight matrices method is a powerful tool for the analysis of genomic mutations. Further, we identified prominent mutational footprints of APOBECA and APOBECB in many human cancers. Mutable motifs attributable to AID are less pronounced but are nevertheless present ubiquitously in cancer genomes.

2. Results

2.1. *Weight Matrices of AID/APOBEC Mutable Motifs*

The information content of AID/APOBEC mutable motifs is shown in Figure 1 (the list and sources of the mutated sequences are shown in Supplementary Table S1). AID/APOBEC cytosine deaminases exhibit substantial variability in terms of their mutable motifs. T in position −1 (number 5 in Figure 1) was the most prominent feature of the APOBEC1, APOBEC3A, and APOBEC3B enzymes, consistent with previous studies (reviewed in [23]). APOBEC3C has a distinct mutable motif with T in position −2. Additionally, APOBEC1 has an excess of T in position −3 (number 3 in Figure 1).

APOBEC3G has a distinct mutation pattern wcCCw (lower case w and c mean substantially lower information content as compared with the upper case, Figure 1), which is a variation of the previously described CCC motif and CCR motif [7,30]. The AID deaminase has the expected context specificity, WRC [16,31].

It is hard to demarcate the mutational signatures of APOBECs using the consensus approach due to the high variability of information content across sites. For example, APOBEC3G has a highly conserved C in positions −4 and −5; however, there is also a less conserved C (and lower information content) in position −3 that may or may not be included in a consensus sequence (Figure 1). We opted to employ the widely used weight matrix technique (see Section 4) in order to avoid uncertainties with the less informative positions.

We compared the nucleotide composition of mutation sites (±5 nucleotides, Supplemental Figure S1) for all the studied AID/APOBEC proteins using the χ^2 test (Table 1). We found that all six AID/APOBEC proteins studied were significantly different with respect to the DNA sequence context of the mutation sites expressed in the form of nucleotide frequency matrices (Table 1). Thus, weight matrices properly represent the DNA sequence context of mutations induced by various AID/APOBEC proteins, as noted in previous studies [5] where a simple consensus approach was used. We aimed to differentiate between the mutable motifs associated with the various AID/APOBEC proteins, although this was not always possible (for example, the sequence contexts of the APOBEC3A, APOBEC3B, and APOBEC3C targets are not as different as other pairwise comparisons, see Table 1).

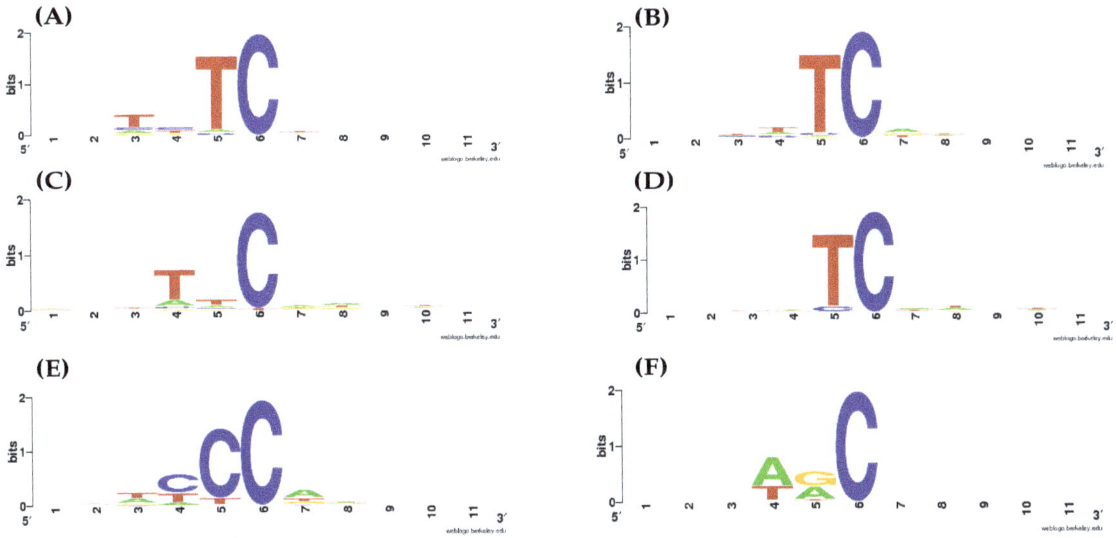

Figure 1. Information content and derived consensus sequences of the DNA context of mutations induced by AID/APOBEC deaminases in yeast genomes (frequencies of nucleotides were used as input). (**A**) APOBEC1, (**B**) APOBEC3A, (**C**) APOBEC3C, (**D**) APOBEC3B, (**E**) APOBEC3G, and (**F**) AID. Position 6 is the position of the somatic mutations. AID/APOBEC weight matrices are shown in Supplementary Figure S1.

Table 1. Pairwise differences between the DNA context (position-specific nucleotide frequencies across ±5 surrounding bases) of the studied AID/APOBEC proteins.

	AID	APOBEC3G	APOBEC3C	APOBEC3B	APOBEC3A
APOBEC1	1986.8	2299.2	203.2	378.6	344.1
APOBEC3A	1674.4	2057.0	138.4	175.7	
APOBEC3B	1764.5	2316.8	175.7		
APOBEC3C	237.2	327.5			
APOBEC3G	2711.8				

The critical χ^2 values = 71.1 (after Bonferroni correction $P = 0.05/15 = 0.0033$, degrees of freedom = 42). The χ^2 test was applied to raw numbers of nucleotides.

We performed four control experiments (for details, see Sections 4.5–4.8): (1) analysis of the sequence context of somatic mutations in mitochondrial DNA as a negative control [32]; (2) analysis of the correlation between the matrices of shuffled sites of mutations and the sites of somatic mutation in cancer cells using the expected false discovery rate approach [33]; (3) analysis of the correlation between matrices of randomly sampled sites from the yeast genome and somatic mutations in cancer cells using the expected false discovery rate approach [33]; and (4) analysis of somatic mutations in human immunoglobulin genes as a positive control [34–36]. The results of all four control experiments (Supplementary Tables S2–S5) strongly support our contention that the weight matrix technique is applicable to the studied AID/APOBECs (for details, see Section 4).

2.2. Analysis of the Correlation between AID/APOBEC Mutable Motifs and Somatic Mutations in Cancer Cells: C:G>T:A Transitions

We examined the correlation of the sites of C:G>T:A mutations in cancers and AID/APOBEC mutable motifs. A correlation between a mutable motif and the DNA context of somatic mutations from the COSMIC database was claimed when the results of two statistical tests (Monte Carlo test and *t*-test, see Section 4) were both significant. A correlation between the mutable motifs of (at least one) deaminase(s) and the sites of somatic C:G>T:A mutations was found for all cancer tissues (Figure 2 and

Supplementary Table S6). AID activity was the most ubiquitous according to the enzyme characteristic signature in various cancer types, whereas the APOBEC1, APOBEC3A, APOBEC3B, and APOBEC3G signatures were detected less frequently, although their signatures were stronger, most notably in breast, lung, cervix, skin, and bladder cancer (Figure 2).

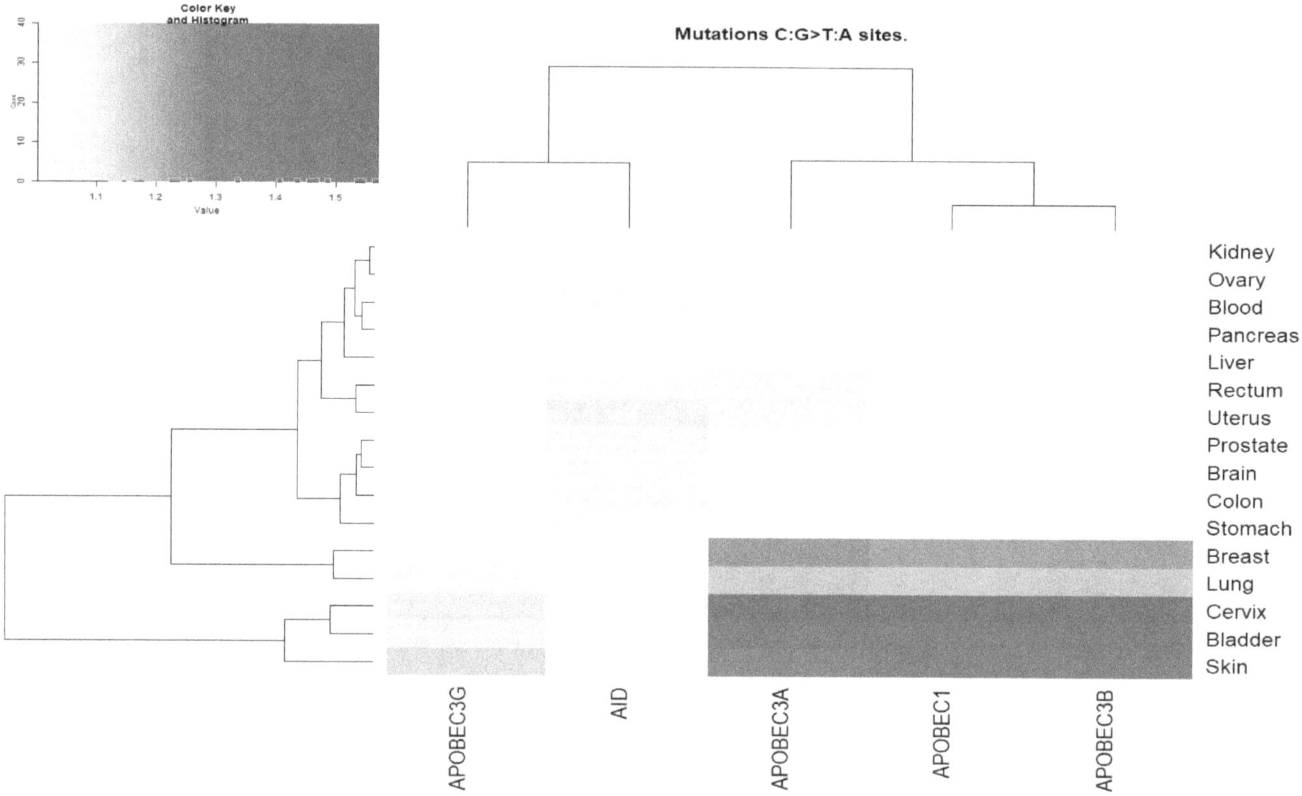

Figure 2. Correlation between AID/APOBEC mutable motifs and the sequence context of somatic C:G>T:A mutations. For the actual data, see Supplementary Table S6. The intensities of the gray color correspond to the ratio values (the ratio being the mean weight of the mutated sites divided by the mean weight of the non-mutated sites). The unweighted pair group method with arithmetic mean (UPGMA) clustering of ratio values for the AID/APOBEC footprints and tissues is shown as dendrograms.

We attempted to estimate the fraction of somatic mutations associated with AID/APOBEC deamination using a mixture of two normal distributions (see Sections 3 and 4 for details). For example, estimated fractions of APOBEC1-associated mutations (0.66, 0.48, 0.74, 0.39, and 0.62) look consistent with the smallest value of 0.39 corresponding to the lowest ratio value (1.064, APOBEC1, lung), although this method sometimes yielded potentially underestimated values (0.17, APOBEC3G, cervix, ratio = 1.113) and overestimated values (0.92, APOBEC3G, bladder, ratio = 1.101) (Supplementary Table S6). The overall distribution of fractions for APOBEC1, APOBEC3A, ABOPECB, and AID deaminases is shown in Supplementary Figure S2. The mean of the fractions in Figure S2 is 0.42 (Supplementary Table S6). This result suggests that a substantial proportion of somatic mutations is associated with AID/APOBEC mutagenesis.

2.3. Analysis of the Correlation between AID/APOBEC Mutable Motifs and Somatic Mutations in Cancer Cells: C:G>G:C and C:G>A:T Transversions

Many C:G > G:C transversions were suggested to be the result of processing abasic sites after the removal of uracils originating via DNA deamination by AID/APOBEC proteins [37]. Consistent with this idea, a significant correlation of these mutations with mutable motifs was found in many cancers (Figure 3 and Supplementary Table S7). The transversions associated with APOBEC1,

APOBEC3A, and APOBEC3B were found to be more abundant in comparison with APOBEC3G and AID, suggesting a role of these three deaminases in generating C:G>G:C somatic mutations in human cancer. The correlation with the three APOBEC motifs was again strongest for breast, bladder, cervix, and lung cancer.

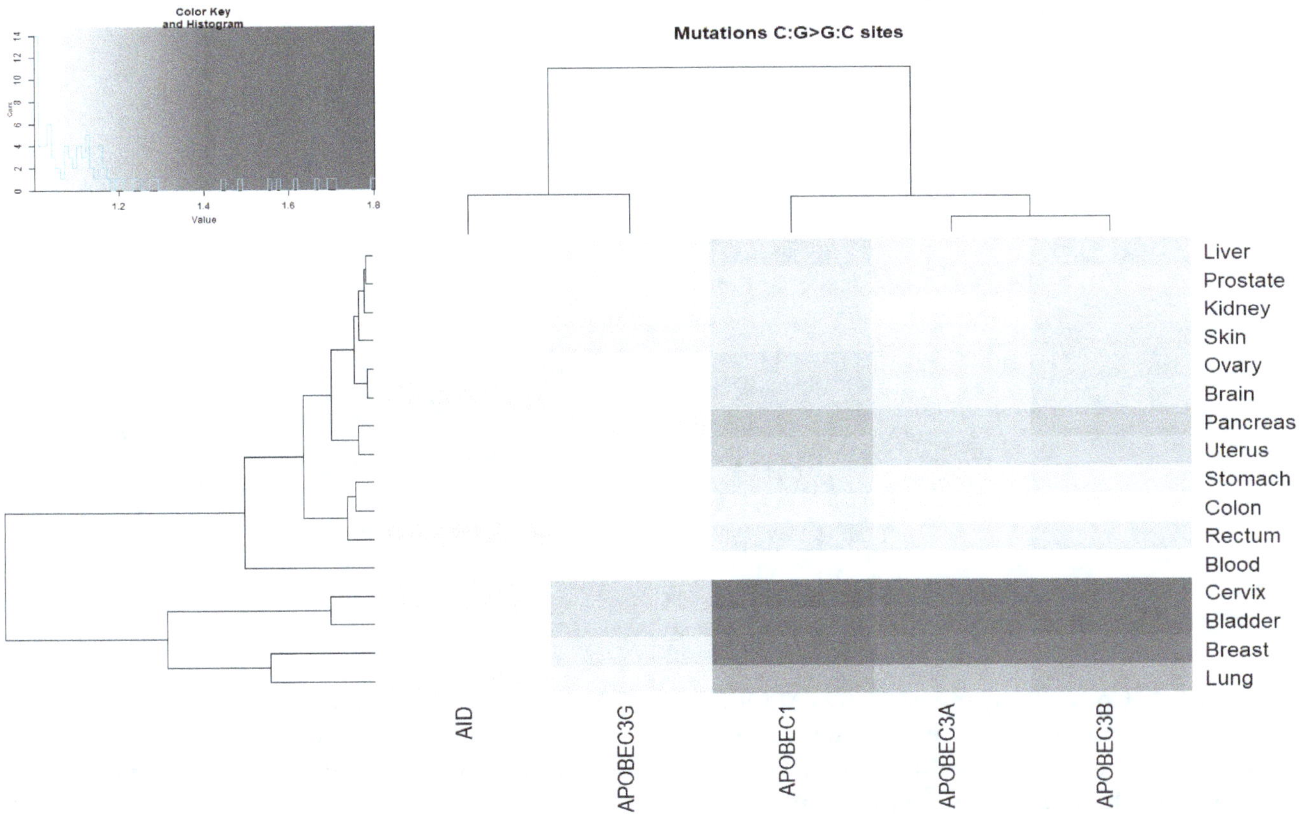

Figure 3. Correlation between AID/APOBEC mutable motifs and the sequence context of somatic C:G>G:C mutations. For actual data, see Supplementary Table S7. The intensities of the gray color correspond to the ratio values (the ratio being the mean weight of the mutated sites divided by the mean weight of the non-mutated sites).

Although it has been proposed that C:G>A:T mutations are a less likely outcome of AID/APOBEC enzymatic action, we found a significant excess of these transversions in many cancers (Figure 4 and Supplementary Table S8), suggesting that a significant portion of C:G>A:T mutations may be caused by processes initiated by deamination by AID/APOBEC enzymes. That the APOBEC3A, APOBEC3B, and APOBEC3G footprints are more abundant in comparison with the APOBEC1 and AID motifs suggests an important role for these three deaminases in generating somatic C:G>A:T mutations in human cancers.

The unweighted pair group method with arithmetic mean (UPGMA) clustering of ratio values for AID/APOBEC footprints and tissues (Figures 2–4) suggests that AID/APOBEC3G form one clade, whereas APOBEC1/3A/3B form another clade according to the distributions of the ratios across tissues (graphs above heatmaps at Figures 2–4). This can be explained by the high similarity of APOBEC1/3A/3B signatures (Figure 1). Breast, bladder, and colon tend to form a separate group according to the distributions of ratios across the AID/APOBEC footprints (graphs above heatmaps at Figures 2–4). In general, these classifications are not consistent, reflecting large variations in transition/transversion ratios (Supplementary Tables S6–S8) and are likely to be a result of variation in the efficiency of DNA repair of such sites in different tissues [5,36,38].

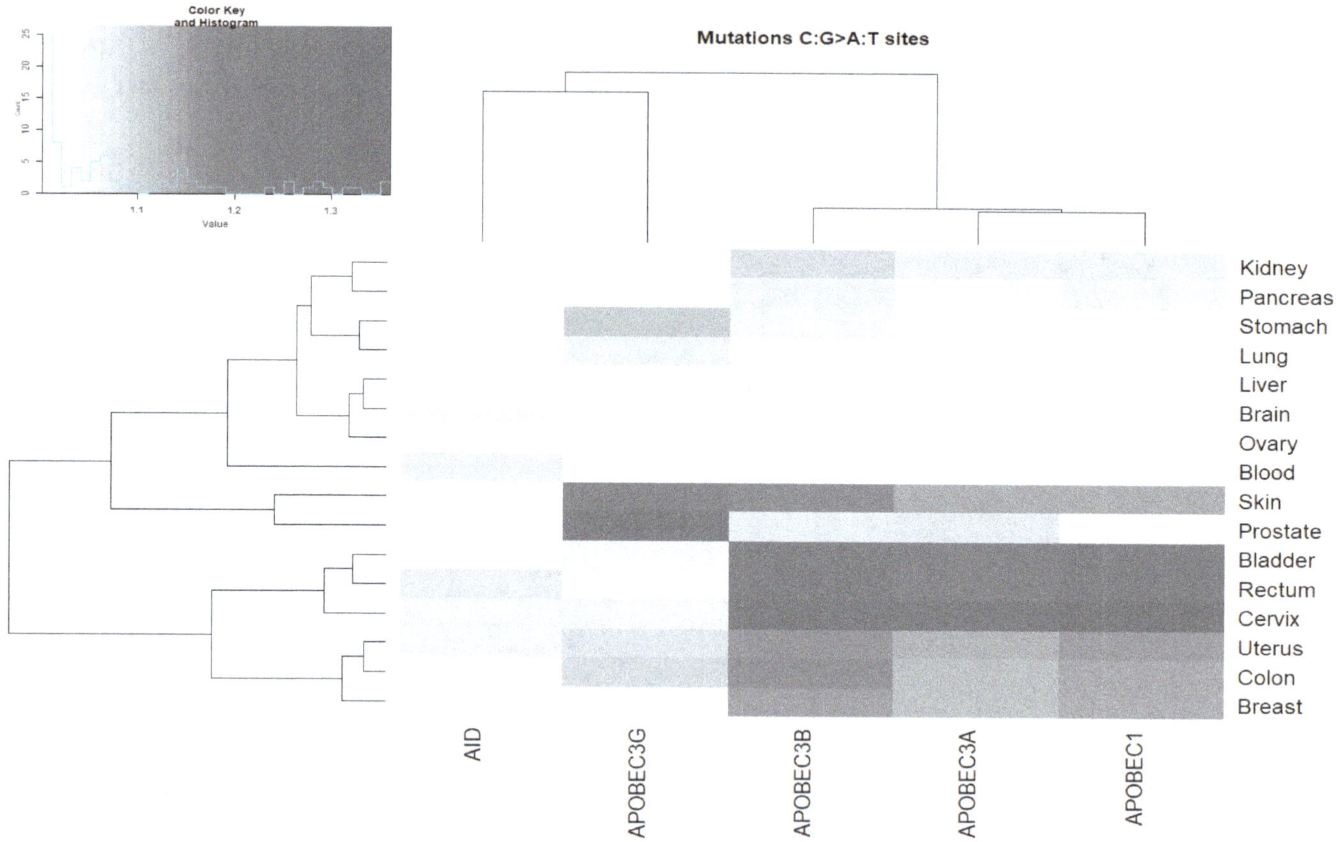

Figure 4. Correlation between AID/APOBEC mutable motifs and the sequence context of somatic C:G>A:T mutations. For actual data, see Supplementary Table S8. The intensities of the gray color correspond to the ratio values (the ratio being the mean weight of the mutated sites divided by the mean weight of the non-mutated sites).

2.4. Analysis of Various Tumor Types in Blood and Skin

Cancers of the blood system were found to be associated with AID and APOBEC3A (Figures 2–4 and Supplementary Tables S6–S8). No other putative associations with APOBEC enzymes were identified. We performed an analysis of two blood cancer subtypes with the highest representation in the COSMIC dataset (see Section 4): acute myeloid leukemia and germinal center B-cell-like (GCB) lymphomas (Table 2). A significant excess of somatic mutations in AID mutable motifs was detected in acute myeloid leukemia (Table 2). In GCB lymphomas, a significant excess of somatic mutations was detected in both AID and APOBEC3A mutable motifs (Table 2). These results suggest that there is variability of mutation context specificity across the same tissue, as seen previously [39].

We also performed an analysis of two skin cancer subtypes with the highest representation in the COSMIC dataset (see Section 4.3) (Table 2): skin cutaneous melanoma and skin adenocarcinoma. Both tumor types yielded somewhat similar results. An overwhelming excess of somatic mutations in APOBEC1 and APOBEC3A/B/G mutable motifs (Table 2) is likely to be due to the known excess of mutations in dipyrimidine dinucleotides (for example, TC) in skin cutaneous melanoma caused by mutagenic UV photoproducts [40]. Accordingly, we interpreted the excess of mutations in the AID/APOBEC3A/B/G contexts (Table 2) to be the result of false positives (as was already suggested by the results of the control experiments; for details, see Section 4.7), but we are also aware of evidence for the direct role of deaminases in skin cancer [41]. We observed a much lower excess of mutations in the mutable motifs observed in skin adenocarcinoma (Table 2). These results are likely to reflect the participation of AID/APOBEC deaminases in mutagenesis, because UV photoproducts do not play any role in the mutagenesis of skin adenocarcinomas [39]. Thus, APOBECs may play a role in a proportion of cases of squamous cell carcinoma [42].

Table 2. Correlation between AID/APOBEC mutable motifs and the context of somatic mutations in C:G sites in various blood and skin tumor types.

Cancer Tissue Type	Number of Mutations	Test	APOBEC1	APOBEC3A	APOBEC3B	APOBEC3G	AID
Blood: acute myeloid leukemia	6844	Ratio	0.920	0.978	0.958	0.977	1.031
		t-test	NSE #	NSE	NSE	NSE	**6.5** *
		MC test					<0.001
		Fraction					
Blood: GCB lymphomas	2747	Ratio	0.967	1.030	0.979	0.980	1.091
		t-test	NSE	**3.4** *	NSE	NSE	**12.3** *
		MC test		<0.001			<0.001
		Fraction		0.208			
Skin: cutaneous melanoma	235043	Ratio	1.388	1.308	1.334	1.138	1.026
		t-test	**321.3** *	**292.8** *	**344.6***	**176.2** *	**35.8** *
		MC test	<0.001	<0.001	<0.001	<0.001	<0.001
		Fraction	0.608		0.508	0.982	0.687
Skin: adeno-carcinoma	780	Ratio	1.045	1.073	1.088	1.075	1.025
		t-test	NSE	**4.4** *	**4.8** *	**4.6** *	NSE
		MC test		<0.001	<0.001	<0.001	
		Fraction		0.213			

#—NSE (no significant excess) indicates the absence of a significant excess of mutations in the mutable motifs, suggesting that there is no association between mutagenesis and the motifs. The significance of any excess was measured using the Student *t* and Monte Carlo (MC) tests. The bold font and asterisk (*) denote that the corresponding $P < 0.002$ (critical value = 3.1); this is a conservative estimate of the critical overall value of the *t*-test having allowed for multiple testing by means of the Bonferroni correction ($4 \times 6 = 24$). The "Ratio" is the mean weight of the mutated sites divided by the mean weight of the non-mutated sites. The predicted fraction of mutations induced by AID/APOBEC proteins ("Fraction") is shown when a significant excess of somatic mutations in the mutable motif comparisons was detected; all cases where there was a significant difference between the observed and expected distributions ($P > 0.05$) were discarded.

The mixture of two normal distributions yielded fairly predictable results (0.168–0.687, Table 2, see Section 2.2) except for the APOBEC3G mutable motifs in skin cutaneous melanoma samples where the fraction of sites potentially associated with the APOBEC3G mutable motifs is extremely large (0.982, Table 2). The distribution of weights for this case is shown in Figure 5A. A putative component (normal distribution) corresponding to the APOBEC3G mutable motifs (large weights, the rightmost distribution) was less obvious compared with Figure 5B, which can be classified as a reasonable result, because the fraction of sites potentially associated with the APOBEC1 mutable motifs (0.65) is close to the mean of the fractions estimated above (0.42, Supplementary Figure S2). This distorted normal distribution (another problem is a much larger number of sites in the last bin compared with the previous bin) may be a reason why two distributions (Figure 5A) were incorrectly classified (mixed together) yielding an obvious overestimate for the APOBEC3G mutable motifs (see Section 3). This is a known problem in classification analyses of this kind [43,44].

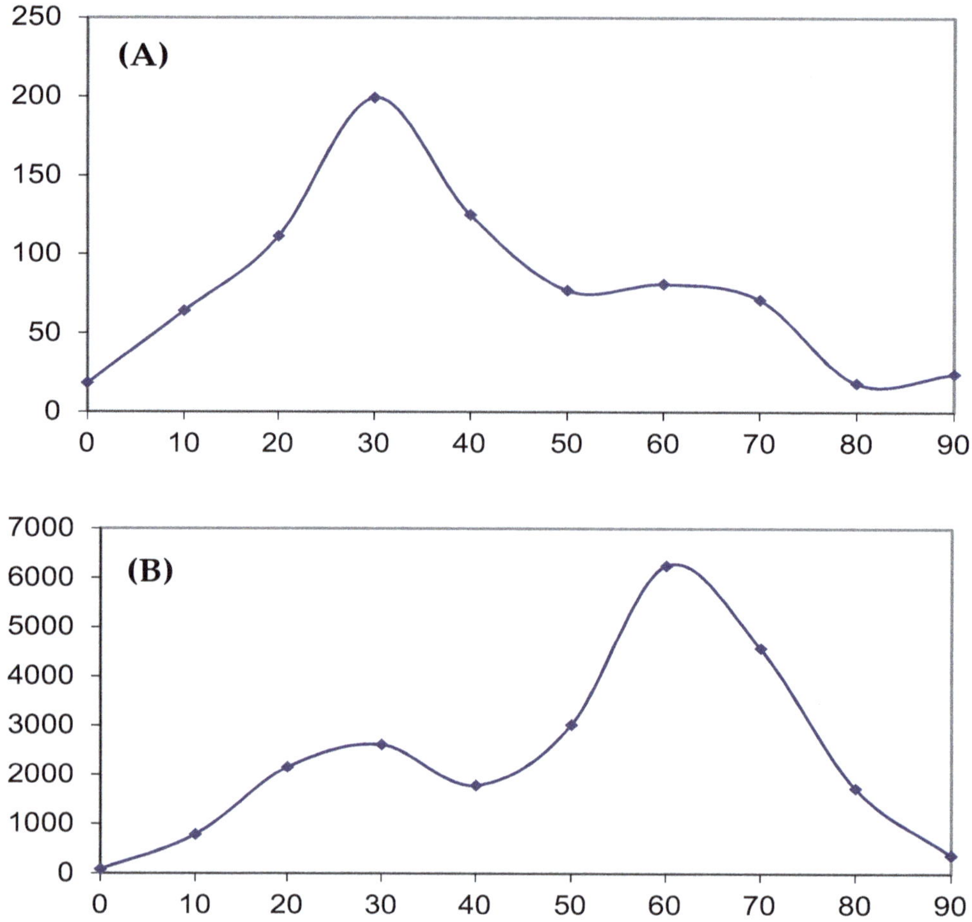

Figure 5. The weight distribution obtained using (**A**) the APOBEC3G weight matrix for skin adenocarcinoma (Table 2) and (**B**) the APOBEC1 weight matrix for bladder tissue (Supplementary Table S6). X axis: 0 stands for 0–9 interval of weights, 1 stands for the 10–19 interval, 2 stands for 20–29, etc.

3. Discussion

The advantage of our approach is that we used a unified computational technique that allowed an objective and accurate comparison of the mutational contribution of various APOBEC enzymes under the same experimental conditions and for the same datasets. We confirm that while the mutational footprints of APOBEC1, APOBEC3A, APOBEC3B, and APOBEC3G are prominent in many cancers, mutable motifs characteristic of the humoral immune response somatic hypermutation machine, AID, are the most widespread feature of the somatic mutation spectra attributed to APOBECs in cancer genomes. It is important to note that the suggested technique does not depend on expert opinion as to the exact consensus sequences and, therefore, objectively represents mutable motifs.

Somatic mutations in all 18 studied cancer types are significantly associated with at least one AID/APOBEC mutable motif. The blood subset of mutations stands apart because only AID mutable motifs are detected (Figures 2–4 and Table 2). Although there are significant differences between the contexts of AID/APOBEC-induced mutations manifested in frequency matrices (Table 1), there are many tissues where mutable sites have been found to be targeted by two or more deaminases (Figures 2–4). In such cases, we cannot reliably differentiate between different deaminases with similar mutable motifs (Figure 1). For example, the frequency matrices of APOBEC1, APOBEC3A, and APOBEC3B are quite similar to each other (Figure 1 and Table 1), and this represents a major problem. To resolve this issue, it may be possible to use additional information, for example, gene expression data. However, the addition of expression data was not particularly informative for the AID and DNA polymerase η mutational footprints [21,39]. The same conclusion was reached in several other studies, because the genomic level of cytosine deamination does not necessarily correlate with the expression of the corresponding AID/APOBEC genes [15,23,45]. For this reason, we did not attempt to compare expression data from different tissue types and relate these data to the results we obtained.

In order to take into account the differences in the base composition between the yeast and human genomes, we used the simplest normalization procedure by taking the frequencies of nucleotides in the non-informative positions −5, −4, +4, and +5 as a null model (Figure 1, see Section 4.7 for details). Although the control experiments suggest that this normalization tends to yield results that are consistent with our expectations (with the exception of bladder, cervix, and skin tumors; see Section 4.7), we cannot exclude the possibility that more sophisticated normalization schemes might be required to generate more accurate results.

In addition, the role of APOBEC3C in mutagenesis remains uncertain and requires further investigation. Another potential methodological problem (at least, for complex computational techniques) is that we have a "positive" set (sites of mutations: sites that contain characteristic features of mutable motifs) and do not have a "negative" set (sites of mutations: sites that do not contain characteristic features of mutable motifs). Randomly sampled sites from yeast chromosomes are far from being a good "negative" set, because distributions of mutations across yeast chromosomes are too sparse and may contain a lot of mutable motifs. This is not a problem for the weight matrix technique, which does not use negative sets as a part of its learning procedures. However, this is the major problem for more sophisticated methods. For example, it is an obstacle for the application of supervised learning methods (e.g., hidden Markov models or support vector machine), because the training of these artificial intelligence (AI) algorithms requires classified or labeled data. However, unsupervised learning methods (such as k-means clustering), which do not need classified data, may be applied to this problem. Another issue is the need to take into account the much higher A:T content of the mutation sites in the yeast genome as compared with the human genome; this should be implemented as a part of a learning procedure.

The results of all the control experiments and somatic mutations in cancers strongly suggest that the weight matrix technique is applicable to various types of mutational signatures. The suggested approach complimented with clustering techniques (Figures 2–4) allows for comparison between the studied enzymes and tissues. The suggested approach can be applied to various exciting questions in cancer genomics, including the underlying causes of the non-uniform distribution of somatic mutations across the human genome and asymmetries of mutagenesis with respect to leading/lagging and non-transcribed/transcribed DNA strands.

We estimated the impact of mutagenesis associated with AID/APOBEC deamination by representing distributions of weights as mixtures of two normal distributions. This approach is based on the method of estimating the protein coding density in a corpus of DNA sequence data, in which a 'protein-coding coding statistic' (which is similar to distributions of weights of somatic mutation contexts) is calculated for a large number of windows for the sequences under study, and the distribution of the statistic is decomposed into two normal distributions, assumed to be the distributions of the coding statistic in the coding and non-coding fractions of the sequence windows [43]. The distribution with the largest mean was assumed to reflect the fraction of protein coding fragments [43]. Similarly, the fraction of sites in a distribution with the largest mean was assumed to be the fraction of mutations induced by the AID/APOBEC enzymes. We noted problems with such an approach for some cases (see Section 2.4). However, the method tends to produce reasonable estimates. Rare deviations from normality caused by the natural boundaries of weight distributions (0 and 100, see the last bin in Figure 5A) is a possible explanation for the problems associated with the use of this classification technique in some cases.

Our analysis suggested that initial deamination events lead to both transitions and transversions. This is already known for somatic mutations initiated by AID in immunoglobulin genes and for APOBEC enzymes in cancer [5,38]. A large variation in transition/transversion ratios (Supplementary Tables S6–S8) is likely to be a result of peculiarities in the relative abundance of proper DNA substrates for deamination and the various efficiency of the DNA repair of such sites [5,36,38]. Overall, our results suggest that AID/APOBEC proteins make a major contribution to several different types of somatic mutations in cancer. The idea that APOBECs can be carcinogenic was originally proposed by Neuberger et al. in early 2000s [46], after the discovery that these proteins can edit DNA [47,48] and, therefore, are by definition mutators. Under normal conditions, deaminases are involved in adaptive (AID) and innate (APOBEC3s) immunity, lipid metabolism (APOBEC1), and possibly even active DNA demethylation [49–51] both in developing and in terminally differentiated cells. Extremely precise, tight, and complex (and therefore, not surprisingly, poorly understood) regulation of AID/APOBEC proteins ensures that in normal cells, they edit cytosines at very specific sites, such as immunoglobulin genes or viral DNA. However, when the regulatory constraints fail, these housekeepers can become much more promiscuous and edit DNA genome-wide.

The overexpression of active APOBECs is highly toxic in human cell lines [18,52], indicating that a precise balance of deaminase production and other factors is required in order to cause non-lethal genome-wide hypermutagenesis and kataegis. This is apparently also true in the case of APOBECs, where only a small fraction of cells with unfettered deaminases and a fine-tuned environment survive and give rise to malignant clones. It is also possible that the sudden overproduction of deaminases in tumor cells with genomes shaped by other mutagenic processes will kill the tumor by extensively damaging its genome, unless the tumor cells can protect themselves against APOBEC.

4. Materials and Methods

4.1. Mutations in Yeast Genomes

Coordinates and types of mutations induced by various APOBEC/AID proteins in yeast were obtained from previously published SNV datasets (see legend to Supplementary Table S1) [37,53–56]. To extract the sequence context of the mutations, we used the getfasta tool from the bedtools package (http://bedtools.readthedocs.org/en/latest/). These datasets are available upon request from I.B.R. The logo description of mutable motifs was constructed using the Weblogo website (http://weblogo.berkeley.edu/logo.cgi).

4.2. Analysis of Mutable Motifs

Several approaches have been developed for the analysis of a set of mutated sequences [27–29]. A mononucleotide weight matrix is a simple and straightforward way to present the structure of a functional signal and to calculate weights for the signal sequence. Each matrix includes information on a normalized frequency of A, T, G, C bases in each of the 10 positions surrounding the detected sites of mutation (5 bases downstream and 5 bases upstream). We calculated the weight matrices for 6f different AID/APOBEC mutational signatures in the yeast genome (Supplementary Table S1).

A simple formula for W(b,j) was used for data analysis: W(b,j) = log2[f(b,j)/e(b)], where f(b,j) is the observed frequency of the nucleotide b in position j and e(b,j) is the expected frequency of the nucleotide b in position j, calculated as the mean nucleotide frequencies of positions −5,−4, +4, +5 for sites of mutations in the yeast genome; the resulting W(b,i) matrices are shown in Supplementary Figure S1.

The matching score S(b1, ..., bL) of a sequence b1, ..., bL is as follows:

$$S(b1, \ldots, bL) = \sum_{j=1}^{L} W(b,j) \quad (1)$$

The matching score between sequence b1, ..., bL and a weight matrix can be further expressed as a percentage:

$$\%\ \text{matching score} = 100 \times (S(b1, \ldots, bL) - Smin)/(Smax - Smin) \quad (2)$$

$$Smin = \sum_{j=1}^{L} \min_{b} W(b,j) \qquad Smax = \sum_{j=1}^{L} \max_{b} W(b,j) \tag{3}$$

Hereafter, we use the term "weight" instead of "% matching score". We used the positions −3:+3 to estimate the weights of the sites.

In addition to the analyses of AID/APOBEC mutational signatures in cancer genomes, we performed a control experiment: we randomly shuffled a dataset of AID/APOBEC contexts in the yeast genome (Supplementary Table S1), keeping position 6 (the position of mutations) intact. Each sequence was shuffled separately; thus, the overall base composition and the base compositions of each sequence were the same. We also performed another control experiment: we randomly extracted sequences from the yeast genome, maintaining the nucleotide composition and the size of sequence sets for each set of mutation sites with AID/APOBEC-induced mutations. Weight matrices were derived from these sampled sites. Where there was a significant difference between an extracted set and the analyzed set (the 2-tailed *t*-test), the sampling procedure was repeated.

4.3. Datasets and Analysis of Somatic Mutations

Somatic mutation data from the ICGC and TCGA cancer genome projects were extracted from the Sanger COSMIC Whole Genome Project v75 (http://cancer.sanger.ac.uk/wgs). The ICGC/TCGA datasets are almost exclusively passenger mutations, and they are unlikely to be subject to selection to promote cellular proliferation. Thus, they are more likely to reflect the original AID/APOBEC mutational spectrum [23]. The tissues and cancer types were defined according to the primary tumor site and the cancer project in question [12,13]. A dataset of somatic mutations in mitochondrial DNA in various cancer types was extracted from [32]. In this set, no excess of mutations in known mutable motifs is to be expected, because the mutation landscape in mitochondrial DNA is shaped by its very specific mode of replication [32]. The mitochondrial mutation set can, therefore, be used as a negative control.

DNA sequences surrounding the mutated nucleotide represent the mutation context. We compared the frequency of known mutable motifs for somatic mutations with the frequency of these motifs in the vicinity of the mutated nucleotide. Specifically, for each base substitution, the 121 bp sequence centered at the mutation was extracted (the DNA neighborhood). We used only the nucleotides immediately flanking the mutations, because the AID/APOBEC enzymes are thought to scan a very limited region of DNA to deaminate (methyl)cytosines in a preferred motif [16,57,58]. This approach does not exclude any specific area of the genome, but rather uses the areas within each sample where mutagenesis has occurred (taking into account the variability in the mutation rates across the human genome) and then evaluates whether the mutagenesis in these samples were enriched for AID/APOBEC motifs [58]. This approach was thoroughly tested, and the high accuracy of the analysis was demonstrated [58]. The mean weight of the mutable motifs (Supplementary Figure S1) in the positions of somatic mutations was compared to the mean weight of the same motifs in the DNA neighborhood using the *t*-test (2-tail test) and Monte Carlo test (MC, 1-tail test) similar to the consensus method, as previously described [58].

4.4. Impact of AID/APOBEC Mutagenesis

In order to estimate the proportion of mutated sites that are likely to be caused by the AID/APOBEC enzymes, we applied a mixture model of two normal distributions [43] to distributions of weights of somatic mutation contexts. An example of such a distribution is shown in Figure 5B. This approach is based on the method of estimating the protein coding density in a corpus of DNA sequence data, in which a 'protein-coding coding statistic' (which is similar to distributions of weights of somatic mutation contexts) is calculated for a large number of windows of the sequence under study. The distribution of the statistic is decomposed into two normal distributions and assumed to be distributions of the coding statistic in the coding and non-coding fractions of the sequence windows [43]. The distribution with the largest mean was assumed to reflect the fraction of protein coding fragments [43]. Similarly, the fraction of sites in a distribution with the largest mean was assumed to be the fraction of mutations induced by the AID/APOBEC enzymes. The results were considered to be reliable only if no significant difference was found between the observed and expected distributions according to the χ^2 test. The suggested classification approach for normal distributions had been tested by Fickett and Guigo and showed good accuracy [43]. All the details of the suggested methodology and underlined statistical Bayesian framework were previously described for analyses of normal and binomial distributions [43,44].

Heatmap visualization analysis for each of the AID/APOBEC pseudo-mutable motifs groups was performed. The R (https://www.R-project.org/) software package heatmap.2 (https://CRAN.R-project.org/package=gplots) was employed to generate the heatmaps for each group. For each group, a specific range of values was established in grayscale representation, from the lowest values to the highest values. For the pseudo-mutable motifs in somatic mutation in the C:G sites group, the range was from 0.01 to 0.84 with intervals between 0.05. Values <0.01 were denoted as white. For the pseudo-mutable motifs in somatic mutation in the C:G>T:A sites group, the range was from 1 to 1.573 with intervals between 0.01. Values <1 were denoted as white. For the pseudo-mutable motifs in somatic mutation in the C:G>C:G sites group, the range was from 1 to 1.802 with intervals between 0.01. Values <1 were denoted as white. For the pseudo-mutable motifs in somatic mutation in the C:G>A:T sites group, the range was from 1 to 1.362 with intervals between 0.02. Values <1 were denoted as white.

4.5. Control Experiment 1: Analysis of Somatic Mutations in Mitochondrial DNA

In the first control experiment, we analyzed the sequence context of somatic mutations in mitochondrial DNA. In this set, no excess of mutations in known mutable motifs was to be expected, because the mutation landscape in mitochondrial DNA is shaped by its very specific mode of replication [32]. Thus, the mitochondrial mutation set can be used as a negative control. No significant excess of AID/APOBEC mutable motifs was found (Supplementary Table S2). This is consistent with a previous study [32]. In all the studied tissues, the ratio of the mean weight of the mutated sites vs. the mean weight of the non-mutated sites was less than or close to 1; this is expected when there is no correlation between mutable motifs and mutation (Supplementary Table S2). We observed only a single case where the Monte Carlo test yielded a significant P-value ($P = 0.031$, APOBEC3B/brain), but this result was not confirmed by use of the *t*-test and is likely to be an isolated false positive. Thus, the weight matrix appears to be a reliable method for the analysis of somatic mutations.

4.6. Control Experiment 2: Correlation between the Matrices of Shuffled Sites of Mutations and the Sites of Somatic Mutation in Cancer Cells

In order to allow for differences in nucleotide content between the yeast and human genomes, we used normalized weight matrices (see above). To test the robustness of the normalization, a simple control experiment was designed: we randomly shuffled the sequences of the AID/APOBEC mutation sites (Supplementary Table S1). We identified rare cases of a significant deviation from the expected value of the ratio (1.0, the ratio is the mean weight of the mutated sites divided by the mean weight of the non-mutated sites), but those cases constituted only 2.6% of all the studied cases (Supplementary Table S3). This result establishes that the weight matrix technique yields an expected proportion of false positives (the expected false discovery rate should be around 5% according to the standard in the field [33]) and hence is robust with respect to the biased nucleotide composition of mutated sites in the yeast genome. However, the results for colon, skin, and stomach cancers may not be reliable for some APOBECs (the fractions of false positives were found to be large, for example, 0.96 for APOBEC3C/skin; Supplementary Table S3). In general, the APOBEC3C weight matrix tends to yield the largest number of false positives, suggesting that this matrix might be problematic. We conclude that such controls should always be performed when starting work with a new mutation set.

4.7. Control Experiment 3: Correlation between Matrices of Randomly Sampled Sites from the Yeast Genome and Somatic Mutations in Cancer Cells

To check for a potential influence of nucleotide content biases and the extent of a correlation between positions in yeast and human genomes, we randomly extracted sequences from the yeast genome, maintaining the nucleotide composition and size of sequence sets for each set of mutation sites. Weight matrices were derived from these sampled sites. We identified numerous examples of a substantial deviation from the expected values that produced significant results that should be considered to be false positives (Figure 6 and Supplementary Table S4), because we did not expect any meaningful association between randomly sampled sites and somatic mutations. The APOBEC3C weight matrix yielded a large number of significant yet spurious results (false positives) for all the studied tissues (Figure 6 and Supplementary Table S4) and therefore cannot be recommended for the analysis of somatic mutation. This effect may have been due to the much smaller number of mutations in the dataset, a lack of highly informative positions and a high A/T content of sites for APOBEC3C (Figure 1). The results for APOBEC3C are likely to be false positives in this and previous control experiments and were included in the Supplementary Materials only.

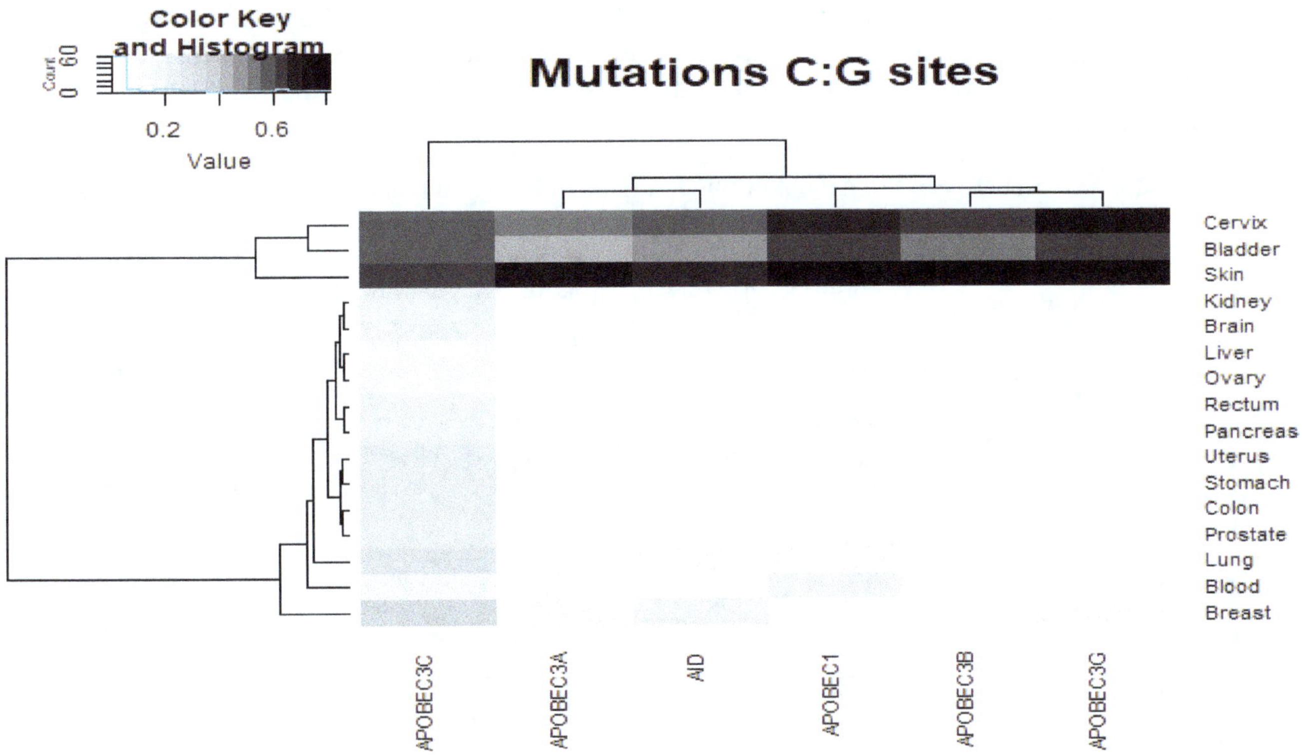

Figure 6. Fraction of random matrices with a significant correlation between AID/APOBEC pseudo-mutable motifs (randomly sampled sites from the yeast genome) and the sequence context of somatic mutations in C:G sites. For the actual data, see Supplementary Table S2. The intensities of the gray color correspond to the fractions of cases with a significant correlation between pseudo-mutable motifs (represented as weight matrices) and the context of somatic mutations in C:G sites.

The analysis of mutations in various tissues suggested that the weight matrix technique may also produce misleading results for bladder, cervix, and skin tumors (Figure 6). The skin tissue consistently produced a high rate of false positives in control experiments 3 and 4; thus, weight matrices should be used with great caution for this tissue. The analysis of nucleotide frequencies for the region ± 3 suggested that skin, cervix, and bladder tumors are characterized by a high frequency of T nucleotides around the sites of mutation (Supplementary Table S5), and this is likely to be a reason for the high rate of false positives. It should be noted that other techniques are also likely to produce a high rate of false positives for these tissues, although this type of control experiment has, to our knowledge, never been performed before except for analysis of somatic mutations in normal tissues [21]. The likely reason for high rates of false positives is that APOBEC mutable motifs tend to be A/T-rich (even C-rich APOBEC3G sites contain excessive amounts of A and T nucleotides in positions −3, +1, +2, and +3; Figure 1 and Supplementary Figure S1). We attempted to take this into account by removing sites with a high A/T content (≥50% A+T in the 10-nucleotide region around sites of somatic mutations, Supplementary Table S4). Although there was a substantial improvement in the accuracy of prediction (rates of false positives were much smaller, Supplementary Table S4), problems with the accuracy of prediction for skin tumors persisted (Supplementary Table S4).

4.8. Control Experiment 4: Analysis of Somatic Mutations in Human Immunoglobulin Genes

Somatic mutations in human immunoglobulin genes are known to be associated with AID mutable motifs [35], and these mutations can be used as a positive control set. Indeed, a significant association between the AID mutable motif and mutations was found in all three studied sets of somatic mutations [34,35] (Table 3), suggesting that the AID weight matrix is a reliable descriptor of AID-induced mutagenesis. The APOBEC1/3A/3B/3G weight matrices did not, however, yield significant results for all the studied cases (Table 3). This is consistent with the absence of any traces of APOBEC1/3A/3B/3G-induced mutation in the somatic hypermutation profiles of immunoglobulin genes [36]. The results of all four control experiments suggested that the weight matrix technique is applicable to studied APOBECs.

Table 3. Correlation between the AID/APOBEC mutable motifs and the sequence context of somatic mutations in fragments of human immunoglobulin genes.

Locus	Number of Mutations	Test	APOBEC1	APOBEC3A	APOBEC3B	APOBEC3G	AID
V_H26	708	Ratio	0.931	0.986	0.919	0.908	1.162
		t-test	NSE #	NSE	NSE	NSE	**11.1** *
		MC test					<0.001
		Fraction					0.477
J_H4 intron, control individuals	177	Ratio	0.927	0.957	0.887	0.870	1.331
		t-test	NSE	NSE	NSE	NSE	**11.9** *
		MC test					<0.001
		Fraction					0.559
J_H4 intron, XP-V patients	235	Ratio	0.981	1.008	0.957	0.930	1.266
		t-test	NSE	NSE	NSE	NSE	**9.6** *
		MC test					<0.001
		Fraction					0.366

#—NSE (no significant excess) indicates the absence of a significant excess of mutations in mutable motifs, suggesting that there is no association between mutagenesis and the motifs. The significance of any excess was measured using the Student *t* and Monte Carlo (MC) tests. The bold font and asterisk (*) denote that the corresponding $P <$ 0.003 (critical value = 3.1); this is a conservative estimate of the critical overall value of the *t*-test having allowed for multiple testing by means of the Bonferroni correction ($3 \times 6 = 18$). The "Ratio" is the mean weight of the mutated sites divided by the mean weight of the non-mutated sites. The predicted fraction of mutations induced by the AID/APOBEC proteins ("Fraction") is shown when a significant excess of somatic mutations in the mutable motif comparisons was detected; all the cases where there was a significant difference between the observed and expected distributions ($P > 0.05$) were discarded.

5. Conclusions

For the first time, we have adopted the weight matrix (sequence profile) approach for the analysis of mutations in cancer genomes, and we provide evidence for this method being a more precise descriptor of mutations than the commonly used sequence consensus approach. Control experiments using shuffled sites and constrained samples of randomly sampled sequences from the yeast genome yielded a low level of false positives.

We confirm that while mutational footprints of APOBEC1, APOBEC3A, APOBEC3B, and APOBEC3G are prominent in many cancers, mutable motifs characteristic of the action of the humoral immune response somatic hypermutation enzyme, AID, are the most widespread feature of the somatic mutation spectra attributed to APOBECs in cancer genomes. The AID and APOBEC3A mutable motifs are the most prominent features of the C:G>T:A transitions that constitute the vast majority of somatic mutations in studied cancers. We also demonstrated an abundance of APOBEC3A/3B/3G mutable motifs in DNA contexts of C:G>A:T transversions. A potential association of AID and APOBEC3A in a certain type of blood cancers is another interesting outcome of our study. Overall, the weight matrix approach revealed that somatic mutations are significantly associated with at least one AID/APOBEC mutable motif in the studied cancer types.

Supplementary Materials:
Figure S1:AID/APOBEC weight matrices W(b,j).itle; Figure S2: The overall distribution of fraction of somatic C:G>T:A mutations associated with AID/APOBEC deamination (APOBEC1, APOBEC3A, ABOPEC3B, and AID deaminases); Table S1: Datasets of mutations induced by overexpression of AID/APOBEC enzymes in the yeast genome; Table S2: Control study: correlation between AID/APOBEC mutable motifs and the context of somatic mutations in C:G sites in mitochondrial DNA; Table S3: Control study: fractions of random matrices with a significant correlation between AID/APOBEC pseudo-mutable motifs (shuffled sites of mutations) and the context of somatic mutations at C:G sites; Table S4: Control study: fraction of random matrices with a significant correlation between AID/APOBEC pseudo-mutable motifs (randomly sampled sites from the yeast genome) and the context of somatic mutations at C:G sites; Table S5: Nucleotide composition of the DNA context of somatic mutations (±3 nucleotides); Table S6: Correlation between AID/APOBEC mutable motifs and the context of C:G>T:A somatic mutations; Table S7: Correlation between AID/APOBEC mutable motifs and the context of C:G>G:C somatic mutations; and Table S8: Correlation between AID/APOBEC mutable motifs and the context of C:G>A:T somatic mutations.

Author Contributions: Conceptualization, I.B.R. and Y.I.P.; Data curation, I.B.R., A.G.L., F.B., I.A.S., and V.N.B.; Formal analysis, I.B.R., A.R.-L., F.B., I.A.S., and V.N.B.; Investigation, I.B.R., A.R.-L., and Y.I.P.; Methodology, I.B.R., A.R.-L., D.N.C., and Y.I.P.; Resources, I.B.R., A.R.-L, F.B., I.A.S., V.N.B., and Y.I.P.; Software, I.B.R., A.R.-L., A.G.L., I.A.S., G.V.G., and V.N.B.; Validation, I.B.R., A.R.-L., I.A.S., G.V.G., and V.N.B.; Original draft, I.B.R., A.R.-L., D.N.C., and Y.I.P.; and Review and editing of the manuscript, I.B.R., A.R.-L., A.G.L., F.B., I.A.S., G.V.G., V.N.B., D.N.C., and Y.I.P.

Acknowledgments: We appreciate the help from Elizabeth Moore (Y.I.P. laboratory) during the study and manuscript writing.

References

1. Weinstein, J.N.; Collisson, E.A.; Mills, G.B.; Shaw, K.R.M.; Ozenberger, B.A.; Ellrott, K.; Shmulevich, I.; Sander, C.; Stuart, J.M. The Cancer Genome Atlas Pan-Cancer analysis project. *Nat. Genet.* **2013**, *45*, 1113–1120.
2. Forbes, S.A.; Beare, D.; Gunasekaran, P.; Leung, K.; Bindal, N.; Boutselakis, H.; Ding, M.; Bamford, S.; Cole, C.; Ward, S.; et al. COSMIC: Exploring the world's knowledge of somatic mutations in human cancer. *Nucleic Acids Res.* **2015**, *43*, D805–D811. [CrossRef] [PubMed]
3. Nakagawa, H.; Fujita, M. Whole genome sequencing analysis for cancer genomics and precision medicine. *Cancer Sci.* **2018**, *109*, 513–522. [CrossRef] [PubMed]
4. Loeb, L.A.; Springgate, C.F.; Battula, N. Errors in DNA replication as a basis of malignant changes. *Cancer Res.* **1974**, *34*, 2311–2321. [PubMed]
5. Roberts, S.A.; Gordenin, D.A. Hypermutation in human cancer genomes: Footprints and mechanisms. *Nat. Rev. Cancer* **2014**, *14*, 786–800. [CrossRef] [PubMed]
6. Bailey, M.H.; Tokheim, C.; Porta-Pardo, E.; Sengupta, S.; Bertrand, D.; Weerasinghe, A.; Colaprico, A.; Wendl, M.C.; Kim, J.; Reardon, B.; et al. Comprehensive characterization of cancer driver genes and mutations. *Cell* **2018**, *173*, 371–385. [CrossRef] [PubMed]
7. Bailey, M.H.; Tokheim, C.; Porta-Pardo, E.; Sengupta, S.; Bertrand, D.; Weerasinghe, A.; Colaprico, A.; Wendl, M.C.; Kim, J.; Reardon, B.; et al. Erratum: Comprehensive characterization of cancer driver genes and mutations. *Cell* **2018**, *174*, 1034–1035. [CrossRef]
8. Martincorena, I.; Roshan, A.; Gerstung, M.; Ellis, P.; Van Loo, P.; McLaren, S.; Wedge, D.C.; Fullam, A.; Alexandrov, L.B.; Tubio, J.M.; et al. Tumor evolution. High burden and pervasive positive selection of somatic mutations in normal human skin. *Science* **2015**, *348*, 880–886. [CrossRef]

9. Martincorena, I.; Raine, K.M.; Gerstung, M.; Dawson, K.J.; Haase, K.; Van Loo, P.; Davies, H.; Stratton, M.R.; Campbell, P.J. Universal patterns of selection in cancer and somatic tissues. *Cell* **2017**, *171*, 1029–1041. [CrossRef]
10. Alexandrov, L.B.; Nik-Zainal, S.; Wedge, D.C.; Aparicio, S.A.; Behjati, S.; Biankin, A.V.; Bignell, G.R.; Bolli, N.; Borg, A.; Borresen-Dale, A.L.; et al. Signatures of mutational processes in human cancer. *Nature* **2013**, *500*, 415–421. [CrossRef]
11. Hutchinson, L. Genetics: Signatures of mutational processes in cancer-a big step closer. *Nat. Rev. Clin. Oncol.* **2013**, *10*, 545. [CrossRef] [PubMed]
12. Alexandrov, L.B.; Stratton, M.R. Mutational signatures: The patterns of somatic mutations hidden in cancer genomes. *Curr. Opin. Genet. Dev.* **2014**, *24*, 52–60. [CrossRef] [PubMed]
13. Goncearenco, A.; Rager, S.L.; Li, M.; Sang, Q.X.; Rogozin, I.B.; Panchenko, A.R. Exploring background mutational processes to decipher cancer genetic heterogeneity. *Nucleic Acids Res.* **2017**, *45*, W514–W522. [CrossRef]
14. Burns, M.B.; Temiz, N.A.; Harris, R.S. Evidence for APOBEC3B mutagenesis in multiple human cancers. *Nat. Genet.* **2013**, *45*, 977–983. [CrossRef] [PubMed]
15. Roberts, S.A.; Lawrence, M.S.; Klimczak, L.J.; Grimm, S.A.; Fargo, D.; Stojanov, P.; Kiezun, A.; Kryukov, G.V.; Carter, S.L.; Saksena, G.; et al. An APOBEC cytidine deaminase mutagenesis pattern is widespread in human cancers. *Nat. Genet.* **2013**, *45*, 970–976. [CrossRef] [PubMed]
16. Pham, P.; Bransteitter, R.; Petruska, J.; Goodman, M.F. Processive AID-catalysed cytosine deamination on single-stranded DNA simulates somatic hypermutation. *Nature* **2003**, *424*, 103–107. [CrossRef] [PubMed]
17. Chan, K.; Gordenin, D.A. Clusters of multiple mutations: Incidence and molecular Mechanisms. *Annu. Rev. Genet.* **2015**, *49*, 243–267. [CrossRef]
18. Burns, M.B.; Lackey, L.; Carpenter, M.A.; Rathore, A.; Land, A.M.; Leonard, B.; Refsland, E.W.; Kotandeniya, D.; Tretyakova, N.; Nikas, J.B.; et al. APOBEC3B is an enzymatic source of mutation in breast cancer. *Nature* **2013**, *494*, 366–370. [CrossRef]
19. Kuong, K.J.; Loeb, L.A. APOBEC3B mutagenesis in cancer. *Nat. Genet.* **2013**, *45*, 964–965. [CrossRef]
20. Franchini, D.M.; Schmitz, K.M.; Petersen-Mahrt, S.K. 5-Methylcytosine DNA demethylation: More than losing a methyl group. *Annu. Rev. Genet.* **2012**, *46*, 419–441. [CrossRef]
21. Rogozin, I.B.; Lada, A.G.; Goncearenco, A.; Green, M.R.; De, S.; Nudelman, G.; Panchenko, A.R.; Koonin, E.V.; Pavlov, Y.I. Activation induced deaminase mutational signature overlaps with CpG methylation sites in follicular lymphoma and other cancers. *Sci. Rep.* **2016**, *6*, 38133. [CrossRef] [PubMed]
22. Alexandrov, L.B.; Nik-Zainal, S.; Wedge, D.C.; Campbell, P.J.; Stratton, M.R. Deciphering signatures of mutational processes operative in human cancer. *Cell Rep.* **2013**, *3*, 246–259. [CrossRef] [PubMed]
23. Rogozin, I.B.; Pavlov, Y.I.; Goncearenco, A.; De, S.; Lada, A.G.; Poliakov, E.; Panchenko, A.R.; Cooper, D.N. Mutational signatures and mutable motifs in cancer genomes. *Brief. Bioinform.* **2017**, *19*, 1085–1101. [CrossRef] [PubMed]
24. Seplyarskiy, V.B.; Soldatov, R.A.; Popadin, K.Y.; Antonarakis, S.E.; Bazykin, G.A.; Nikolaev, S.I. APOBEC-induced mutations in human cancers are strongly enriched on the lagging DNA strand during replication. *Genome Res.* **2016**, *26*, 174–182. [CrossRef] [PubMed]
25. Haradhvala, N.J.; Polak, P.; Stojanov, P.; Covington, K.R.; Shinbrot, E.; Hess, J.M.; Rheinbay, E.; Kim, J.; Maruvka, Y.E.; Braunstein, L.Z.; et al. Mutational strand asymmetries in cancer genomes reveal mechanisms of DNA damage and repair. *Cell* **2016**, *164*, 538–549. [CrossRef] [PubMed]
26. Temiz, N.A.; Donohue, D.E.; Bacolla, A.; Vasquez, K.M.; Cooper, D.N.; Mudunuri, U.; Ivanic, J.; Cer, R.Z.; Yi, M.; Stephens, R.M.; et al. The somatic autosomal mutation matrix in cancer genomes. *Hum. Genet.* **2015**, *134*, 851–864. [CrossRef] [PubMed]
27. Staden, R. Computer methods to locate signals in nucleic acid sequences. *Nucleic Acids Res.* **1984**, *12*, 505–519. [CrossRef]
28. Gelfand, M.S. Prediction of function in DNA sequence analysis. *J. Comput. Biol.: J. Comput. Mol. Cell Biol.* **1995**, *2*, 87–115. [CrossRef]
29. Rogozin, I.B.; Milanesi, L. Analysis of donor splice sites in different eukaryotic organisms. *J. Mol. Evol.* **1997**, *45*, 50–59. [CrossRef]

30. Bishop, K.N.; Holmes, R.K.; Sheehy, A.M.; Davidson, N.O.; Cho, S.J.; Malim, M.H. Cytidine deamination of retroviral DNA by diverse APOBEC proteins. *Curr. Biol.* **2004**, *14*, 1392–1396. [CrossRef]
31. Rogozin, I.B.; Pavlov, Y.I. The cytidine deaminase AID exhibits similar functional properties in yeast and mammals. *Mol. Immunol.* **2006**, *43*, 1481–1484. [CrossRef] [PubMed]
32. Ju, Y.S.; Alexandrov, L.B.; Gerstung, M.; Martincorena, I.; Nik-Zainal, S.; Ramakrishna, M.; Davies, H.R.; Papaemmanuil, E.; Gundem, G.; Shlien, A.; et al. Origins and functional consequences of somatic mitochondrial DNA mutations in human cancer. *eLife* **2014**, *3*, e02935. [CrossRef] [PubMed]
33. Benjamini, Y.; Hochberg, Y. Controlling the false discovery rate: A practical and powerful approach to multiple testing. *J. R. Stat. Soc. Ser. B (Methodol.)* **1995**, *57*, 289–300. [CrossRef]
34. Milstein, C.; Neuberger, M.S.; Staden, R. Both DNA strands of antibody genes are hypermutation targets. *Proc. Natl. Acad. Sci. USA* **1998**, *95*, 8791–8794. [CrossRef] [PubMed]
35. Mayorov, V.I.; Rogozin, I.B.; Adkison, L.R.; Frahm, C.R.; Kunkel, T.A.; Pavlov, Y.I. Expression of human AID in yeast induces mutations in context similar to the context of somatic hypermutation at G-C pairs in immunoglobulin genes. *BMC Immunol.* **2005**, *6*, 10. [CrossRef] [PubMed]
36. Zanotti, K.J.; Gearhart, P.J. Antibody diversification caused by disrupted mismatch repair and promiscuous DNA polymerases. *DNA Repair* **2016**, *38*, 110–116. [CrossRef] [PubMed]
37. Taylor, B.J.; Nik-Zainal, S.; Wu, Y.L.; Stebbings, L.A.; Raine, K.; Campbell, P.J.; Rada, C.; Stratton, M.R.; Neuberger, M.S. DNA deaminases induce break-associated mutation showers with implication of APOBEC3B and 3A in breast cancer kataegis. *eLife* **2013**, *2*, e00534. [CrossRef]
38. Neuberger, M.S.; Rada, C. Somatic hypermutation: Activation-induced deaminase for C/G followed by polymerase eta for A/T. *J. Exp. Med.* **2007**, *204*, 7–10. [CrossRef]
39. Rogozin, I.B.; Goncearenco, A.; Lada, A.G.; De, S.; Yurchenko, V.; Nudelman, G.; Panchenko, A.R.; Cooper, D.N.; Pavlov, Y.I. DNA polymerase eta mutational signatures are found in a variety of different types of cancer. *Cell Cycle* **2018**, *17*, 348–355. [CrossRef]
40. Saini, N.; Roberts, S.A.; Klimczak, L.J.; Chan, K.; Grimm, S.A.; Dai, S.; Fargo, D.C.; Boyer, J.C.; Kaufmann, W.K.; Taylor, J.A.; et al. The impact of environmental and endogenous damage on somatic mutation load in human skin fibroblasts. *PLoS Genet.* **2016**, *12*, e1006385. [CrossRef]
41. Pham, P.; Landolph, A.; Mendez, C.; Li, N.; Goodman, M.F. A biochemical analysis linking APOBEC3A to disparate HIV-1 restriction and skin cancer. *J. Biol. Chem.* **2013**, *288*, 29294–29304. [CrossRef] [PubMed]
42. Cho, R.J.; Alexandrov, L.B.; den Breems, N.Y.; Atanasova, V.S.; Farshchian, M.; Purdom, E.; Nguyen, T.N.; Coarfa, C.; Rajapakshe, K.; Prisco, M.; et al. APOBEC mutation drives early-onset squamous cell carcinomas in recessive dystrophic epidermolysis bullosa. *Sci. Transl. Med.* **2018**, *10*, eaas9668. [CrossRef] [PubMed]
43. Fickett, J.W.; Guigo, R. Estimation of protein coding density in a corpus of DNA sequence data. *Nucleic Acid Res.* **1993**, *21*, 2837–2844. [CrossRef] [PubMed]
44. Glazko, G.B.; Milanesi, L.; Rogozin, I.B. The subclass approach for mutational spectrum analysis: Application of the SEM algorithm. *J. Theor. Biol.* **1998**, *192*, 475–487. [CrossRef] [PubMed]
45. Siriwardena, S.U.; Perera, M.L.W.; Senevirathne, V.; Stewart, J.; Bhagwat, A.S. A tumor promoting phorbol ester causes a large increase in APOBEC3A and a moderate increase in APOBEC3B expression in a normal human keratinocyte cell line without increasing genomic uracils. *Mol. Cell. Biol.* **2018**, *39*, e00238-18. [CrossRef] [PubMed]
46. Neuberger, M.S.; Harris, R.S.; Di Noia, J.; Petersen-Mahrt, S.K. Immunity through DNA deamination. *Trends Biochem. Sci.* **2003**, *28*, 305–312. [CrossRef]
47. Harris, R.S.; Petersen-Mahrt, S.K.; Neuberger, M.S. RNA editing enzyme APOBEC1 and some of its homologs can act as DNA mutators. *Mol. Cell* **2002**, *10*, 1247–1253. [CrossRef]
48. Petersen-Mahrt, S.K.; Harris, R.S.; Neuberger, M.S. AID mutates *E. coli* suggesting a DNA deamination mechanism for antibody diversification. *Nature* **2002**, *418*, 99–103. [CrossRef]
49. Bhagwat, A.S. DNA-cytosine deaminases: From antibody maturation to antiviral defense. *DNA Repair* **2004**, *3*, 85–89. [CrossRef]
50. Franchini, D.M.; Petersen-Mahrt, S.K. AID and APOBEC deaminases: Balancing DNA damage in epigenetics and immunity. *Epigenomics* **2014**, *6*, 427–443. [CrossRef]
51. Rebhandl, S.; Huemer, M.; Greil, R.; Geisberger, R. AID/APOBEC deaminases and cancer. *Oncoscience* **2015**, *2*, 320–333. [CrossRef] [PubMed]

52. Landry, S.; Narvaiza, I.; Linfesty, D.C.; Weitzman, M.D. APOBEC3A can activate the DNA damage response and cause cell-cycle arrest. *Embo Rep.* **2011**, *12*, 444–450. [CrossRef] [PubMed]
53. Taylor, B.J.; Wu, Y.L.; Rada, C. Active RNAP pre-initiation sites are highly mutated by cytidine deaminases in yeast, with AID targeting small RNA genes. *eLife* **2014**, *3*, e03553. [CrossRef] [PubMed]
54. Lada, A.G.; Kliver, S.F.; Dhar, A.; Polev, D.E.; Masharsky, A.E.; Rogozin, I.B.; Pavlov, Y.I. Disruption of transcriptional coactivator Sub1 leads to genome-wide re-distribution of clustered mutations induced by APOBEC in active yeast genes. *PLoS Genet.* **2015**, *11*, e1005217. [CrossRef] [PubMed]
55. Lada, A.G.; Krick, C.F.; Kozmin, S.G.; Mayorov, V.I.; Karpova, T.S.; Rogozin, I.B.; Pavlov, Y.I. Mutator effects and mutation signatures of editing deaminases produced in bacteria and yeast. *Biochemistry* **2011**, *76*, 131–146. [CrossRef] [PubMed]
56. Lada, A.G.; Stepchenkova, E.I.; Zhuk, A.S.; Kliver, S.F.; Rogozin, I.B.; Polev, D.E.; Dhar, A.; Pavlov, Y.I. Recombination is responsible for the increased recovery of drug-resistant mutants with hypermutated genomes in resting yeast diploids expressing APOBEC deaminases. *Front. Genet.* **2017**, *8*, 202. [CrossRef] [PubMed]
57. Shi, K.; Carpenter, M.A.; Banerjee, S.; Shaban, N.M.; Kurahashi, K.; Salamango, D.J.; McCann, J.L.; Starrett, G.J.; Duffy, J.V.; Demir, O.; et al. Structural basis for targeted DNA cytosine deamination and mutagenesis by APOBEC3A and APOBEC3B. *Nat. Struct. Mol. Biol.* **2017**, *24*, 131–139. [CrossRef]
58. Nik-Zainal, S.; Wedge, D.C.; Alexandrov, L.B.; Petljak, M.; Butler, A.P.; Bolli, N.; Davies, H.R.; Knappskog, S.; Martin, S.; Papaemmanuil, E.; et al. Association of a germline copy number polymorphism of APOBEC3A and APOBEC3B with burden of putative APOBEC-dependent mutations in breast cancer. *Nat. Genet.* **2014**, *46*, 487–491. [CrossRef]

10

Genomic Profiling of the Steroidogenic Acute Regulatory Protein in Breast Cancer: In Silico Assessments and a Mechanistic Perspective

Pulak R. Manna [1,*], Ahsen U. Ahmed [1], Shengping Yang [2], Madhusudhanan Narasimhan [3], Joëlle Cohen-Tannoudji [4], Andrzej T. Slominski [5,6] and Kevin Pruitt [1]

1 Departments of Immunology and Molecular Microbiology, School of Medicine, Texas Tech University Health Sciences Center, Lubbock, TX 79430, USA; ahsen.ahmed@ttuhsc.edu (A.U.A.); kevin.pruitt@ttuhsc.edu (K.P.)
2 Internal Medicine, School of Medicine, Texas Tech University Health Sciences Center, Lubbock, TX 79430, USA; shengping.yang@ttuhsc.edu
3 Pharmacology and Neuroscience, School of Medicine, Texas Tech University Health Sciences Center, Lubbock, TX 79430, USA; madhu.narasimhan@ttuhsc.edu
4 Physiologie de l'axe gonadotrope U1133, Institut National de la Santé et de la Recherche Médicale, CNRS, Biologie Fonctionnelle et Adaptative UMR 8251, Université Paris Diderot, 75205 Paris, France; tannoudji@univ-paris-diderot.fr
5 Department of Dermatology and Laboratory Medicine, Comprehensive Cancer Center, Cancer Chemoprevention Program, University of Alabama at Birmingham, Birmingham, AL 35294, USA; aslominski@uabmc.edu
6 Veterans Administration Medical Center, Birmingham, AL 35294, USA
* Correspondence: pulak.manna@ttuhsc.edu;

Abstract: Cancer is a multifactorial condition with aberrant growth of cells. A substantial number of cancers, breast in particular, are hormone sensitive and evolve due to malfunction in the steroidogenic machinery. Breast cancer, one of the most prevalent form of cancers in women, is primarily stimulated by estrogens. Steroid hormones are made from cholesterol, and regulation of steroid/estrogen biosynthesis is essentially influenced by the steroidogenic acute regulatory (StAR) protein. Although the impact of StAR in breast cancer remains a mystery, we recently reported that StAR protein is abundantly expressed in hormone sensitive breast cancer, but not in its non-cancerous counterpart. Herein, we analyzed genomic profiles, hormone receptor expression, mutation, and survival for StAR and steroidogenic enzyme genes in a variety of hormone sensitive cancers. These profiles were specifically assessed in breast cancer, exploiting The Cancer Genome Atlas (TCGA) datasets. Whereas StAR and key steroidogenic enzyme genes evaluated (*CYP11A1*, *HSD3B*, *CYP17A1*, *CYP19A1*, and *HSD17B*) were altered to varying levels in these hormone responsive cancers, amplification of the *StAR* gene was correlated with poor overall survival of patients afflicted with breast cancer. Amplification of the *StAR* gene and its correlation to survival was also verified in a number of breast cancer studies. Additionally, TCGA breast cancer tumors associated with aberrant high expression of *StAR* mRNA were found to be an unfavorable risk factor for survival of patients with breast cancer. Further analyses of tumors, nodal status, and metastases of breast cancer tumors expressing *StAR* mRNA displayed cancer deaths in stage specific manners. The majority of these tumors were found to express estrogen and progesterone receptors, signifying a link between StAR and luminal subtype breast cancer. Collectively, analyses of genomic and molecular profiles of key steroidogenic factors provide novel insights that StAR plays an important role in the biologic behavior and/or pathogenesis of hormone sensitive breast cancer.

Keywords: hormone sensitive cancers; breast cancer; StAR; estrogen; steroidogenic enzymes

1. Introduction

The rate-limiting step in the regulation of steroid hormone biosynthesis is the transport of the substrate of all steroid hormones, cholesterol, from the outer to the inner mitochondrial membrane, a process that is predominantly mediated by the steroidogenic acute regulatory (StAR; also called STARD1) protein [1–4]. There is wealth of information that regulation of steroid biosynthesis is mediated by mechanisms that enhance the transcription, translation, or activity of StAR [2,4–6]. Noteworthy, whereas phosphorylation of StAR is associated with the optimal cholesterol transferring ability of the StAR protein in steroid biosynthesis, mutations in the *StAR* gene results in a protein that is nonfunctional and inactive in transporting cholesterol. In almost every system studied, agents/factors that influence StAR expression also influence steroid biosynthesis through endocrine, autocrine, and paracrine regulation in a variety of classical and non-classical steroidogenic tissues [2,4,7–11]. Following the transport of cholesterol, by StAR, to the inner mitochondrial membrane, the P450 side chain cleavage (P450scc) enzyme, encoded by the *CYP11A1* gene, catalyzes the first enzymatic step in steroidogenesis i.e., the conversion of cholesterol to pregnenolone [4,6]. In addition, CYP11A1 converts 7-dehydrocholesterol to 7-dehydropregneolone and activates vitamin D, emphasizing the importance of StAR to transport other substrates for non-canonical activity of CYP11A1 [12,13]. The first steroid, pregnenolone, is then metabolized to various sex steroids by a series of enzymes in target tissues. These enzymes include 3β-hydroxysteroid dehydrogenase (3β-HSD), 17α-monooxygenase, 17α-hydroxylase, 17,20-lyase (P45017α), aromatase, and 17β-HSD, which are encoded by the *HSD3B*, *CYP17A1*, *CYP19A1*, and *HSD17B* genes, respectively [4,8].

Steroid hormones are synthesized not only in endocrine tissues, but also in a variety of extra-gonadal/adrenal tissues, and they play crucial roles in diverse processes, ranging from development to homeostasis to carcinogenesis [4,10,11,14–16]. Of note, StAR mediates steroid biosynthesis by controlling the transport of cholesterol and, thus, its entry to the mitochondrial inner membrane is a key event in influencing various cholesterol/steroid led functions. Conversely, inappropriate regulation of StAR, involving cholesterol transport, might influence hormone dependent disorders. Accordingly, cholesterol and its metabolites have been shown to be involved in the etiology of a number of cancers [17,18]. Moreover, dysregulation of androgen and estrogen biosynthesis has long been implicated in the pathogenesis a variety of hormone sensitive cancers [16,19].

One of the most common malignancies in women is breast cancer, which is activated by estrogens, especially 17β-estradiol (E2), and it accounts for over one-fourth of all cancer cases [16,20–22]. The American Cancer Society estimated that 266,120 women were expected to be diagnosed with invasive breast cancer, with 40,920 deaths in 2018. Breast cancers are classified into four subtypes, i.e., luminal A, luminal B, HER2/ErbB2+ (human epidermal growth factor receptor 2/the erythroblastosis oncogene-B2 positive), and TNBC (triple negative breast cancer), based on estrogen receptor (ER), progesterone receptor (PR), and HER2 expression [23]. Hormone sensitive breast cancers predominantly express ER, especially ERα, and/or PR, and account for ~80% of all breast cancer cases. The remaining 15–20% cancers include HER2+ that expresses HER2, and TNBC that does not express ER, PR, and HER2 [24,25]. In this connection, it is worth noting that expression of the StAR protein has been shown to be markedly high in ER+/PR+ breast cancer, modest in TNBC, but little to none in normal mammary epithelial cells [5]. Additionally, accumulation of E2 mirrored StAR protein expression in both noncancerous and cancerous breast cell lines, suggesting that StAR plays a key role in the development of ER+/PR+ breast cancer. To obtain more insight into the association of StAR in breast cancer, genomic profiling of StAR and key steroidogenic enzyme genes were analyzed by exploiting two publicly available research databases: The Cancer Genome Atlas (TCGA, provisional for different cancer types) and cBioPortal (for independent breast cancer studies).

2. Materials and Methods

2.1. TCGA Hormone Responsive Cancer Tumors and Their Correlation to Copy Number Alterations of StAR and Steroidogenic Enzyme Genes

TCGA genomic research databases were assessed for the following hormone sensitive cancers: breast (1080 tumors), colorectal (616 tumors), melanoma (367 tumors), ovarian (579 tumors), pancreatic (184 tumors), prostate (492 tumors), and uterine endometrial (539 tumors) [26–29]. These tumors were analyzed for DNA copy number alterations (CNAs) for StAR and key steroidogenic enzyme genes using the GISTIC 2.0. algorithm. CNA data were categorized as high-level amplification (+2 copies), gain (+1 copy), diploid (normal/no change), homozygous deletion (−2 copies), and hemizygous deletion (−1 copy). These analyses were performed using UCSC Xena [30] and/or cBioPortal Cancer Genomics [31,32] platforms. StAR CNA data were further evaluated for their correlation to StAR mRNA expression with RNA-Seq data, using the RSEM algorithm [33]. The correlation between StAR CNA and StAR mRNA levels was verified by Spearman's rank coefficient analysis.

2.2. Expression of ER, PR, and HER2 in Breast Cancer Tumors

The predictive immunohistochemical (IHC) markers, employed in clinical settings to classify breast cancer tumors into biologically distinct subtypes with unique pathogenesis, were examined. The use of IHC to assess ER, PR, and HER2 expression status in breast cancer has been routinely performed in clinics. IHC based tumor classification was analyzed for ER, PR, and HER2 expression using TCGA breast cancer datasets. These receptors were also evaluated in a number of breast cancer publications and/or projects that are available in cBioPortal website [31,32].

2.3. Amplification of the StAR Gene in Breast Cancer Studies

Amplification of the *StAR* gene was assessed in a variety of breast cancer publications/projects with cBioPortal browser. In particular, *StAR* gene amplification was analyzed in the following breast cancer studies: METABRIC (Molecular Taxonomy of Breast Cancer International Consortium), *Nature Communication* [34], (2173 tumors); breast cancer patient xenografts [35], (29 tumors); breast invasive carcinoma [36], (TCGA Cell 2015, 816 tumors); breast invasive carcinoma, [27], (TCGA Provisional; *Nature* 2012, 1080 tumors); metastatic breast cancer, *PLoS Medicine* [37], (216 tumors); and metastatic breast cancer (MBC) project (TCGA 2017, 103 tumors). These studies include mixed tumor types with variable numbers, in which amplification of the *StAR* gene and its correlation to overall survival, were evaluated, using available datasets.

2.4. Mutational Portraits of the StAR Gene in TCGA Hormone Responsive Cancers

Mutation in the *StAR* gene was examined in different hormone responsive cancers by analyzing exome sequencing, utilizing TCGA datasets. Mutational analyses were limited for functional forms. Intronic, silent, or other forms of mutations were not considered. These analyses were performed using UCSC Xena platform [30]. Gene mutation frequency is described as a percentage of total number of tumors.

2.5. Expression of StAR mRNA in TCGA Breast Cancer Tumors and Their Correlation to TNM Stages

Expression of StAR mRNA, evaluated from RNA-Seq data, available for breast cancer tumors, was downloaded from TCGA and UCSC Xena websites. StAR mRNA expressed as upper quartile-normalized fragments per kilobase of transcript per million mapped reads (fpkm+uq+1), generated by TCGA, was plotted using the Box and Whisker plot [38]. The Box and Whisker plot depicts normal distribution of StAR mRNA and determines the median and quartiles in a statistical population.

The T (tumor), N (node), and M (metastasis) staging, is a globally recognized system for defining the extent of stage and/or spread of solid tumors for prognosis and treatment [39,40]. The TNM staging of TCGA breast cancer tumors, expressing StAR mRNA, was performed using the American Joint

Committee on cancer classifications [39,40]. StAR mRNA/RNA-Seq data analyzed for various purposes are provided as an Excel file under Supplemental Materials.

2.6. *Generation of Kaplan-Meier Curves and Overall Survival Analyses*

Kaplan-Meier curve is frequently used to determine survival analysis for clinical outcomes such as recovery rates, probability of death, and disappearance of a tumor [41]. Utilizing TCGA and/or cBioportal breast cancer tumor CNA data, Kaplan-Meier survival curves were generated using with (high level amplification) and without (diploid) amplification [42–44] for *StAR, CYP11A1, HSD3B1, CYP17A1, CYP19A1, HSD17B1,* and *HSD17B2* genes. For StAR, survival curve was also generated with and without (all tumors excluding homozygous deletion) amplification. Both *HSD17B1* and *HSD17B2* gene isoforms evaluated were based on their association with breast cancer [45]. Additionally, Kaplan-Meier survival curves were generated by dividing tumors into non-overlapping upper and lower groups based on two reports, with StAR mRNA values up to 50th percentile as low and above 50th as high [46]; and up to 25th percentile as low and above 25th percentile as high [47,48].

2.7. *Statistical Analysis*

Statistical analyses were performed using GraphPad Prism software (GraphPad, San Diego, CA, USA). Data represented are the mean ± SEM and analyzed using one-way analysis of variance (ANOVA) followed by post-hoc test. Spearman's rank coefficient analysis was performed to determine the correlation between StAR CNA and StAR mRNA levels. The analysis of overall survival between groups was performed by log-rank Mantel-Cox method. A p-value less than 0.05 was considered statistically significant.

3. Results

3.1. *Assessment of StAR CNAs in Various Hormone Sensitive Cancers*

Gene amplification, comprising oncogene activation, is a fundamental event in tumor progression [42]. The hypothesis that estrogen and/or androgen sensitive cancers involve gain of function of StAR in the transport of cholesterol, and thereby influence hormone sensitive cancers, was examined. Utilizing TCGA datasets, StAR CNA data were analyzed in a variety of hormone dependent cancers (Table 1). Breast cancer CNA data for StAR demonstrated ~13% high level amplification (138 tumors), ~25% gain (268 tumors), ~38% diploid (406 tumors), ~23% hemizygous deletion (252 tumors), and ~1.5% homozygous deletion (16 tumors). Tumor numbers altered in each category are shown in parentheses. Analysis of colorectal cancer CNA data for StAR resulted in ~2.5%, ~30%, ~44%, ~23%, and ~8% high level amplification, gain, diploid, hemizygous deletion, and homozygous deletion, respectively. Whereas StAR CNA data were found to be altered at varying levels, high level amplification was observed at 4.4% in pancreatic cancer. Likewise, melanoma, ovarian, prostate, and uterine endometrial cancer CNA data for StAR displayed ~0.3%, ~3.5%, ~2.9%, and ~1.9% high level amplification in these malignant tumors, respectively (Table 1). These data are consistent with previous detection of StAR in peripheral tissues and malignant tumors [4,49]. Higher amplification of the *StAR* gene (~13%) was next evaluated for its impact on breast cancer.

Table 1. DNA copy number alterations of the steroidogenic acute regulatory (*StAR*) gene in different hormone responsive cancers.

CNAs	Breast *N* (%)	Colorectal *N* (%)	Melanoma *N* (%)	Ovarian *N* (%)	Pancreatic *N* (%)	Prostate *N* (%)	Uterine Endometrial *N* (%)
Homozygous Deletion	16 (1.48)	8 (1.30)	3 (0.82)	7 (1.21)	0 (0.00)	32 (6.50)	7 (1.30)
Hemizygous Deletion	252 (23.33)	140 (22.73)	69 (18.80)	215 (37.13)	42 (22.83)	133 (27.03)	66 (12.24)
Diploid	406 (37.59)	271 (43.99)	184 (50.14)	220 (38.00)	109 (59.24)	258 (52.44)	345 (64.01)
Gain	268 (24.81)	182 (29.55)	110 (29.97)	117 (20.21)	25 (13.59)	55 (11.18)	111 (20.59)
High Level Amplification	138 (12.78)	15 (2.44)	1 (0.27)	20 (3.45)	8 (4.35)	14 (2.85)	10 (1.86)
Total Number of Tumors	1080	616	367	579	184	492	539

StAR CNA data were assessed for the following cancer tumors: breast (1080 cases), colorectal (616 cases), melanoma (367 cases), ovarian (579 cases), pancreatic (184 cases), prostate (492 cases), and uterine endometrial (539 cases). The CNA level was categorized as homozygous deletion, hemizygous deletion, diploid, gain, and high level amplification, as described under Section 2. *N* (%) = number of tumors with percentages in parentheses.

3.2. Expression of ER, PR and HER2 in TCGA Breast Cancer Tumors

To assess breast cancer subtype(s) in TCGA tumor datasets, expression of ER, PR and HER2 was examined. IHC data revealed differential expression of ER (74% positive, 21% negative, 5% unknown), PR (64% positive, 31% negative, 5% unknown), and HER2 (15% positive, 51% negative, 34% unknown) (Figure 1). These results indicate that TCGA breast cancer tumors are mostly ER+/PR+, representing they are largely luminal subtypes.

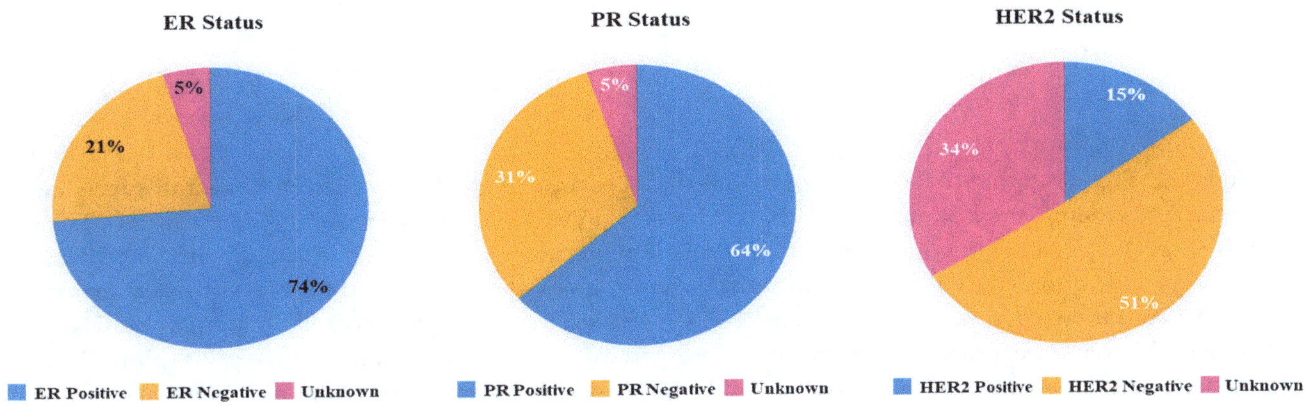

Figure 1. Expression of ER, PR and HER2 in The Cancer Genome Atlas (TCGA) breast cancer tumors. These tumors were previously stained with specific IHC markers in a clinical setting to classify into biologically distinct subtypes. Pie charts illustrate ER, PR, and HER2 expression in breast cancer tumors, which are presented as percentage of total numbers. Expression of these receptors was categorized as positive, negative, and unknown. The unknown category includes tumors in which IHC analysis was either not done or indeterminate or equivocal or data was not available.

3.3. Amplification of the StAR Gene in Breast Cancer and Its Correlation to Overall Survival

Utilizing TCGA breast cancer data cohort, amplification of the *StAR* gene was examined for cancer survival. As illustrated in Figure 2A, StAR CNA data in different categories were positively correlated with StAR mRNA expression (RNA-Seq data). The correlation between StAR CNA and StAR mRNA levels was verified with Spearman's correlation coefficient, i.e., 0.463. The analysis of Kaplan-Meier curve demonstrated that amplification of the *StAR* gene (~13%) was correlated with poor survival of breast cancer patients (p-value = 0.020). The median survival rate was noticeably reduced with amplification of the *StAR* gene when compared without amplification (Figure 2B). Similarly, the survival of breast cancer was affected (p-value = 0.045) when Kaplan-Meier curve was generated with and without (in which all tumors, excluding homozygous deletion, was included) *StAR* gene amplification (Figure 2C).

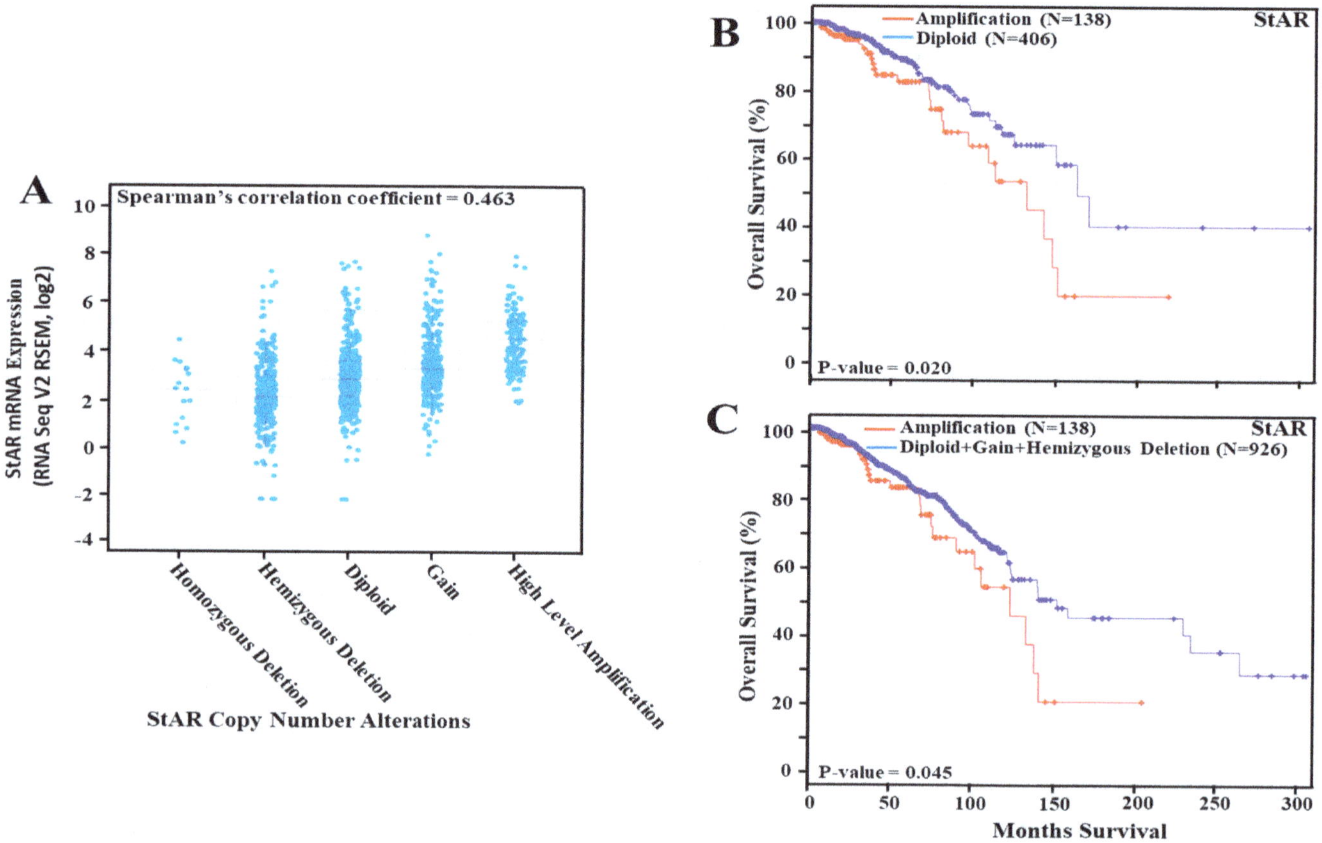

Figure 2. Frequency of StAR CNA data in breast cancer tumors and its correlation to overall survival. StAR CNA data were obtained from TCGA breast cancer tumor datasets with 1080 tumors. The CNA level was categorized as homozygous deletion, hemizygous deletion, diploid, gain, and high level amplification (**A**), utilizing cBioPortal browser, as described under Section 2. Breast cancer RNA-Seq data were assessed for StAR mRNA expression that positively correlated with StAR CNA data in different categories (**A**), which were presented in Y-axis and X-axis, respectively. Amplification of the *StAR* gene was evaluated for overall breast cancer survival (**B**,**C**). Kaplan-Meier curve was generated with TCGA breast cancer tumor CNA data, using with amplification (138 tumors) vs. without amplification (diploid, 406 tumors; **B**), or with a category (926 tumors; **C**) excluding homozygous deletion (16 tumors) of the *StAR* gene. Red and blue lines in panels B and C represent with and without amplification of the *StAR* gene, respectively.

3.4. StAR Gene Amplification, Hormone Receptor Expression, and Their Correlation to Cancer Survival in a Number of Breast Cancer Studies

To better understand involvement of *StAR* gene amplification in breast cancer deaths, genomic data from a number of publications/projects, as available in cBioPortal, were analyzed. As depicted in Figure 3A, amplification of the *StAR* gene was observed between 12% and 26% in all breast cancer studies examined. Specifically, amplification of the *StAR* gene was 26% in a breast cancer patient xenografts study, 12% in breast cancer METABRIC, and 13% and 14% in two independent publications associated with breast invasive carcinomas, and 15% each in two independent metastatic breast cancer studies (specified in Section 2).

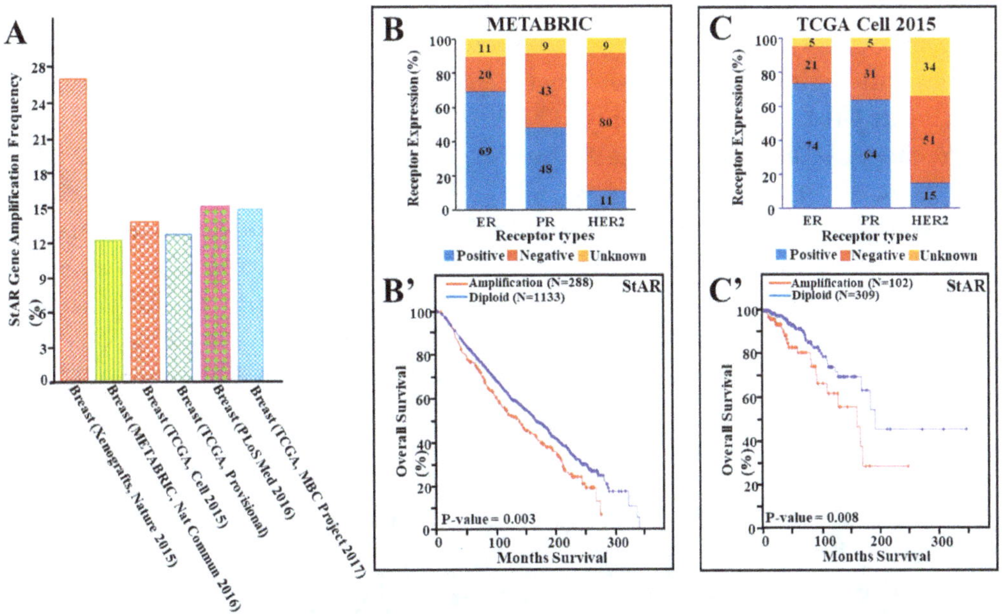

Figure 3. Amplification of the *StAR* gene, expression of hormone receptors, and their correlation to breast cancer survival in a number of publications/projects. Amplification of the *StAR* gene in different breast cancer studies, as available in cBioPortal, was analyzed. (**A**), amplification of the *StAR* gene was evaluated in the following breast cancer studies: breast cancer patient xenografts, Nature 2015 (29 tumors), [35]; breast METABRIC, *Nature Communication* 2016 (2173 tumors) [34]; breast TCGA Cell 2015, (816 tumors), [36]: TCGA Provisional (1080 tumors), [27]; breast *PLoS Medicine* 2016 (216 tumors), [37]; and TCGA Metastatic Breast Cancer (MBC) Project 2017 (103 tumors). Receptor expression was categorized as positive, negative, and unknown, and presented as percentages of total number of tumors (**B**,**C**), as described in the legend of Figure 1. Levels of ER, PR, and HER2 expression and their correlation to overall survival were analyzed for METABRIC (**B**,**B′**) and TCGA Cell 2015 (**C**,**C′**) studies. Kaplan-Meier survival curves were generated with METABRIC (red line, 288 tumors; blue line, 1133 tumors) and *Cell* 2015 (red line, 102 tumors; blue line, 309 tumors) CNA data, using tumors with amplification and without amplification (diploid) of the *StAR* gene.

In additional analyses, ER, PR, and HER2 expression, amplification of the *StAR* gene and its correlation to overall survival, were evaluated. In METABRIC study, breast cancer tumors (2173 tumors) were 69% ER+, 48% PR+, and 80% HER−, representing a mixed subtype, in which amplification of the *StAR* gene (~12%) affected the survival (p-value = 0.003) of breast cancer (Figure 3B,B′). In a breast invasive carcinoma study (Cell 2015, 816 tumors), amplification of the *StAR* gene (~14%), associated with 74% ER+, 64% PR+, and 51% HER2− (15% HER2+), was found to correlate (p-value = 0.008) with poor breast cancer survival (Figure 3C,C′). These data corroborate the findings presented in Figure 2B,C, and demonstrate that amplification of the *StAR* gene is correlated with poor survival of patients with luminal subtype breast cancer. Survival data were not available for other studies included in Figure 3A.

3.5. Amplification of Steroidogenic Enzyme Genes and Their Correlation to Overall Breast Cancer Survival

Estrogen plays an important role in stimulating breast cancer. The involvement of key steroidogenic enzyme genes (Supplementary Figure S1) to estrogen synthesis was next evaluated for their association to breast cancer survival utilizing TCGA data cohort. The data presented in Figure 4A–F illustrate bar graphs of different CNA frequencies (high level amplification (red), gain (blue), hemizygous deletion (green), and homozygous deletion (pink) for *CYP11A1*, *CYP17A1*, *HSD3B1*, *CYP19A1*, *HSD17B1*, and *HSD17B2* enzyme genes in different hormone sensitive cancers. Diploid category is not shown in these bar diagrams for easier visualization. CNA data demonstrate that the *CYP11A1* gene was amplified at ~1.5%, ~1.4%, ~3%, ~1.6%, and ~1.1% in breast, melanoma, ovarian, pancreatic, and uterine endometrial cancers, respectively (Figure 4A). No amplification of the *CYP11A1* gene was observed in prostate and colorectal cancers. The *CYP17A1* gene was amplified less than 1% in all cancer types analyzed (Figure 4B). Amplification of the *HSD3B1* gene was highest (~5%) in melanoma and none in colorectal cancer (Figure 4C). In breast cancer, this gene was amplified at ~2.3%. Amplification of the *CYP19A1* gene (aromatase) was ~1%, ~0.5%, ~0.3%, ~0.2%, ~1.6%, 0%, and ~0.2% in breast, colorectal, melanoma, ovarian, pancreatic, prostate, and uterine endometrial cancers, respectively (Figure 4D). Additionally, both *HSD17B1* and *HSD17B2* gene isoforms were found to be amplified minimally (0–1.4%) in different hormone sensitive cancers studied (Figure 4E,F). These *HSD17B1* and *HSD17B2* isoforms were amplified at ~1.4% and ~0.6% in breast cancer, respectively. These results are in support of previous studies that demonstrated upregulation of aberrant steroidogenesis during tumor progression [49,50].

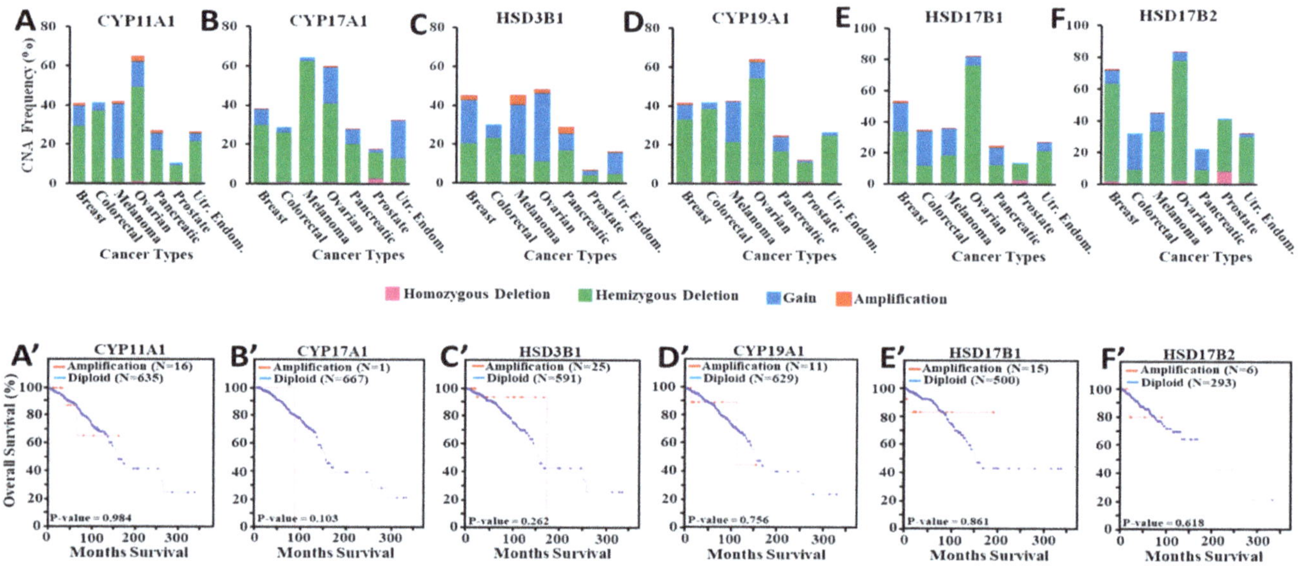

Figure 4. Analyses of CNA data for various steroidogenic enzyme genes in different hormone sensitive cancers and their correlation to breast cancer survival. TCGA CNA data analyzed for different cancers were the following: breast cancer tumors (1080 cases), colorectal (616 cases), melanoma (367 cases), ovarian (579 cases), pancreatic (184 cases), prostate (492 cases), and uterine endometrial (539 cases). Bar graphs illustrate CNA data for steroidogenic enzyme genes: *CYP11A1* (**A**), *CYP17A1* (**B**), *HSD3B1* (**C**), *CYP19A1* (**D**), *HSD17B1* (**E**), and *HSD17B2* (**F**). Amplification of these genes was analyzed for overall breast cancer survival (**A′–F′**). Kaplan-Meier survival curves were generated with and without (diploid) amplification of the following steroidogenic enzyme genes: *CYP11A1* (**A′**; red line, 16 tumors; blue line, 635 tumors), *CYP17A1* (**B′**; red line, 1 tumor; blue line, 667 tumors), *HSD3B1* (**C′**; red line, 25 tumors; blue line, 591 tumors), *CYP19A1* (**D′**; red line, 11 tumors; blue line, 629 tumors), *HSD17B1* (**E′**; red line, 15 tumors; blue line, 500 tumors), and *HSD17B2* (**F′**; red line, 6 tumors; blue line, 293 tumors). Red and blue lines represent with and without amplification of target genes, respectively. Utr. Endom., Uterine Endometrial.

The amplification of these steroidogenic enzyme genes in breast cancer survival was next evaluated. As determined by Kaplan-Meier survival analyses, amplification of the *CYP11A1* gene was not associated (p-value = 0.984) with breast cancer survival (Figure 4A′). Similarly, both *CYP17A1* and *HSD3B1* gene amplifications were not found to affect the survival of breast cancer, in which p-values were 0.103 and 0.262, respectively (Figure 4B′,C′). Kaplan-Meier survival analysis revealed that amplification of the *CYP19A1* gene was not correlated (p-value = 0.756) with breast cancer survival (Figure 4D′). Additionally, amplification of both *HSD17B1* and *HSD17B2* gene isoforms did not affect the survival of breast cancer, where p-values were 0.861 and 0.618, respectively (Figure 4E′,F′). These data indicate that none of these steroidogenic enzyme genes were either substantially amplified or affected the survival of ER+/PR+ breast cancer.

3.6. Assessment of StAR Gene Mutation in Hormone Sensitive Cancers

TCGA hormone responsive cancer datasets were analyzed for identifying mutation(s) in the *StAR* gene, which has been shown to affect the biological activity of the StAR protein in steroid biosynthesis [4,51]. As determined by exome sequencing, no mutations in the *StAR* gene were observed in breast (982 tumors) and prostate (499 tumors) cancers, suggesting StAR is functionally active in mobilizing cholesterol to the mitochondria. However, one mutation in the *StAR* gene was identified in each of the following cancers: colorectal (one out of 223 tumors; 0.45%), pancreatic (one out of 150 tumors; 0.67%), and ovarian (one out of 316 tumors; 0.32%). In melanoma and uterine endometrial carcinomas, five (368 tumors; 1.36%) and four (248 tumors; 1.61%) mutations were observed in the *StAR* gene, respectively (Supplementary Figure S2). The absence of mutation in the *StAR* gene, especially in breast cancer, suggests that amplification of the *StAR* gene is culpable in the transport of excess cholesterol to the inner mitochondrial membrane, resulting in increased estrogen synthesis which would promote tumorigenesis.

3.7. Expression of StAR mRNA in TCGA Breast Cancer Tumors and Its Association to Overall Survival

TCGA breast cancer tumor datasets were assessed for StAR mRNA expression. As illustrated by the Box and Whisker plot, StAR mRNA expression was represented as fkpm+uq+1 (obtained from RNA-Seq data), in which normal distribution across the population was visualized as 25th (9.114) and 75th (11.32) percentiles with a median of 10.2 (Figure 5A).

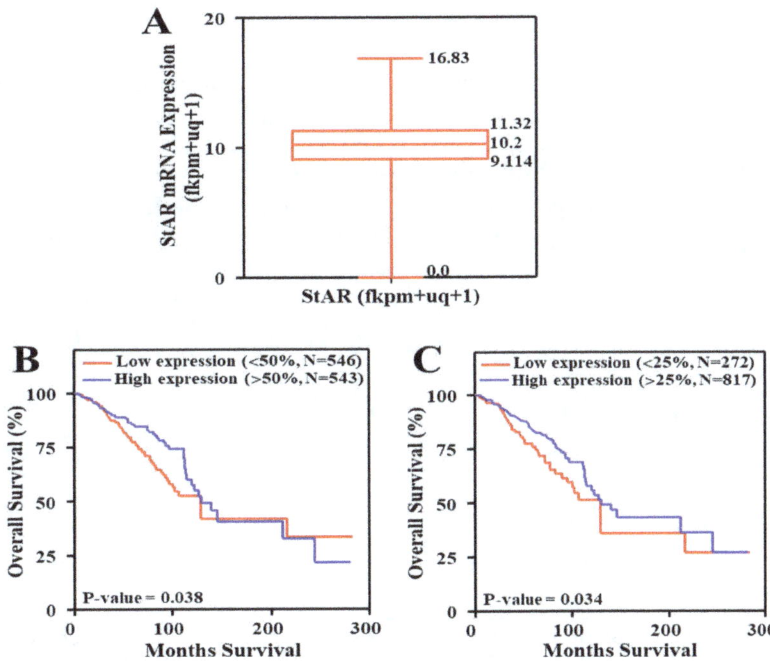

Figure 5. Expression of StAR mRNA in TCGA breast cancer tumors using the Box and Whisker Plot, and generation of Kaplan-Meier curves with low vs. high StAR levels. StAR mRNA expression was illustrated as fkpm+uq+1, generated by TCGA (1089 tumors), and visualized with the Box and Whisker Plot (**A**), as described in Section 2. Shown are 25th (9.114) and 75th (11.32) percentiles with a median of 10.2 (indicated by a horizontal line). Kaplan-Meier survival curves were generated with StAR mRNA values up to 50th percentile (<10.2; 546 tumors) as low and above 50th percentile (>10.2; 543 tumors) as high (**B**), and up to 25th percentile as low (<9.114; 272 tumors) and above 25th percentile (>9.114; 817 tumors) as high (**C**). Red and blue lines represent low and high StAR mRNA expression, respectively.

To better understand the involvement of StAR in breast cancer, TCGA breast cancer tumors expressing StAR mRNA were verified for survival analyses with two different quartile combinations. As depicted in Figure 5B, Kaplan-Meier curve generated with StAR mRNA values up to 50th percentile (<10.2) as low and above 50th percentile (>10.2) as high [46], was found to correlate with poor survival (p-value = 0.038) of patients with breast cancer. In a different category, StAR mRNA values up to 25th percentile (<9.114) as low and above 25th percentile (>9.114) as high [48], showed qualitatively similar effect ($p = 0.034$) on the survival of breast cancer (Figure 5C). These data suggest that higher expression of StAR mRNA can be a risk factor for poor survival of patients with breast cancer.

3.8. TNM Staging and Its Correlation to Breast Cancer Deaths

To obtain more insight in to the impact of StAR in breast cancer deaths, TCGA breast cancer tumors expressing StAR mRNA were analyzed in conjunction with the TNM staging. Specifically, different TNM stages were evaluated with low and high StAR mRNA levels with two quantile combinations as those utilized in Figure 5B,C. The results presented in Table 2 demonstrate TNM stage specific effects of tumors and their correlation to breast cancer deaths. These results show that breast cancer deaths were found to be coordinately associated with not only to increased tumor sizes, but also to lymph nodes in stage dependent manners. Additionally, tumor metastasis (M1) markedly affected the survival of breast cancer when compared with no metastasis (M0) in both low and high categories (Table 2). Specifically, the results obtained with TNM stages confirm the Kaplan-Meier survival data presented in Figure 5B,C. Altogether, genomic analyses of key steroidogenic factors, within the context of TCGA breast cancer datasets, indicated that aberrant amplification/ expression of the *StAR* gene is involved, at least in part, in poor survival of ER+/PR+ breast cancer patients. These results are in support of our recent finding that demonstrated that StAR protein is abundantly expressed in hormone sensitive breast cancer [5].

Table 2. T, N, M staging of TCGA breast cancer tumors segregated for low and high StAR mRNA expression based on two different quartile combinations, and their correlation to patient deaths.

TNM Staging	Low Expression (<50%)			High Expression (>50%)			Low Expression (<25%)			High Expression (>25%)		
	Tumor Nos.	Death Nos.	% Deaths	Tumor Nos.	Death Nos.	% Deaths	Tumor Nos.	Death Nos.	% Deaths	Tumor Nos.	Death Nos.	% Deaths
T1	120	17	14.2	158	16	10.1	54	8	14.8	224	25	11.2
T2	336	44	13.1	294	33	11.2	169	25	14.8	461	52	11.3
T3	63	11	17.5	75	14	18.7	32	9	28.1	106	16	15.1
T4	26	8	30.8	14	7	50	16	5	31.3	24	10	41.7
N0	257	22	8.6	257	22	8.6	120	15	12.5	394	29	7.4
N1	169	31	18.3	190	28	14.7	91	19	20.1	268	40	14.9
N2	75	16	21.3	45	6	13.3	38	6	15.8	82	16	19.5
N3	33	5	15.2	45	12	26.7	16	4	25.0	60	11	18.3
M0	459	62	13.5	621	32	5.2	224	26	11.6	672	83	12.4
M1	13	10	76.9	8	5	62.5	4	2	50	12	9	75.0

TCGA breast cancer tumors expressing low and high StAR mRNA levels (as specified) were categorized based on tumor sizes (T1–T4), nodal variations (N0–N3), and metastasis and non-metastasis (M0–M1), as described in Section 2.

4. Discussion

Abnormality in gene expression is responsible for anomalous growth of cells connecting tumor progression. The majority of the human genome is transcribed, but not translated, and gene amplification, involving oncogene activation, is a fundamental event in cancers. Hormone responsive cancers, especially breast cancer, are most common globally. Since StAR plays an indispensable role in the regulation of steroidogenesis, its expression must be finely regulated to appropriate functioning of steroid led activities. Conversely, dysregulation of steroid biosynthesis has been implicated in the pathophysiology of a number of relevant cancers. While StAR's involvement in breast malignancy remains obscure, we recently reported that both StAR protein expression and E2 synthesis are profoundly higher in ER+/PR+ breast cancer cell lines, when compared their levels with either non-cancerous mammary epithelial cells or TNBC [5]. By analyzing genomic profiles of StAR and steroidogenic enzyme genes for several hormone sensitive cancers, our data extend previous observations and provide novel insight that aberrant high amplification/expression of the *StAR* gene is correlated with poor survival of patients with breast cancer.

The comprehensive analyses of TCGA and cBioPortal research datasets for various hormone responsive cancers demonstrate that *StAR* gene is amplified (associated with a positive correlation between StAR CNA and StAR mRNA levels), but not mutated, in luminal subtype breast cancer. Specifically, the association of StAR with ER+/PR+ breast cancer indicates that StAR acts as a tumor promoter in the most prevalent hormone sensitive breast cancer. Several lines of evidence demonstrate a close correlation between StAR mRNA and StAR protein synthesis which parallels the synthesis of steroids in a variety of target tissues [4,7,10,52]. The involvement of StAR in breast cancer appeared specific, as translocator protein (TSPO), a mitochondrial factor involved in steroidogenesis [53,54], was not connected (*TSPO* gene was amplified at 0.7% with a p-value = 0.540) with cancer deaths (data not illustrated). The mechanism accounting for estrogen sensitive ovarian and endometrial cancers, connecting mutations in the *StAR* gene, remains unclear, and may involve one or more compensatory event(s), including involvement of StAR related lipid transfer proteins 3-6 (STARD3-6) and/or other factors involved in cholesterol trafficking [55,56]. Of note, the late endosomal membrane protein STARD3 (also known as metastatic lymph node 64), with ~37% C-terminal homology to StAR, was initially cloned as a gene amplified in the breast, gastric, and esophageal cancers [57,58]. It has previously been shown that overexpression of STARD3 is associated with increased cholesterol biosynthesis in HER2+ breast cancer subtype [59,60]. Regardless of the influence of these transporters, cholesterol and its oxygenated derivatives were demonstrated to be involved in the pathophysiology of a number of hormone sensitive malignancies, including breast cancer [17,18]. Studies have also reported that both cholesterol and its metabolites, including 27-hydroxycholesterol (27-HC) and 6-oxocholestan-diol, are capable to accelerate and/or enhance breast tumorigenesis [17,61,62]. Noteworthy, 27-HC is a ligand for ER and liver X receptor (LXR), in which the effects of 27-HC on tumor formation and growth are dependent on ER, while the action of this oxysterol involves LXR in tumor metastasis in mouse breast cancer models [17]. Whereas an overwhelming amount of evidence indicates the involvement of cholesterol in hormone sensitive breast cancer, epidemiologic findings are contradictory, requiring future studies to assess whether total cholesterol and its metabolites, high-density lipoprotein, or low-density lipoprotein influence cancer development and progression.

Almost all proteins in eukaryotic cells are modified by various post-translational modifications (PTMs) that influence protein function. We recently identified that StAR is a novel acetylated protein in ER+ breast cancer cells, in which three acetyl lysine residues were recognized endogenously, surmising they contribute to higher accumulation E2 in these cells [5]. It is plausible that both higher expression and activity of StAR facilitate abnormal cholesterol delivery to the mitochondrial inner membrane and, as a consequence, precursor availability for estrogen in promoting breast tumorigenesis. This reinforces the notion that estrogen levels in the majority of hormone sensitive malignant breast tumors can be 10–30 times higher than those found in either circulation or non-cancerous counterparts [16,21,63,64]. Previously, we [14,65,66] and others [67,68] have reported that cAMP mediated mechanisms phosphorylate StAR and this PTM enhances the optimal cholesterol transferring ability of the StAR protein in steroid biosynthesis. Despite the regulatory events involved, the impact of StAR to serve as a risk factor in affecting the survival of ER+/PR+ breast cancer opens up a new avenue in breast cancer research.

A notable aspect of the present findings is that amplification of the *CYP19A1* gene (aromatase), within the context of TCGA data cohort, was not correlated with breast cancer death [16], even though aromatase is the rate-limiting enzyme in estrogen biosynthesis. Expression of aromatase has been shown to be high in both non-cancerous and cancerous breast cell lines, suggesting its relevance in a number of physiological and pathophysiological events [5,69]. There is increasing evidence that enhanced expression/activity of aromatase is one of the key events for elevated intra-tumoral production of estrogen in malignant breast tissues [16,21,70,71]. Estrogen is also produced by the action of the 17β-HSD enzyme, and CNA data revealed that the *HSD17B* gene was neither significantly amplified nor connected with the survival of hormone sensitive breast cancer. These data imply that StAR mediated delivery of excess cholesterol, resulting in a substantial increase in estrogen accumulation, appears to be a fundamental event in the development of hormone sensitive breast cancer. In accordance with this, preliminary data obtained reveal that the expression of both StAR mRNA and StAR protein was markedly high in transgenic (Tg) mouse models of breast cancer, activated by MMTV promoter driven cNeu and H-Ras oncogenes, and polyomavirus, in comparison to nearly undetectable level of StAR in normal Tg mammary tissue.

Estrogen is primarily produced in the ovaries via the classical steroidogenic pathway through the synthesis of androstenedione and testosterone from cholesterol (in which StAR plays a permissive role) in the theca cells. These androgens are then converted to estrogens in granulosa cells. In peri- and post-menopausal women, extra ovarian tissues become a major source for estrogen synthesis [72]. This transition is critical since most hormone sensitive cancers, including breast, occur over the age of 50, in which estrogens synthesized in peripheral tissues are believed to play pivotal roles [63,64]. The plasma androgen level in post-menopausal women, with the loss of ovarian estrogen production, remains stable for years. Utilizing the non-classical pathway, these androgens are converted to estrogens in peripheral tissues. In addition to peripheral estrogen that reaches the tumor site through systemic circulation, estrogen is also synthesized locally in malignant breast tumors [16,21,63,64]. Breast cancer tumors in TCGA datasets were predominantly ER+/PR+, in which aberrant high expression of *StAR* mRNA, was found to affect poor survival of breast cancer. Further analyses of these tumors, expressing StAR mRNA, demonstrated increasing patterns of breast cancer deaths with advanced TNM stages. It should be noted, however, while breast cancer deaths were steadily increased with various TNM stages, they were not coordinately associated with StAR mRNA expression, which could be due to tumor numbers, tumor stages, or involvement of additional factors.

5. Conclusions

Analyses of molecular genomic profiling of steroidogenic factors associated with TCGA and cBioPortal research datasets revealed that abundant amplification and/or expression of the StAR gene is connected with poor survival of patients with luminal subtype breast cancer. This is in support of our recent report that demonstrated that StAR protein, concomitant with E2 synthesis, is markedly expressed in ER+/PR+ breast cancer, in comparison to nearly undetectable to modest StAR and E2 levels in non-cancerous mammary epithelial cells [5]. Based on these data (albeit limited), it is highly likely that StAR facilitates abnormal delivery of cholesterol to the inner mitochondria, resulting in adequate availability of precursors for E2 overproduction, which could be a plausible mechanism in the development and growth of hormone sensitive breast cancer. Furthermore, the results of in silico analyses, together with our in vitro data reported recently, attest that StAR can serve as a novel prognostic marker in ER+/PR+ breast cancer, whereas its inhibition, involving E2 synthesis, by a number of histone deacetylase inhibitors, might have therapeutic implications in the prevention/treatment of this devastating disease. The present data indicating the involvement of the classical pathway in intra-tumoral androgen/estrogen synthesis points to an additional new mechanism in growth and development of ER+/PR+ breast and/or other pertinent cancers, even though overexpression of aromatase, resulting in an increase in estrogen synthesis through the non-classical pathway is well established. Whereas *StAR* gene is highly amplified/expressed in hormone sensitive breast cancer, its association with HER2 and TNBC subtypes remains to be elucidated.

Author Contributions: Conceptualization, P.R.M.; Methodology, P.R.M., A.U.A., S.Y. and M.N.; Project Administration and Supervision, P.R.M.; Validation, P.R.M., A.U.A., S.Y. and M.N.; Formal Analysis, P.R.M., A.U.A., S.Y., M.N., J.C.-T., A.T.S. and K.P.; Investigation, P.R.M., A.U.A., S.Y., A.T.S. and M.N.; Writing—Original Draft Preparation, P.R.M.; Visualization, P.R.M., A.U.A., M.N., J.C.-T., A.T.S. and K.P.; Funding acquisition, A.T.S. and K.P.; Writing—Review & Editing, P.R.M., A.U.A., S.Y., M.N., J.C.-T., A.T.S. and K.P.

Acknowledgments: The authors would like to acknowledge the utilization of TCGA (https://tcga-data.nci.nih.gov), cBioPortal (http://www.cbioportal.org), and UCSC Xena (http://www.xenabrowser.net) research network datasets in this study.

References

1. Manna, P.R.; Stocco, D.M. Regulation of the steroidogenic acute regulatory protein expression: Functional and physiological consequences. *Curr. Drug Targets Immune Endocr. Metabol. Disord.* **2005**, *5*, 93–108. [CrossRef] [PubMed]
2. Manna, P.R.; Dyson, M.T.; Stocco, D.M. Regulation of the steroidogenic acute regulatory protein gene expression: Present and future perspectives. *Mol. Hum. Reprod.* **2009**, *15*, 321–333. [CrossRef]
3. Papadopoulos, V.; Miller, W.L. Role of mitochondria in steroidogenesis. *Best Pract. Res. Clin. Endocrinol. Metab.* **2012**, *26*, 771–790. [PubMed]
4. Manna, P.R.; Stetson, C.L.; Slominski, A.T.; Pruitt, K. Role of the steroidogenic acute regulatory protein in health and disease. *Endocrine* **2016**, *51*, 7–21. [CrossRef] [PubMed]
5. Manna, P.R.; Ahmed, A.U.; Vartak, D.; Molehin, D.; Pruitt, K. Overexpression of the steroidogenic acute regulatory protein in breast cancer: Regulation by histone deacetylase inhibition. *Biochem. Biophys. Res. Commun.* **2019**, *509*, 476–482. [CrossRef] [PubMed]
6. Miller, W.L.; Bose, H.S. Early steps in steroidogenesis: Intracellular cholesterol trafficking. *J. Lipid Res.* **2011**, *52*, 2111–2135. [CrossRef]
7. Manna, P.R.; Dyson, M.T.; Eubank, D.W.; Clark, B.J.; Lalli, E.; Sassone-Corsi, P.; Zeleznik, A.J.; Stocco, D.M. Regulation of steroidogenesis and the steroidogenic acute regulatory protein by a member of the cAMP response-element binding protein family. *Mol. Endocrinol.* **2002**, *16*, 184–199. [CrossRef] [PubMed]
8. Miller, W.L.; Auchus, R.J. The molecular biology, biochemistry, and physiology of human steroidogenesis and its disorders. *Endocr. Rev.* **2011**, *32*, 81–151. [CrossRef]
9. Manna, P.R.; Cohen-Tannoudji, J.; Counis, R.; Garner, C.W.; Huhtaniemi, I.; Kraemer, F.B.; Stocco, D.M. Mechanisms of action of hormone sensitive lipase in mouse Leydig cells: Its role in the regulation of the steroidogenic acute regulatory protein. *J. Biol. Chem.* **2013**, *288*, 8505–8518. [CrossRef] [PubMed]
10. Manna, P.R.; Stetson, C.L.; Daugherty, C.; Shimizu, I.; Syapin, P.J.; Garrel, G.; Cohen-Tannoudji, J.; Huhtaniemi, I.; Slominski, A.T.; Pruitt, K.; et al. Up-regulation of steroid biosynthesis by retinoid signaling: Implications for aging. *Mech. Ageing. Dev.* **2015**, *150*, 74–82. [CrossRef] [PubMed]
11. Slominski, A.T.; Manna, P.R.; Tuckey, R.C. On the role of skin in the regulation of local and systemic steroidogenic activities. *Steroids* **2015**, *103*, 72–88. [CrossRef] [PubMed]
12. Slominski, A.; Semak, I.; Zjawiony, J.; Wortsman, J.; Li, W.; Szczesniewski, A.; Tuckey, R.C. The cytochrome P450scc system opens an alternate pathway of vitamin D3 metabolism. *FEBS J.* **2005**, *272*, 4080–4090. [CrossRef]
13. Slominski, A.T.; Li, W.; Kim, T.K.; Semak, I.; Wang, J.; Zjawiony, J.K.; Tuckey, R.C. Novel activities of CYP11A1 and their potential physiological significance. *J. Steroid Biochem. Mol. Biol.* **2015**, *151*, 25–37. [CrossRef] [PubMed]
14. Manna, P.R.; Slominski, A.T.; King, S.R.; Stetson, C.L.; Stocco, D.M. Synergistic Activation of Steroidogenic Acute Regulatory Protein Expression and Steroid Biosynthesis by Retinoids: Involvement of cAMP/PKA Signaling. *Endocrinology* **2014**, *155*, 576–591. [CrossRef]
15. Slominski, A.T.; Manna, P.R.; Tuckey, R.C. Cutaneous glucocorticosteroidogenesis: Securing local homeostasis and the skin integrity. *Exp. Dermatol.* **2014**, *23*, 369–374. [CrossRef]
16. Manna, P.R.; Molehin, D.; Ahmed, A.U. Dysregulation of Aromatase in Breast, Endometrial, and Ovarian Cancers: An Overview of Therapeutic Strategies. *Prog. Mol. Biol. Transl. Sci.* **2016**, *144*, 487–537. [PubMed]
17. Nelson, E.R.; Wardell, S.E.; Jasper, J.S.; Park, S.; Suchindran, S.; Howe, M.K.; Carver, N.J.; Pillai, R.V.; Sullivan, P.M.; Sondhi, V.; et al. 27-Hydroxycholesterol links hypercholesterolemia and breast cancer pathophysiology. *Science* **2013**, *342*, 1094–1098. [CrossRef] [PubMed]

18. Silvente-Poirot, S.; Dalenc, F.; Poirot, M. The Effects of Cholesterol-Derived Oncometabolites on Nuclear Receptor Function in Cancer. *Cancer Res.* **2018**, *78*, 4803–4808. [CrossRef]
19. Brodie, A.; Njar, V.; Macedo, L.F.; Vasaitis, T.S.; Sabnis, G. The Coffey Lecture: Steroidogenic enzyme inhibitors and hormone dependent cancer. *Urol. Oncol.* **2009**, *27*, 53–63. [CrossRef]
20. Richie, R.C.; Swanson, J.O. Breast cancer: A review of the literature. *J. Insur. Med.* **2003**, *35*, 85–101.
21. Bulun, S.E.; Lin, Z.; Zhao, H.; Lu, M.; Amin, S.; Reierstad, S.; Chen, D. Regulation of aromatase expression in breast cancer tissue. *Ann. N. Y. Acad. Sci.* **2009**, *1155*, 121–131. [CrossRef]
22. Folkerd, E.; Dowsett, M. Sex hormones and breast cancer risk and prognosis. *Breast* **2013**, *22* (Suppl. 2), S38–S43. [CrossRef]
23. Cheang, M.C.; Martin, M.; Nielsen, T.O.; Prat, A.; Voduc, D.; Rodriguez-Lescure, A.; Ruiz, A.; Chia, S.; Shepherd, L.; Ruiz-Borrego, M.; et al. Defining breast cancer intrinsic subtypes by quantitative receptor expression. *Oncologist* **2015**, *20*, 474–482. [CrossRef] [PubMed]
24. Prat, A.; Pineda, E.; Adamo, B.; Galvan, P.; Fernandez, A.; Gaba, L.; Diez, M.; Viladot, M.; Arance, A.; Munoz, M. Clinical implications of the intrinsic molecular subtypes of breast cancer. *Breast* **2015**, *24* (Suppl. 2), S26–S35. [CrossRef]
25. Dai, X.; Li, T.; Bai, Z.; Yang, Y.; Liu, X.; Zhan, J.; Shi, B. Breast cancer intrinsic subtype classification, clinical use and future trends. *Am. J. Cancer Res.* **2015**, *5*, 2929–2943.
26. Cancer Genome Atlas Research Network. Integrated genomic analyses of ovarian carcinoma. *Nature* **2011**, *474*, 609–615. [CrossRef]
27. Cancer Genome Atlas Network. Comprehensive molecular portraits of human breast tumours. *Nature* **2012**, *490*, 61–70. [CrossRef] [PubMed]
28. Cancer Genome Atlas, N. Comprehensive molecular characterization of human colon and rectal cancer. *Nature* **2012**, *487*, 330–337. [CrossRef] [PubMed]
29. Kandoth, C.; Schultz, N.; Cherniack, A.D.; Akbani, R.; Liu, Y.; Shen, H.; Robertson, A.G.; Pashtan, I.; Shen, R.; Benz, C.C.; et al. Integrated genomic characterization of endometrial carcinoma. *Nature* **2013**, *497*, 67–73.
30. Casper, J.; Zweig, A.S.; Villarreal, C.; Tyner, C.; Speir, M.L.; Rosenbloom, K.R.; Raney, B.J.; Lee, C.M.; Lee, B.T.; Karolchik, D.; et al. The UCSC Genome Browser database: 2018 update. *Nucleic Acids Res.* **2018**, *46*, D762–D769. [PubMed]
31. Cerami, E.; Gao, J.; Dogrusoz, U.; Gross, B.E.; Sumer, S.O.; Aksoy, B.A.; Jacobsen, A.; Byrne, C.J.; Heuer, M.L.; Larsson, E.; et al. The cBio cancer genomics portal: An open platform for exploring multidimensional cancer genomics data. *Cancer Discov.* **2012**, *2*, 401–404. [CrossRef] [PubMed]
32. Gao, J.; Aksoy, B.A.; Dogrusoz, U.; Dresdner, G.; Gross, B.; Sumer, S.O.; Sun, Y.; Jacobsen, A.; Sinha, R.; Larsson, E.; et al. Integrative analysis of complex cancer genomics and clinical profiles using the cBioPortal. *Sci. Signal.* **2013**, *6*, pl1. [CrossRef]
33. Li, B.; Dewey, C.N. RSEM: Accurate transcript quantification from RNA-Seq data with or without a reference genome. *BMC Bioinform.* **2011**, *12*, 323. [CrossRef] [PubMed]
34. Pereira, B.; Chin, S.F.; Rueda, O.M.; Vollan, H.K.; Provenzano, E.; Bardwell, H.A.; Pugh, M.; Jones, L.; Russell, R.; Sammut, S.J. The somatic mutation profiles of 2,433 breast cancers refines their genomic and transcriptomic landscapes. *Nat. Commun.* **2016**, *7*, 11479. [CrossRef]
35. Eirew, P.; Steif, A.; Khattra, J.; Ha, G.; Yap, D.; Farahani, H.; Gelmon, K.; Chia, S.; Mar, C.; Wan, A.; et al. Dynamics of genomic clones in breast cancer patient xenografts at single-cell resolution. *Nature* **2015**, *518*, 422–426. [CrossRef] [PubMed]
36. Ciriello, G.; Gatza, M.L.; Beck, A.H.; Wilkerson, M.D.; Rhie, S.K.; Pastore, A.; Zhang, H.; McLellan, M.; Yau, C.; Kandoth, C.; et al. Comprehensive Molecular Portraits of Invasive Lobular Breast Cancer. *Cell* **2015**, *163*, 506–519. [CrossRef] [PubMed]
37. Lefebvre, C.; Bachelot, T.; Filleron, T.; Pedrero, M.; Campone, M.; Soria, J.C.; Massard, C.; Levy, C.; Arnedos, M.; Lacroix-Triki, M.; et al. Mutational Profile of Metastatic Breast Cancers: A Retrospective Analysis. *PLoS Med.* **2016**, *13*, e1002201. [CrossRef]
38. Bullard, J.H.; Purdom, E.; Hansen, K.D.; Dudoit, S. Evaluation of statistical methods for normalization and differential expression in mRNA-Seq experiments. *BMC Bioinform.* **2010**, *11*, 94. [CrossRef]
39. O'Sullivan, B.; Brierley, J.; Byrd, D.; Bosman, F.; Kehoe, S.; Kossary, C.; Pineros, M.; Van Eycken, E.; Weir, H.K.; Gospodarowicz, M. The TNM classification of malignant tumours-towards common understanding and reasonable expectations. *Lancet Oncol.* **2017**, *18*, 849–851. [CrossRef]

40. Lydiatt, W.M.; Patel, S.G.; O'Sullivan, B.; Brandwein, M.S.; Ridge, J.A.; Migliacci, J.C.; Loomis, A.M.; Shah, J.P. Head and Neck cancers-major changes in the American Joint Committee on cancer eighth edition cancer staging manual. *CA Cancer J. Clin.* **2017**, *67*, 122–137. [CrossRef]
41. Sedgwick, P. How to read a Kaplan-Meier survival plot. *BMJ* **2014**, *349*, g5608. [CrossRef] [PubMed]
42. Slamon, D.J.; Clark, G.M.; Wong, S.G.; Levin, W.J.; Ullrich, A.; McGuire, W.L. Human breast cancer: Correlation of relapse and survival with amplification of the HER-2/neu oncogene. *Science* **1987**, *235*, 177–182. [CrossRef]
43. Schneiderman, J.; London, W.B.; Brodeur, G.M.; Castleberry, R.P.; Look, A.T.; Cohn, S.L. Clinical significance of MYCN amplification and ploidy in favorable-stage neuroblastoma: A report from the Children's Oncology Group. *J. Clin. Oncol.* **2008**, *26*, 913–918. [CrossRef] [PubMed]
44. Liu, L.; Kimball, S.; Liu, H.; Holowatyj, A.; Yang, Z.Q. Genetic alterations of histone lysine methyltransferases and their significance in breast cancer. *Oncotarget* **2015**, *6*, 2466–2482. [CrossRef] [PubMed]
45. Hilborn, E.; Stal, O.; Jansson, A. Estrogen and androgen-converting enzymes 17beta-hydroxysteroid dehydrogenase and their involvement in cancer: With a special focus on 17beta-hydroxysteroid dehydrogenase type 1, 2, and breast cancer. *Oncotarget* **2017**, *8*, 30552–30562. [CrossRef] [PubMed]
46. Giovannetti, E.; Wang, Q.; Avan, A.; Funel, N.; Lagerweij, T.; Lee, J.H.; Caretti, V.; van der Velde, A.; Boggi, U.; Wang, Y.; et al. Role of CYB5A in pancreatic cancer prognosis and autophagy modulation. *J. Natl. Cancer Inst.* **2014**, *106*, djt346. [CrossRef] [PubMed]
47. Yoshihara, K.; Shahmoradgoli, M.; Martinez, E.; Vegesna, R.; Kim, H.; Torres-Garcia, W.; Trevino, V.; Shen, H.; Laird, P.W.; Levine, D.A.; et al. Inferring tumour purity and stromal and immune cell admixture from expression data. *Nat. Commun.* **2013**, *4*, 2612. [CrossRef]
48. Geng, X.; Liu, Y.; Diersch, S.; Kotzsch, M.; Grill, S.; Weichert, W.; Kiechle, M.; Magdolen, V.; Dorn, J. Clinical relevance of kallikrein-related peptidase 9, 10, 11, and 15 mRNA expression in advanced high-grade serous ovarian cancer. *PLoS ONE* **2017**, *12*, e0186847. [CrossRef]
49. Slominski, A.T.; Zmijewski, M.A.; Semak, I.; Zbytek, B.; Pisarchik, A.; Li, W.; Zjawiony, J.; Tuckey, R.C. Cytochromes p450 and skin cancer: Role of local endocrine pathways. *Anticancer Agents Med. Chem.* **2014**, *14*, 77–96. [CrossRef]
50. Slominski, A.; Gomez-Sanchez, C.E.; Foecking, M.F.; Wortsman, J. Metabolism of progesterone to DOC, corticosterone and 18OHDOC in cultured human melanoma cells. *FEBS Lett.* **1999**, *455*, 364–366. [CrossRef]
51. Camats, N.; Pandey, A.V.; Fernandez-Cancio, M.; Fernandez, J.M.; Ortega, A.M.; Udhane, S.; Andaluz, P.; Audi, L.; Fluck, C.E. STAR splicing mutations cause the severe phenotype of lipoid congenital adrenal hyperplasia: Insights from a novel splice mutation and review of reported cases. *Clin. Endocrinol.* **2014**, *80*, 191–199. [CrossRef]
52. Miller, W.L. Steroidogenic acute regulatory protein (StAR), a novel mitochondrial cholesterol transporter. *Biochim. Biophys. Acta* **2007**, *1771*, 663–676. [CrossRef]
53. Papadopoulos, V.; Aghazadeh, Y.; Fan, J.; Campioli, E.; Zirkin, B.; Midzak, A. Translocator protein-mediated pharmacology of cholesterol transport and steroidogenesis. *Mol. Cell. Endocrinol.* **2015**, *408*, 90–98. [CrossRef]
54. Fan, J.; Wang, K.; Zirkin, B.; Papadopoulos, V. CRISPR/Cas9Mediated Tspo Gene Mutations Lead to Reduced Mitochondrial Membrane Potential and Steroid Formation in MA-10 Mouse Tumor Leydig Cells. *Endocrinology* **2018**, *159*, 1130–1146. [CrossRef]
55. Strauss, J.F., 3rd; Kishida, T.; Christenson, LK.; Fujimoto, T.; Hiroi, H. START domain proteins and the intracellular trafficking of cholesterol in steroidogenic cells. *Mol. Cell. Endocrinol.* **2003**, *202*, 59–65. [CrossRef]
56. Alpy, F.; Legueux, F.; Bianchetti, L.; Tomasetto, C. START domain-containing proteins: A review of their role in lipid transport and exchange. *Med. Sci. Paris* **2009**, *25*, 181–191.
57. Tomasetto, C.; Regnier, C.; Moog-Lutz, C.; Mattei, M.G.; Chenard, M.P.; Lidereau, R.; Basset, P.; Rio, M.C. Identification of four novel human genes amplified and overexpressed in breast carcinoma and localized to the q11-q21.3 region of chromosome 17. *Genomics* **1995**, *28*, 367–376. [CrossRef]
58. Akiyama, N.; Sasaki, H.; Ishizuka, T.; Kishi, T.; Sakamoto, H.; Onda, M.; Hirai, H.; Yazaki, Y.; Sugimura, T.; Terada, M. Isolation of a candidate gene, CAB1, for cholesterol transport to mitochondria from the c-ERBB-2 amplicon by a modified cDNA selection method. *Cancer Res.* **1997**, *57*, 3548–3553.
59. Alpy, F.; Boulay, A.; Moog-Lutz, C.; Andarawewa, K.L.; Degot, S.; Stoll, I.; Rio, M.C.; Tomasetto, C. Metastatic lymph node 64 (MLN64), a gene overexpressed in breast cancers, is regulated by Sp/KLF transcription factors. *Oncogene* **2003**, *22*, 3770–3780. [CrossRef]

60. Vassilev, B.; Sihto, H.; Li, S.; Holtta-Vuori, M.; Ilola, J.; Lundin, J.; Isola, J.; Kellokumpu-Lehtinen, P.L.; Joensuu, H.; Ikonen, E. Elevated levels of StAR-related lipid transfer protein 3 alter cholesterol balance and adhesiveness of breast cancer cells: Potential mechanisms contributing to progression of HER2-positive breast cancers. *Am. J. Pathol.* **2015**, *185*, 987–1000. [CrossRef]
61. Llaverias, G.; Danilo, C.; Mercier, I.; Daumer, K.; Capozza, F.; Williams, T.M.; Sotgia, F.; Lisanti, M.P.; Frank, P.G. Role of cholesterol in the development and progression of breast cancer. *Am. J. Pathol.* **2011**, *178*, 402–412. [CrossRef]
62. Voisin, M.; de Medina, P.; Mallinger, A.; Dalenc, F.; Huc-Claustre, E.; Leignadier, J.; Serhan, N.; Soules, R.; Segala, G.; Mougel, A.; et al. Identification of a tumor-promoter cholesterol metabolite in human breast cancers acting through the glucocorticoid receptor. *Proc. Natl. Acad. Sci. USA* **2017**, *114*, E9346–E9355. [CrossRef] [PubMed]
63. Simpson, E.; Santen, R.J. Celebrating 75 years of oestradiol. *J. Mol. Endocrinol.* **2015**, *55*, T1–T20. [CrossRef]
64. Zhao, H.; Zhou, L.; Shangguan, A.J.; Bulun, S.E. Aromatase expression and regulation in breast and endometrial cancer. *J. Mol. Endocrinol.* **2016**, *57*, 19–33. [CrossRef]
65. Manna, P.R.; Chandrala, S.P.; King, S.R.; Jo, Y.; Counis, R.; Huhtaniemi, I.T.; Stocco, D.M. Molecular mechanisms of insulin-like growth factor-I mediated regulation of the steroidogenic acute regulatory protein in mouse leydig cells. *Mol. Endocrinol.* **2006**, *20*, 362–378. [CrossRef]
66. Manna, P.R.; Soh, J.W.; Stocco, D.M. The involvement of specific PKC isoenzymes in phorbol ester-mediated regulation of steroidogenic acute regulatory protein expression and steroid synthesis in mouse Leydig cells. *Endocrinology* **2011**, *152*, 313–325. [CrossRef]
67. Arakane, F.; King, S.R.; Du, Y.; Kallen, C.B.; Walsh, L.P.; Watari, H.; Stocco, D.M.; Strauss, J.F., 3rd. Phosphorylation of steroidogenic acute regulatory protein (StAR) modulates its steroidogenic activity. *J. Biol. Chem.* **1997**, *272*, 32656–32662. [CrossRef]
68. Clark, B.J.; Ranganathan, V.; Combs, R. Steroidogenic acute regulatory protein expression is dependent upon post-translational effects of cAMP-dependent protein kinase A. *Mol. Cell. Endocrinol.* **2001**, *173*, 183–192. [CrossRef]
69. Castro-Piedras, I.; Sharma, M.; den Bakker, M.; Molehin, D.; Martinez, E.G.; Vartak, D.; Pruitt, W.M.; Deitrick, J.; Almodovar, S.; Pruitt, K. DVL1 and DVL3 differentially localize to CYP19A1 promoters and regulate aromatase mRNA in breast cancer cells. *Oncotarget* **2018**, *9*, 35639–35654. [CrossRef]
70. Simpson, E.R.; Misso, M.; Hewitt, K.N.; Hill, R.A.; Boon, W.C.; Jones, M.E.; Kovacic, A.; Zhou, J.; Clyne, C.D. Estrogen–the good, the bad, and the unexpected. *Endocr. Rev.* **2005**, *26*, 322–330. [CrossRef] [PubMed]
71. Molehin, D.; Castro-Piedras, I.; Sharma, M.; Sennoune, S.R.; Arena, D.; Manna, P.R.; Pruitt, K. Aromatase Acetylation Patterns and Altered Activity in Response to Sirtuin Inhibition. *Mol. Cancer Res.* **2018**, *16*, 1530–1542. [CrossRef] [PubMed]
72. Bulun, S.E.; Lin, Z.; Imir, G.; Amin, S.; Demura, M.; Yilmaz, B.; Martin, R.; Utsunomiya, H.; Thung, S.; Gurates, B.; et al. Regulation of aromatase expression in estrogen-responsive breast and uterine disease: From bench to treatment. *Pharmacol. Rev.* **2005**, *57*, 359–383. [CrossRef] [PubMed]

11

False Discovery Rate Control in Cancer Biomarker Selection Using Knockoffs

Arlina Shen [1,†], Han Fu [2,†,‡], Kevin He [2] and Hui Jiang [2,*]

1 The Blake School, 511 Kenwood Pkwy, Minneapolis, MN 55403, USA; ahshen20@blakeschool.org
2 Department of Biostatistics, University of Michigan, 1415 Washington Heights, Ann Arbor, MI 48109, USA; fu.607@osu.edu (H.F.); kevinhe@umich.edu (K.H.)
* Correspondence: jianghui@umich.edu;
† These authors contributed equally to this work.
‡ Current address: Department of Statistics, Ohio State University, 1958 Neil Ave, Columbus, OH 43210, USA.

Abstract: The discovery of biomarkers that are informative for cancer risk assessment, diagnosis, prognosis and treatment predictions is crucial. Recent advances in high-throughput genomics make it plausible to select biomarkers from the vast number of human genes in an unbiased manner. Yet, control of false discoveries is challenging given the large number of genes versus the relatively small number of patients in a typical cancer study. To ensure that most of the discoveries are true, we employ a knockoff procedure to control false discoveries. Our method is general and flexible, accommodating arbitrary covariate distributions, linear and nonlinear associations, and survival models. In simulations, our method compares favorably to the alternatives; its utility of identifying important genes in real clinical applications is demonstrated by the identification of seven genes associated with Breslow thickness in skin cutaneous melanoma patients.

Keywords: cancer biomarker; diseases genes; variable selection; false discovery rate; knockoffs

---

1. Introduction

The discovery of biomarkers that are informative for cancer risk assessment, diagnosis, prognosis and treatment predictions is crucial. Many biomarkers have been proven to be very informative for clinical usage, with prominent examples such as BRCA1 and HER2 in breast cancer [1,2], EGFR in non-small-cell lung carcinoma [3] and PSA in prostate cancer [4]. Recent advances in high-throughput genomics make it plausible to select biomarkers from the vast number of human genes in an unbiased manner. For instance, genes associated with disease-related clinical outcomes can be identified by linking a patient's gene expression to the disease progression [5] or other disease phenotypes. Furthermore, by understanding the regulatory roles of these associated genes on various cancers, treatment strategies may be developed. For these reasons, many gene signatures have been discovered for a variety of cancers.

However, many challenges exist for the selection of genes from the high-throughput and high-dimensional expression data at a genomic scale. Besides computational challenges due to the large size of data, a critical statistical difficulty is the control of false discoveries of all identified genes mainly due to the large number of genes versus the relatively small number of patients in a typical cancer study. The conventional method for genomic data analysis is known as univariate analysis, that is, exploring the relationship of the disease-related outcomes with one gene at a time. Due to its simplicity and intuitiveness, univariate analysis has been widely used in gene selection. However, high correlations exist among genes induced by co-expression activities, and hence genes correlated with disease-related genes are also correlated with disease outcomes (a.k.a. spurious correlation). Therefore they will be selected via univariate analysis, leading to high false discoveries. Another issue of univariate analysis is its low statistical power of identifying any disease-related genes due to the multiplicity of hypothesis testing [6] as well as noise that is unaccounted for. That is, relatively fewer genes that are truly associated with the outcome will be identified from univariate analysis than that with multivariate analysis. For the reasons above, penalized multivariate analysis approaches such as the lasso regression [7] and its extensions such as penalized generalized linear models and the Cox proportional hazard model with elastic-net penalty [8,9] have been applied recently to genomic data analysis [10,11]. Nevertheless, because cross-valuation is typically used for the selection of the optimal tuning parameters, such approaches often fail to control false discoveries [12]. This aspect has been clearly illustrated in our simulations in Section 3.1.

For prediction purposes, genes with spurious correlations to the disease outcomes may be useful. However, they are unsuitable when the goal is to understand the disease etiology, or to identify potential treatment targets, where genes that are genuinely associated with the disease are required. In other words, when the number of false discoveries is high, the discoveries are not scientifically replicable. Due to the high cost to experimentally validate the selected genes, there is an urgent need to control for false discoveries in gene selection procedures. The false discovery rate (FDR) [13], defined as the expected proportion of false discoveries among all discoveries, is a widely used method to control for false discoveries in genomic studies, due to its high statistical power compared with conventional methods that control for family-wise error rates (FWER) such as the Bonferroni correction. Controlling for FDR leads to limited proportion of non-true findings among all findings produced by a given analysis and discovery procedure, which translates to reliable scientific discoveries as well as reduced attempts and costs to validate non-true findings. The importance of controlling for the false discovery rate in lasso regression has also been recognized. Recently, [12] proposed a bootstrap/resampling method to control the FDR in lasso type variable selection. The smoothness of the limiting distributions of the bootstrap, which is the standard assumption for the bootstrap, is needed for such methods [14]. In [15], a knockoff procedure was introduced to control the FDR in linear regression when the number of variables is not too large; knockoff variables are constructed to mimic the correlation structure found within the existing variables. In a follow-up paper [16], the method was further expanded to a general framework and a high-dimensional situation for Gaussian variables was studied extensively. However, there is still a gap between the generally simple knockoff framework and the complicated data structures in real world applications.

In this paper, we propose several novel strategies based on the knockoff framework for variable selection subject to control for the false discovery rate. The proposed method is general and flexible, accommodating arbitrary covariate distributions, linear and nonlinear associations, and survival models. Simulation experiments and a real data example on gene identification for Breslow thickness in skin cutaneous melanoma patients demonstrate the utility of the proposed method.

2. Methodology

In many practical situations, identification of a set of explanatory variables which are truly associated with the response is a primary interest in investigation. This is particularly true in biomedical research when genes are selected from a pool of candidate genes that are potentially associated with a disease. To assure that most of the discoveries are true and replicable, one must know whether the false discovery rate, or the expected fraction of false discoveries among all discoveries, as defined in Definition 1, is acceptable or too large. In other words, the false discovery rate in this discovery process needs to be controlled at a desirable level.

Definition 1 (False discovery). *Let S be the true set of variables associated with an outcome, and $\hat{S}$ be the set of variables selected based on a dataset. The false discovery proportion (FDP) is defined as the proportion of false discoveries among all discoveries, i.e., $FDP := |\hat{S} \setminus S| / |\hat{S}|$, where $|\cdot|$ is the size of a set, with the convention $0/0 = 0$. The false discovery rate (FDR) [13] is defined as the expectation of FDP, i.e., $FDR := E[FDP]$.*

The method proposed in this paper is based on the knockoff framework first proposed in [15] and later generalized in [16]. The knockoff framework provides a recipe for building algorithms to control for FDR in variable selection. Under certain mild conditions, the FDR can be theoretically guaranteed to be controlled at a pre-specified level. The key contribution of the knockoff framework is the introduction of the concept of knockoff variables, as defined in Definition 2.

Definition 2 (Knockoff variables). *A set of random variables* $(\widetilde{X}_1, \cdots, \widetilde{X}_p)$ *is said to be model-free knockoffs [16] for* $(X_1, \cdots, X_p)$ *with respect to response* Y *if they are constructed without looking at* Y*, and for any* $j \in \{1, \cdots, p\}$*, the pair* $(X_j, \widetilde{X}_j)$ *is exchangeable conditioned on all the other variables* $(\widetilde{X}_1, \cdots \widetilde{X}_p)$ *and* $(X_1, \cdots, X_p)$ *excluding* $(X_j, \widetilde{X}_j)$.

In layman's terms, each knockoff variable $\widetilde{X}_j$ can be considered as a "fake" duplicate of the corresponding variable X_j, in that the relationship between $\widetilde{X}_j$ and all the other variables and their knockoffs excluding X_j is indistinguishable from the relationship between X_j and all the other variables and their knockoffs excluding $\widetilde{X}_j$. Furthermore, the knockoff variables are constructed without using the outcome variable, and therefore are guaranteed not to be associated with the outcome. As a result, in a variable selection procedure, a knockoff variable $\widetilde{X}_j$ has equal chance of being selected as the "original" variable X_j when X_j is not associated with the outcome, which makes the knockoff variables robust benchmarks for FDR control. In this paper, we propose several novel strategies based on the knockoff framework for variable selection subject to control for the false discovery rate.

2.1. Construction of Model-Free Knockoff Variables

The first step for variable selection based on the knockoff framework is to construct knockoff variables. In [15,16], algorithms for constructing knockoff variables for low and high dimensional multivariate Gaussian distributions were proposed, respectively. In particular, an approximated algorithm was proposed in [16] to construct knockoffs by sampling from a multivariate Gaussian distribution with the same first two moments as that of the original variables. When the joint distribution of the original variables is known, the conditional distributions can be derived, based on which random samples can be drawn directly and can be used as knockoffs.

Although built on a multivariate Gaussian distribution, the performance of the knockoff variables constructed using the algorithm in [16] is reported to be quite robust against deviations from the Gaussian assumption, as long as the first two moments are approximated well. We also have the same observations in our experiments (See Appendix C). Therefore, we use the algorithm in [16] for the construction of knockoff variables for all the simulated and real data experiments in this paper, unless otherwise noted. Moreover, we propose another algorithm for constructing knockoff variables without the Gaussian assumption with much higher computational burden (See Appendix A), which may be used in situations when the Gaussian assumption is severely violated.

2.2. Model-Free Statistics

The knockoff framework guarantees that the FDR is controlled at a desirable level for variable selection. However, the statistical power for variable selection depends on the specific statistic being used in the knockoff framework. In [16], the lasso coefficient difference (LCD) statistic was proposed and shown to be very powerful for variable selection based on the lasso regression model. However, it assumes a linear relationship between the response variable and the predictors. When such relationship does not hold, the statistical power will be compromised. In this section, we propose two novel statistics to accommodate arbitrary relationships between the response and predictor variables, thereby realizing our goal of model-free variable selection. In contrast to the lasso regression model in [16], we incorporate machine learning techniques, such as support vector regression [17] and boosting [18], to allow for more flexible and complex model settings.

2.2.1. Difference in R-Squared (DRS) Statistic

Intuitively, variable importance can be measured by the amount of variability of the response data explained by each specific variable. In practice, we can define a statistic named difference in R-squared (DRS) based on the difference between the R^2 value achieved by the full model and that by a partial model where one predictor variable is excluded at a time. See Appendix B for details.

2.2.2. Risk Reduction in Boosting (RRB) Statistic

This statistic stems from the `mboost` R package which implements a functional gradient descent algorithm for model-based boosting. This method uses component-wise least squares estimates or regression trees as base-learners to optimize general risk functions. The algorithm is quite flexible in that it allows for various kinds of base-learners to be used, for example, linear, P-spline, and tree based base-learners, as well as a variety of loss functions and corresponding risk functions to be optimized. In a fitted boosting model, the accumulated in-bag risk reductions per boosting step for each base-learner or variable can be used to reflect variable importance. The amount of risk reduction can be provided by a function called varimp in the `mboost` R package with appealing computing efficiency. Similar to DRS, the risk reduction in boosting (RRB) statistic W_j can be constructed by the difference between the risk reduction of variable X_j and that of its corresponding knockoff $\widetilde{X}_j$. Again, W_j here attains the anti-symmetry property and a symmetric distribution under the null hypothesis. The high flexibility of the boosting method allows us to model arbitrarily complex relationships between y and $(X, \widetilde{X})$. The computational efficiency also makes this statistic favorable for our high-dimensional variable selection purpose. In our simulations, compared with the DRS statistic, we found that the RRB statistic achieves better performance in terms of FDR control and of statistical power for variable selection (See Appendix C), with much lower computational burden. Therefore, we use the RRB statistic for all the simulated and real data experiments in this paper, unless otherwise noted.

2.3. Nonlinear Screening

As genomic datasets are often high-dimensional, that is, the number of genes p is much larger than the sample size n, computing the statistics W_j for each variable X_j will take a lot of time. Here, we propose a nonlinear screening strategy to accelerate this procedure. In particular, when $2p > n$, we perform univariate fitting of y to each X_j as well as $\widetilde{X}_j$, using nonlinear regression based on B-splines. In particular, we rank all the variables and their knockoffs based on the L_2 norm of the block-wise gradient vector. The top variables are corresponding to the steepest descent directions, which minimizes the direction derivative, and hence, provides the largest decrease in the linear approximation of the objective function. We then retain the top n variables for computing their W_j's subsequently using a chosen statistic, and set the W_j's for all the remaining $2p - n$ variables to be zero. In our simulations, we found that this nonlinear screening strategy can substantially reduce computational time while maintaining the FDR control as well as statistical power for variable selection (See Appendix C). Therefore, we use this nonlinear screening strategy for all the simulated and real data experiments in this paper, unless otherwise noted.

3. Results

3.1. Simulations

We first use simulation studies to evaluate the performance of our proposed method against two other existing methods: the knockoff method with lasso coefficient difference (LCD) [16] and lasso regression [7] with cross-validation (CV), a widely used variable selection approach. In simulations, we examine several situations to demonstrate that the proposed method performs well in terms of FDR control with increased statistical power. These simulations support the usage of the proposed method for analyzing a real dataset in Section 3.2. All simulations are performed in R.

In particular, we consider three cases of linear and nonlinear associations as well as survival models. In each case, we apply our proposal of using the boosting method with P-spline base-learners to approximate linear or nonlinear associations. We use the knockoff construction algorithm introduced in [16], the RRB statistic described in Section 2.2.2, and the nonlinear screening described in Section 2.3. Specifically, we use the mboost R package to fit y against the augmented design matrix $(X, \widetilde{X})$. For fitting lasso penalized models in the knockoff with the LCD method of [16] and in lasso regression with cross-validation, we use the glmnet R package [8,9] with five-fold cross-validation for selection of the regularization parameter of lasso in simulations for linear (Section 3.1.1) and nonlinear (Section 3.1.2) associations and the Cox proportional hazards regression [19] in simulations for survival analysis (Section 3.1.3).

3.1.1. Linear Associations

The first simulation study focuses on linear associations in regression. In particular, the data were simulated from a linear regression model

$$Y = \sum_{j=1}^{p} X_j \beta_j + \varepsilon, \quad \varepsilon \sim N(0, \sigma^2), \tag{1}$$

in which $\mathbf{X} = (X_1, \cdots, X_p)^T$ is distributed according to a p-dimensional Gaussian distribution $N(\mathbf{0}, \mathbf{\Sigma})$, with the ij-th element of $\mathbf{\Sigma}$ being $\rho^{|i-j|}$, following an auto-regressive variance structure with the auto-regressive coefficient ρ. Moreover, $\mathbf{X}$ and ε are independent. Of p variables, we randomly choose k variables $X_{j_1}, \cdots, X_{j_k}$ and set the corresponding $\beta_{j_l} = \zeta_{j_l} A$, where A, called amplitude, is a varying magnitude given in Figure 1, ζ_{j_l} is a random sign, and $\beta_j = 0$ if $j \notin \{j_1, \ldots, j_k\}$. The amplitude represents the association strength (e.g., correlation) between a biomarker and the outcome. In this case, we simulate $p = 2000$, $k = 10$, $\rho = 0.3$, and $\sigma^2 = 1$ from (1) with sample size $n = 300$. This mimics the real data analysis in Section 3.2. We use the multivariate Gaussian distribution for its simplicity in simulating correlated covariates and the fact that the knockoff framework is robust against deviations from this distributional assumption, as long as the first two moments are approximated well [16]. Furthermore, the relationship between outcome and covariates can be arbitrary.

As suggested by Figure 1, the FDR is controlled around our target value of 20% for the proposed method (knockoff + mboost). The FDR for the knockoff + LCD method is slightly higher. In contrast, the FDR of the lasso + CV method is so high that the discovery is unreliable. All three methods have similar statistical power, and power increases and gets close to 1 as the signal strength gets stronger. A statistical power of 1 means the ideal situation that all genes that are truly associated with the outcome are identified. Although Lasso + CV has the highest power, it is not desirable for discovery, given the uncontrollable FDR levels. Thus, lasso + CV is not a suitable approach for gene selection.

As will be seen in the cases of nonlinear associations (Section 3.1.2) and survival models (Section 3.1.3), the proposed method becomes more powerful when the model assumption of linear associations is violated.

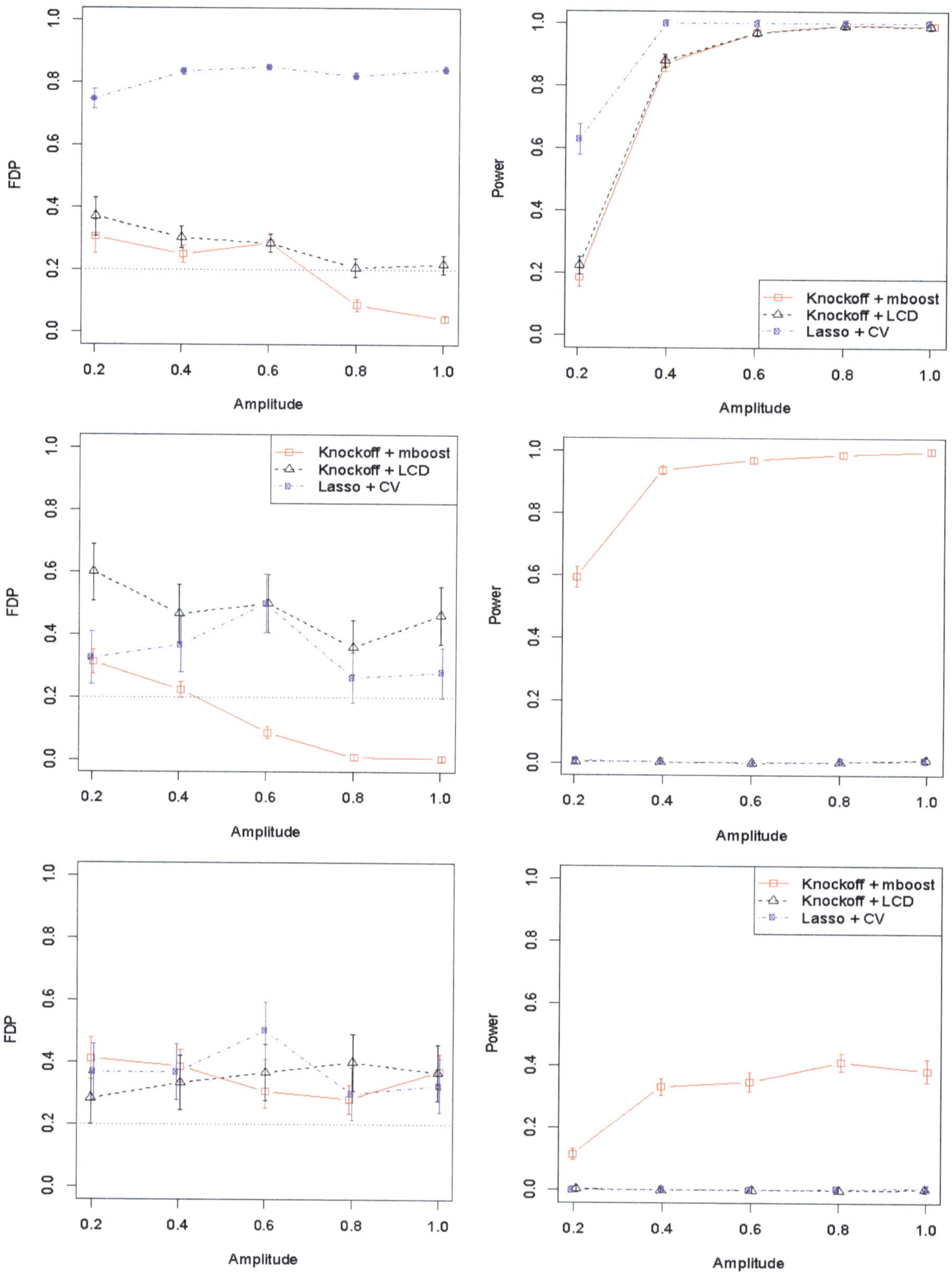

Figure 1. Simulation results for linear associations (**top panel**), nonlinear associations (**middle panel**) and survival analysis (**bottom panel**). Left panel: averaged false discovery proportion (FDP, the empirical version of FDR) and the standard error bars for knockoff variable selection with mboost (red), lasso coefficient difference (LCD) (black) and lasso regression with cross-validation (CV) (blue) as a function of amplitude (association strength (e.g., correlation) between a biomarker and the outcome) based on 30 simulation replications. The reference lines indicate the target false discovery rate of 20%. Right panel: corresponding empirical statistical power of the three methods.

3.1.2. Nonlinear Associations

Our second simulation study deals with nonlinear relationships in regression, in which we again compare the proposed knockoff + mboost method with the knockoff + LCD method of [16] as well as lasso + CV. Here, we replace $\sum_{j=1}^{p} X_j\beta_j$ in (1) by $\sum_{j=1}^{p} X_j^2\beta_j$ to accommodate nonlinear associations. All other settings are the same as in Section 3.1.1.

As indicated in Figure 1, the FDR for the proposed method (knock + mboost) is controlled under the target value of 20%, as marked by the horizontal dotted line, whereas the FDRs for the other two methods are above the target level. In terms of statistical power, the proposed method is much better than the other two methods, which assume a linear predictor while the proposed method is more flexible without such assumptions.

3.1.3. Survival Analysis

Our third simulation study concerns the Cox proportional hazards regression [19] with a nonlinear predictor $\sum_{j=1}^{p} X_j^2\beta_j$ as in Section 3.1.2. Specifically, we generate y from the Cox model with a baseline hazard rate equals to 0.002 and a hazard rate of censoring equals to 0.004. The event time follows a Weibull distribution with the shape parameter equals to 1 and scale parameter equals to the baseline hazard rate multiplied by the exponential of the predictor, i.e., $\exp(\sum_{j=1}^{p} X_j^2\beta_j)$. The censoring time is also sampled from a Weibull distribution with the shape parameter equals to 1 and scale parameter equals to the hazard rate of censoring. The actual observation time is the smaller value between the event and censoring times.

As shown in Figure 1, all three methods roughly achieve the objective of controlling the FDR at the desired level of 20% with slight inflation. The proposed method exhibits much higher power than the other two as was the case in Section 3.1.2.

Based on the simulation studies, we conclude that the proposed method performs well for linear and nonlinear associations as well as survival models. In practice, we do not need to assume linear or non-linear association between the biomarkers and the outcome, and our method will identify biomarkers with high statistical power and well controlled FDR regardless of the type of association that is present in the dataset.

3.2. *Cancer Data*

In this section we apply our proposed method as described in Section 3.1 to a real dataset from a cancer study for the identification of genes that are associated with clinical outcomes. We investigate a skin cutaneous melanoma (SKCM) dataset, which contains the expression levels of 20,531 genes from 355 melanoma patients measured by RNA-Seq. The dataset is a part of The Cancer Genome Atlas (TCGA) project and publicly available from the TCGA data portal at https://portal.gdc.cancer.gov/. The aim is to identify a set of genes associated with the clinical variable of interest, called Breslow thickness.

Due to the large number of genes and the relatively small sample size, to expedite computation while enhancing the accuracy of identification, we apply a filtering rule to select genes whose mean expression levels exceed 1 normalized transcripts per million (TPM) and the q-value (corrected using the BH procedure [13]) from univariate correlation tests with the response less than 0.2. This leaves us 4171 genes to which to apply our method with the log-transformed Breslow thickness as the response. The predictor variables are measured in log-transformed gene expression values (in TPM).

In this case, at a target FDR of 20%, our method identifies seven genes BOLA1 (BolA Family Member 1), CLDN16 (Claudin 16), EBF2 (EBF Transcription Factor 2), KCTD16 (Potassium Channel Tetramerization Domain Containing 16), KRT14 (Keratin 14), LOC100240735 (Uncharacterized LOC100240735), and MAP4K4 (Mitogen-Activated Protein Kinase 4). In the literature, the CLDN (Claudin) gene family is known to be associated with tumor suppressor genes; for example, hypermethylation of the CLDN11 promoter occurs frequently in malignant melanoma of the skin [20], which may encode a novel melanoma-specific tumor suppressor gene [21]. CLDN16 has been found to be associated with breast [22], thyroid [23], ovarian [24] and lung [25] cancers. Our finding suggests that CLDN16 is also associated with cutaneous melanoma of the skin, which seems consistent with the role of CLDN in terms of tumor suppression. Moreover, MAP4k4 belongs to the mammalian STE20/MAP4K family, which is often overexpressed in many types of human cancer and cancer cell lines, including malignant melanoma [26], because of its crucial role in transformation, invasiveness, adhesion, and cell migration [27]. KRT14 has been found to be associated with melanoma [28]. EBF2 has been found to be associated with prostate [29], bone [30], hematological and epithelial [31] cancers. KCTD16 has been found to be associated with thyroid cancer [32], while KCTD12, a member of the KCTD family, has been found to be associated with uveal melanoma [33]. BOLA1 and LOC100240735 (an RNA gene) are not known to be associated with any malignancies. To further understand the roles of these genes in melanoma, experimental follow-up studies are needed.

As a comparison, we also run Lasso + CV on the same dataset, for which a total of 140 genes are identified. Five of the seven genes identified by Knockoff + mboost are also identified by Lasso + CV. The two genes not identified by Lasso + CV are KRT14 and LOC100240735. Given the high false discovery rates of Lasso + CV in simulations (top-left panel of Figure 1), we expect a large proportion of these 140 genes to be false positives.

Furthermore, to demonstrate the performance of our approach in non-Gaussian data, we randomly pick 500 genes and assign 10 random genes among them to be truly associated genes with the remaining 490 genes to be null genes. We then randomly assign coefficients for the 10 truly associated genes by sampling from $Uniform(1,5)$ with a random sign. To make the problem even more challenging and to demonstrate the ability of our approach working with non-quantitative data, we dichotomize the resulting linear predictor $Y = \sum_{j=1}^{p} X_j\beta_j$ at the median of its distribution so that the outcomes are binary (i.e., two groups of equal sizes). After running Knockoff + mboost at a target FDR level of 20%, a total of seven genes are identified, with five true positives and two false positives, which corresponds to an FDP of 28.6% and a statistical power of 50%.

4. Discussion

An advantage of our method is that no prior specification of the type of association (i.e., linear or non-linear) is needed, which is usually unknown for a given dataset. The knockoff construction algorithm in [16] is based on Gaussian assumption. Nevertheless, it seems robust for non-Gaussian data in our experiments. We also present a knockoff construction algorithm which does not require the Gaussian assumption in case such assumption is severely violated.

The statistical power depends both on the statistic being used and the correlation structure among covariates, which was also noted in [16]. As the correlation among covariates increases, the statistical power decreases. Therefore, a future research direction may be developing methods for the detection of highly correlated gene clusters that are associated with the outcome of interest. Furthermore, due to the high computational cost of building the knockoff variables, right now we can only practically use our method with up to around 5000 pre-selected genes. Thus, developing more efficient computational algorithms for building knockoff variables may be another future research direction.

The datasets and R programs for producing the results in this paper are available at http://www-personal.umich.edu/~jianghui/knockoff/.

5. Conclusions

The results in this paper demonstrate that our proposed approach can provide reliable false discovery rate control for variable selection in various statistical models. Such rigorous false discovery rate control is crucial for improving replicability of the findings and avoiding wasting resources for attempts to validate false discoveries. With additional enhancements, our method offers a promising avenue to identify reliable gene markers in cancer studies.

Author Contributions: Conceptualization, H.J.; methodology, K.H. and H.J.; formal analysis, A.S., H.F., K.H. and H.J.; writing-original draft preparation, A.S. and H.F.; writing-review and editing, K.H. and H.J.; supervision, K.H. and H.J.; project administration, H.J.; funding acquisition, H.J.

Acknowledgments: We thank National Cancer Institute and National Human Genome Research Institute for making the TCGA data portal available, and thank Yang Shi at Augusta University for the skin cutaneous melanoma dataset. Thanks to the reviewers for their valuable comments, and to Megan Ludwig at the UM-CMB and Kirsten Herold at the UM-SPH Writing Lab for their helpful suggestions.

Abbreviations

The following abbreviations are used in this manuscript:

FDR	False Discovery Rate
FWER	Family-Wise Error Rate
LCD	Lasso Coefficient Difference
SKCM	Skin Cutaneous Melanoma
TCGA	The Cancer Genome Atlas
TPM	Transcripts Per Million

Appendix A New Algorithm for Model-Free Knockoff Variable Construction

We propose a new algorithm for constructing knockoff variables without Gaussian assumption, by obtaining the conditional distributions empirically through regression models, regardless of the joint distribution of the covariates. Knockoff construction is independent from the response and the form of associations between response and covariates. Our proposal is to generate random samples from the conditional distributions by simply permuting the residuals, assuming that the residuals are approximately independently and identically distributed. Details of the algorithm are summarized in Algorithm A.1.

Algorithm A.1 (Algorithm for construction of model-free knockoff variables).

For each covariate X_j, $j = 1, \cdots, p$,

(1) Fit X_j on $(X_{-j}, \widetilde{X}_{1:j-1})$ with a regression model, where X_{-j} denotes $(X_1, \cdots, X_{j-1}, X_{j+1}, \cdots, X_p)$ and $\widetilde{X}_{1:j-1}$ represents existing knockoffs. No knockoffs are taken into consideration for X_1.

(2) Compute residuals $\varepsilon = (\varepsilon_1, \cdots, \varepsilon_n)$ by subtracting the predicted value for X_j from the corresponding observed values, i.e., $\varepsilon_l = X_{jl} - \hat{X}_{jl}, l = 1, \ldots, n$, where $\hat{X}_{jl}$ is the predicted value of X_{jl} by the regression model.

(3) Permute the residuals randomly, denoted by the permuted residuals $\varepsilon^* = (\varepsilon_1^*, \cdots, \varepsilon_n^*)$.

(4) Construct knockoff variable $\widetilde{X}_j$ by adding the corresponding permuted residual to the predicted value for X_j, i.e., $\widetilde{X}_{jl} = \hat{X}_{jl} + \varepsilon_l^*, l = 1, \ldots, n$.

(5) Proceed to the next covariate until all knockoffs are constructed.

Unlike [15,16], our proposed algorithm does not assume the multivariate Gaussian joint distributions of the covariates. The only requirement is the independence of the residuals, which may require an appropriate choice of regression model for fitting. For example, lasso [7] would be a good choice when X_j is linearly dependent on $(X_{-j}, \widetilde{X}_{1:j-1})$, and supervised machine learning techniques like support vector regression [17] and gradient boosting [18] are flexible enough to approximate nonlinear functional dependence. To avoid the problem of over-fitting, we may use K-fold cross-validation on test sets for prediction in subsequent calculations. Cross-validation may also help select optimal tuning parameters in the regression model and thus enable the method to be well adaptive to the observed covariate data.

Given the construction algorithm, we can generate knockoff variables from an arbitrary distribution, thus, effectively increasing the level of flexibility on the covariate distribution. For instance, for a binary response, we can simply replace the aforementioned regression models by classification models and then permute the binary response within the same prediction group to generate random samples for knockoffs.

The drawback of Algorithm A.1 is an increased computational burden. In our simulations, we noticed that the moments-based knockoff construction algorithm proposed in [16] is not very sensitive to the multivariate Gaussian assumption, and achieve similar performance as our regression-based knockoff construction algorithm in most cases (See Appendix C). Therefore, to save computing times, we use the algorithm in [16] for all the simulations and real data experiments, unless otherwise noted. Nevertheless, our regression-based knockoff construction algorithm has the potential to be used in broader scenarios, including situations when the Gaussian assumption is severely violated.

Appendix B Difference in R-Squared (DRS) Statistic

Algorithm B.1 gives the complete procedure for calculating the DRS statistics.

Algorithm B.1 (The DRS algorithm).

(1) Fit y with $(X, \widetilde{X})$ using a prediction model and obtain R^2, where $X = (X_i, \ldots, X_p)$ contains the original predictor variables and $\widetilde{X} = (\widetilde{X}_1, \ldots, \widetilde{X}_p)$ contains the corresponding knockoff variables. $(X, \widetilde{X})$ is considered as an augmented design matrix with $2p$ columns.

(2) For each variable or knockoff variable in $(X, \widetilde{X})$, $j = 1, \ldots, 2p$, fit y with $(X, \widetilde{X})$ excluding the j-th variable with the same prediction model as in step 1) and obtain R_j^2. Calculate the absolute value of the difference between the two R-squared values, $Z_j = \left|R^2 - R_j^2\right|$, $j = 1, \ldots, 2p$, and record it as the importance score for the j-th variable (or knockoff variable).

(3) For $j = 1, \ldots, p$, the DRS statistic for X_j can be derived as $W_j = Z_j - Z_{j+p}$, that is, the difference in Z between a variable and its knockoff.

The anti-symmetry requirement for feature statistics in [16] is fulfilled by the way we construct the DRS statistic. A large positive value of W_j provides evidence that variable X_j is strongly associated with the response y, while the statistic for a null variable is equally likely to take on a small positive or negative value, i.e., to have a symmetric distribution around zero. Similar to Algorithm A.1, we can apply various prediction methods for fitting in steps (1) and (2), for example, lasso for the linear relationship between y and $(X, \widetilde{X})$, and supervised machine learning techniques such as support vector regression and gradient boosting for nonlinear associations. To avoid the problem of over-fitting, we can use K-fold cross-validation and summarize the predictive power of the models by mean squared prediction error which can produce a cross-validated R^2. Cross-validation can also help select the tuning parameters in the prediction model and thereby enable the method to be well adaptive to the observed data.

Appendix C Additional Simulations

We conduct additional simulation experiments to compare four approaches: (1) knockoff construction using Gaussian based algorithm in [16] with RRB statistics in Section 2.2.2 (named Knockoff + mboost), (2) knockoff construction using model-free algorithm in Appendix A with RRB statistics (named Model-free knockoff + mboost), (3) knockoff construction using Gaussian based algorithm with DRS statistics in Appendix B (named Knockoff + DRS), and (4) knockoff construction using Gaussian based algorithm with RRB statistics but without nonlinear screening in Section 2.3 (named Knockoff + mboost + no screening). The simulation setting is similar to that of Section 3.1.1, except that here we exponentiate each element of the design matrix X, so that the covariates follow multivariate log-normal distribution. Furthermore, to save computing time, we let $n = 100$ and $p = 100$. The comparison results are shown in Figure A1. We can see that except for Knockoff + DRS which has an inflated FDP and a lower power, all three other methods have similar performance.

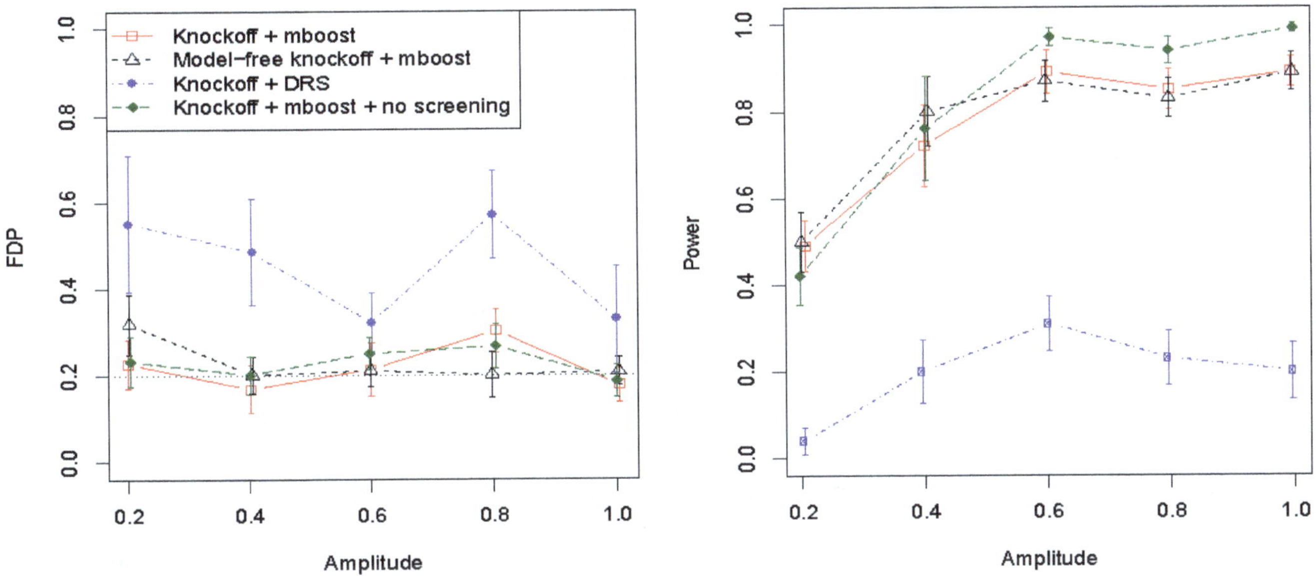

Figure A1. Simulation results for linear associations with log-normal covariates. Left panel: averaged false discovery proportion (FDP, the empirical version of FDR) and the standard error bars for knockoff variable selection with Knockoff with mboost (red), Model-free knockoff with mboost (black), Knockoff with DRS (blue) and Knockoff with mboost without screening (dark green) as a function of amplitude (association strength (e.g., correlation) between a biomarker and the outcome) based on 10 simulation replications. The reference lines indicate the target false discovery rate of 20%. Right panel: corresponding empirical statistical power of the four methods.

References

1. Miki, Y.; Swensen, J.; Shattuck-Eidens, D.; Futreal, P.A.; Harshman, K.; Tavtigian, S.; Liu, Q.; Cochran, C.; Bennett, L.M.; Ding, W.; et al. A strong candidate for the breast and ovarian cancer susceptibility gene BRCA1. *Science* **1994**, *266*, 66–71. [CrossRef] [PubMed]
2. Slamon, D.J.; Leyland-Jones, B.; Shak, S.; Fuchs, H.; Paton, V.; Bajamonde, A.; Fleming, T.; Eiermann, W.; Wolter, J.; Pegram, M.; et al. Use of chemotherapy plus a monoclonal antibody against HER2 for metastatic breast cancer that overexpresses HER2. *N. Engl. J. Med.* **2001**, *344*, 783–792. [CrossRef] [PubMed]
3. Paez, J.G.; Jänne, P.A.; Lee, J.C.; Tracy, S.; Greulich, H.; Gabriel, S.; Herman, P.; Kaye, F.J.; Lindeman, N.; Boggon, T.J.; et al. EGFR mutations in lung cancer: correlation with clinical response to gefitinib therapy. *Science* **2004**, *304*, 1497–1500. [CrossRef] [PubMed]
4. Catalona, W.J.; Smith, D.S.; Ratliff, T.L.; Dodds, K.M.; Coplen, D.E.; Yuan, J.J.; Petros, J.A.; Andriole, G.L. Measurement of prostate-specific antigen in serum as a screening test for prostate cancer. *N. Engl. J. Med.* **1991**, *324*, 1156–1161. [CrossRef]
5. Shaughnessy, J.D.; Zhan, F.; Burington, B.E.; Huang, Y.; Colla, S.; Hanamura, I.; Stewart, J.P.; Kordsmeier, B.; Randolph, C.; Williams, D.R.; et al. A validated gene expression model of high-risk multiple myeloma is defined by deregulated expression of genes mapping to chromosome 1. *Blood* **2007**, *109*, 2276–2284. [CrossRef]
6. Sun, S.; Hood, M.; Scott, L.; Peng, Q.; Mukherjee, S.; Tung, J.; Zhou, X. Differential expression analysis for RNAseq using Poisson mixed models. *Nucleic Acids Res.* **2017**, *45*, e106. [CrossRef]

7. Tibshirani, R. Regression shrinkage and selection via the lasso. *J. R. Stat. Soc. Ser. B (Methodol.)* **1996**, *58*, 267–288. [CrossRef]
8. Friedman, J.; Hastie, T.; Tibshirani, R. Regularization paths for generalized linear models via coordinate descent. *J. Stat. Softw.* **2010**, *33*, 1. [CrossRef]
9. Simon, N.; Friedman, J.; Hastie, T.; Tibshirani, R. Regularization paths for Coxars proportional hazards model via coordinate descent. *J. Stat. Softw.* **2011**, *39*, 1. [CrossRef] [PubMed]
10. Ayers, K.L.; Cordell, H.J. SNP selection in genome-wide and candidate gene studies via penalized logistic regression. *Genet. Epidemiol.* **2010**, *34*, 879–891. [CrossRef]
11. Wu, T.T.; Chen, Y.F.; Hastie, T.; Sobel, E.; Lange, K. Genome-wide association analysis by lasso penalized logistic regression. *Bioinformatics* **2009**, *25*, 714–721. [CrossRef]
12. He, K.; Zhou, X.; Jiang, H.; Wen, X.; Li, Y. False discovery control for penalized variable selections with high-dimensional covariates. *Stat. Appl. Genet. Mol. Biol.* **2018**, *17*. [CrossRef]
13. Benjamini, Y.; Hochberg, Y. Controlling the false discovery rate: A practical and powerful approach to multiple testing. *J. R. Stat. Soc. Ser. B (Methodol.)* **1995**, *57*, 289–300. [CrossRef]
14. Efron, B. Estimation and accuracy after model selection. *J. Am. Stat. Assoc.* **2014**, *109*, 991–1007. [CrossRef] [PubMed]
15. Barber, R.F.; Candès, E.J. Controlling the false discovery rate via knockoffs. *Ann. Stat.* **2015**, *43*, 2055–2085. [CrossRef]
16. Candes, E.; Fan, Y.; Janson, L.; Lv, J. Panning for gold:'model-X' knockoffs for high dimensional controlled variable selection. *J. R. Stat. Soc. Ser. B (Stat. Methodol.)* **2018**, *80*, 551–577. [CrossRef]
17. Cortes, C.; Vapnik, V. Support-vector networks. *Mach. Learn.* **1995**, *20*, 273–297. [CrossRef]
18. Friedman, J.H. Greedy function approximation: A gradient boosting machine. *Ann. Stat.* **2001**, 1189–1232. [CrossRef]
19. Cox, D.R. Regression models and life-tables. *J. R. Stat. Soc. Ser. B (Methodol.)* **1972**, *34*, 187–202. [CrossRef]
20. Gao, L.; Smit, M.A.; van den Oord, J.J.; Goeman, J.J.; Verdegaal, E.M.; van der Burg, S.H.; Stas, M.; Beck, S.; Gruis, N.A.; Tensen, C.P.; et al. Genome-wide promoter methylation analysis identifies epigenetic silencing of MAPK 13 in primary cutaneous melanoma. *Pigment Cell Melanoma Res.* **2013**, *26*, 542–554. [CrossRef]
21. Walesch, S.; Richter, A.; Helmbold, P.; Dammann, R. Claudin11 promoter hypermethylation is frequent in malignant melanoma of the skin, but uncommon in nevus cell nevi. *Cancers* **2015**, *7*, 1233–1243. [CrossRef]
22. Kuo, S.J.; Chien, S.Y.; Lin, C.; Chan, S.E.; Tsai, H.T.; Chen, D.R. Significant elevation of CLDN16 and HAPLN3 gene expression in human breast cancer. *Oncol. Rep.* **2010**, *24*, 759–766.
23. Gomez-Rueda, H.; Palacios-Corona, R.; Gutiérrez-Hermosillo, H.; Trevino, V. A robust biomarker of differential correlations improves the diagnosis of cytologically indeterminate thyroid cancers. *Int. J. Mol. Med.* **2016**, *37*, 1355–1362. [CrossRef] [PubMed]
24. Rangel, L.B.; Sherman-Baust, C.A.; Wernyj, R.P.; Schwartz, D.R.; Cho, K.R.; Morin, P.J. Characterization of novel human ovarian cancer-specific transcripts (HOSTs) identified by serial analysis of gene expression. *Oncogene* **2003**, *22*, 7225. [CrossRef] [PubMed]
25. Fan, J.; Zhu, M.; Wang, Y.; Li, Z.; Zhang, J.; Wang, L.; Sun, Q.; Dai, J.; Jin, G.; Hu, Z.; et al. Genome-wide analysis of expression quantitative trait loci identified potential lung cancer susceptibility variants among Asian populations. *Carcinogenesis* **2019**. [CrossRef]
26. Collins, C.S.; Hong, J.; Sapinoso, L.; Zhou, Y.; Liu, Z.; Micklash, K.; Schultz, P.G.; Hampton, G.M. A small interfering RNA screen for modulators of tumor cell motility identifies MAP4K4 as a promigratory kinase. *Proc. Natl. Acad. Sci. USA* **2006**, *103*, 3775–3780. [CrossRef] [PubMed]
27. Liang, J.J.; Wang, H.; Rashid, A.; Tan, T.H.; Hwang, R.F.; Hamilton, S.R.; Abbruzzese, J.L.; Evans, D.B.; Wang, H. Expression of MAP4K4 is associated with worse prognosis in patients with stage II pancreatic ductal adenocarcinoma. *Clin. Cancer Res.* **2008**, *14*, 7043–7049. [CrossRef]
28. Wang, L.X.; Li, Y.; Chen, G.Z. Network-based co-expression analysis for exploring the potential diagnostic biomarkers of metastatic melanoma. *PLoS ONE* **2018**, *13*, e0190447. [CrossRef]
29. Nikitina, A.S.; Sharova, E.I.; Danilenko, S.A.; Butusova, T.B.; Vasiliev, A.O.; Govorov, A.V.; Prilepskaya, E.A.; Pushkar, D.Y.; Kostryukova, E.S. Novel RNA biomarkers of prostate cancer revealed by RNA-seq analysis of formalin-fixed samples obtained from Russian patients. *Oncotarget* **2017**, *8*, 32990. [CrossRef]

30. Patiño-García, A.; Zalacain, M.; Folio, C.; Zandueta, C.; Sierrasesúmaga, L.; San Julián, M.; Toledo, G.; De Las Rivas, J.; Lecanda, F. Profiling of Chemonaive Osteosarcoma and Paired-Normal Cells Identifies EBF2 as a Mediator of Osteoprotegerin Inhibition to Tumor Necrosis Factor–Related Apoptosis-Inducing Ligand–Induced Apoptosis. *Clin. Cancer Res.* **2009**, *15*, 5082–5091. [CrossRef]
31. Dunwell, T.; Hesson, L.; Rauch, T.A.; Wang, L.; Clark, R.E.; Dallol, A.; Gentle, D.; Catchpoole, D.; Maher, E.R.; Pfeifer, G.P.; et al. A genome-wide screen identifies frequently methylated genes in haematological and epithelial cancers. *Mol. Cancer* **2010**, *9*, 44. [CrossRef]
32. Cai, W.Y.; Chen, X.; Chen, L.P.; Li, Q.; Du, X.J.; Zhou, Y.Y. Role of differentially expressed genes and long non-coding RNAs in papillary thyroid carcinoma diagnosis, progression, and prognosis. *J. Cell. Biochem.* **2018**, *119*, 8249–8259. [CrossRef]
33. Luo, L.; Cui, J.; Feng, Z.; Li, Y.; Wang, M.; Cai, Y.; Wu, Y.; Jin, J. Lentiviral-mediated overexpression of KCTD12 inhibits the proliferation of human uveal melanoma OCM-1 cells. *Oncol. Rep.* **2017**, *37*, 871–878. [CrossRef]

12

Mining of Self-Organizing Map Gene-Expression Portraits Reveals Prognostic Stratification of HPV-Positive Head and Neck Squamous Cell Carcinoma

Laura D. Locati [1,†], Mara S. Serafini [2,†], Maria F. Iannò [2], Andrea Carenzo [2], Ester Orlandi [3], Carlo Resteghini [1], Stefano Cavalieri [1], Paolo Bossi [1], Silvana Canevari [2], Lisa Licitra [1,4] and Loris De Cecco [2,*]

1 Head and Neck Medical Oncology Department, Fondazione IRCCS Istituto Nazionale dei Tumori di Milano, 20133 Milan, Italy
2 Integrated Biology Platform, Department of Applied Research and Technology Development, Fondazione IRCCS Istituto Nazionale dei Tumori di Milano, 20133 Milan, Italy
3 Radiation Oncology Department, Fondazione IRCCS Istituto Nazionale dei Tumori di Milano, 20133 Milan, Italy
4 Department of Oncology, University of Milan, 20122 Milan, Italy
* Correspondence: loris.dececco@istitutotumori.mi.it
† Authors contributed equally to this paper.

Abstract: Patients (pts) with head and neck squamous cell carcinoma (HNSCC) have different epidemiologic, clinical, and outcome behaviors in relation to human papillomavirus (HPV) infection status, with HPV-positive patients having a 70% reduction in their risk of death. Little is known about the molecular heterogeneity in HPV-related cases. In the present study, we aim to disclose the molecular subtypes with potential biological and clinical relevance. Through a literature review, 11 studies were retrieved with a total of 346 gene-expression data points from HPV-positive HNSCC pts. Meta-analysis and self-organizing map (SOM) approaches were used to disclose relevant meta-gene portraits. Unsupervised consensus clustering provided evidence of three biological subtypes in HPV-positive HNSCC: Cl1, immune-related; Cl2, epithelial–mesenchymal transition-related; Cl3, proliferation-related. This stratification has a prognostic relevance, with Cl1 having the best outcome, Cl2 the worst, and Cl3 an intermediate survival rate. Compared to recent literature, which identified immune and keratinocyte subtypes in HPV-related HNSCC, we confirmed the former and we separated the latter into two clusters with different biological and prognostic characteristics. At present, this paper reports the largest meta-analysis of HPV-positive HNSCC studies and offers a promising molecular subtype classification. Upon further validation, this stratification could improve patient selection and pave the way for the development of a precision medicine therapeutic approach.

Keywords: self-organizing map; head and neck cancer; treatment de-escalation; HP; molecular subtypes; tumor microenvironment

---

1. Introduction

Worldwide, head and neck squamous cell carcinoma (HNSCC) affects more than 550,000 patient cases/year with around 380,000 deaths annually [1]. Traditionally, alcohol exposure and tobacco smoking are identified as exogenous risk factors. However, human papillomavirus (HPV) infection, caused predominantly by HPV type 16, is currently recognized as an independent causal factor for the development of HNSCC. Since the 1990s, there was a significant increase in HPV-related HNSCC in western countries, whilst the incidence of HPV-negative HNSCC is globally declining [2,3], in parallel with the decline in tobacco smoking rates. This high incidence of HPV-positive cases establishes HNSCC as one of the most common HPV-related cancers, second only to cervical cancer [4]. Moreover, it is estimated that the annual incidence could increase and eventually surpass the annual incidence of cervical cancer by 2020. Previous epidemiological studies showed that around 25% of all HNSCCs are related to HPV infection, with a tendency for the oropharynx (OPSCC) to be the specific site, compared to infection in other sites (oral cavity, larynx, and hypopharynx) [5]. It is known that HPV-related HNSCC patients have different epidemiologic and clinical behaviors in comparison with HPV-negative HNSCC patients, allowing the identification of HPV-positive HNSCC as a specific distinct disease with peculiar prognostic characteristics [6]. In fact, HPV-positive HNSCC is diagnosed at a younger age than HPV-negative HNSCC, and the five-year survival rate for HPV-positive HNSCC is 60–90% as compared with 20–70% for HPV-negative HNSCC [7], conferring a more favorable prognosis for HPV-positive HNSCC patients. The differences in outcomes between HPV-positive and HPV-negative tumors were already provided, and a multitude of molecular differences comparing HPV-negative and HPV-positive HNSCC patients were reported [8–10]. However, a clear biological picture behind their broad diversity is not yet elucidated. Moreover, considering the better prognosis of HPV-positive HNSCC patients compared with their HPV-negative HNSCC counterparts and the median younger age of patients at diagnosis, the question about how to treat HPV-positive patients requires an answer. De-escalation of treatment protocols, for this subgroup of patients, is currently ongoing [11], with the final aim being to reduce the intensity of treatments (both chemoradiation and surgery) and the burden of treatment-related toxicities over the next few years. A further investigation on HPV-related HNSCC is needed. As already reported in the literature, in addition to the diversity of HPV-positive HNSCC compared with HPV-negative HNSCC, it is possible to also observe an intrinsic biological heterogeneity in the HPV-positive HNSCC. In particular, we refer to Keck et al. [12], who identified two different clusters on the basis of their gene expression, and to Zhang et al. [13], who classified these two groups as HPV-positive immune-related (HPV-IMU) and HPV-positive with keratinocyte differentiation (HPV-KRT) HNSCC. Both of these studies had the ability to explore the biology related to HPV infection, unfortunately without showing a significant survival difference.

High-throughput technologies allow the assessment of thousands of features, posing challenges to data analysis. To deal with increased data complexity, researchers apply machine learning approaches to improve biological knowledge via intuitive visualization, even at single-sample resolution. This allows questions, such as biomarker discovery and functional biological information mining, to be addressed. A particular method, self-organizing maps (SOM), provides important benefits including dimension reduction, multidimensional scaling, visualization capabilities over alternative methods such as non-negative matrix factorization, and hierarchical clustering [14]. SOM gained immediate attention in the bioinformatics field, and early microarray studies reported its application [15,16]. Since then, a number of studies on different cancer types proved its robustness [17,18].

In the present analysis, we focused our attention on HPV-positive HNSCC with annotated gene expression data and clinical annotations by exploiting a meta-analysis approach. We applied the SOM machine learning method on a total of 346 HPV-positive tumor samples. This allowed us to dissect the molecular heterogeneity of the disease and to make suggestions for de-escalation treatment.

2. Results

2.1. Case Material

In order to dissect the molecular heterogeneity in HPV-positive HNSCC, 11 eligible published studies reporting gene expression data were selected for a systematic survey (Table S1, Supplementary Materials). Of these studies, all but one utilized microarray technology for gene expression analysis, and, in the majority of cases, HPV status was assessed with qPCR or HPV genotyping. The resulting meta-analysis dataset, containing 346 samples and 8254 EntrezID genes, was used for the genomic analysis. HPV infection was assessed by p16 immunohistochemistry (IHC) (13 cases, 4%) or DNA or RNA from HPV testing (333, 96%) (Table S1, Supplementary Materials). All the methods used are recognized and utilized in clinical practice [19].

According to the clinical information (Table 1), a male preponderance (83%) and median age of 58.7 years (range, 35–87) were observed, in line with the epidemiological data reported in the literature. The main subsite of origin was the oropharynx (68%), followed by the oral cavity (17%), larynx (6%), and hypopharynx (3%). Stages, assessed following malignant tumor classification system (TNM edition 7, American Joint Committee on Cancer, AJCC), were divided into stages I–II (35), stages III–IV (229), and information not available (82). Locally advanced stages (III–IV) were the most represented (66%), followed by not available (24%) and early stages (I–II; 10%). Survival data were available for 197 cases (57%) and not present for 149 cases (43%). Smoking habits were reported for 245 patients (169 smokers, 76 never smokers), and were unknown for 101 patients (Table 1).

Table 1. Demographic and clinical data of the head and neck squamous cell carcinoma (HNSCC) human papillomavirus (HPV)-positive patients entered in the meta-analysis.

Characteristics	No.	%
Age, years		
(median; range)	57 (35–87)	77%
Not available	78	23%
Gender (male:female ratio)	287/59	83%/17%
Subsite		
Oropharynx	235	68%
Oral cavity	59	17%
Larynx	20	6%
Hypopharynx	10	3%
Not available	22	6%
Stage according to TNM edition 7		
Stage I–II	35	10%
Stage III–IV	229	66%
Not available	82	24%
Smoking		
Smoker	169	49%
Not smoker	76	22%
Not available	101	29%
Availability of follow-up data		
Yes	197	57%
No	149	43%
Total	**346**	100%

2.2. *HPV-Positive HNSCC Tumor Clusters: First-Level Self-Organizing Map (SOM) and Unsupervised Clustering Analysis*

We applied the SOM machine learning algorithm to convert the meta-analysis dataset into a matrix of meta-gene expression data. Starting from the 8254 genes, we imposed the log-intensity variation p-value < 0.01, and a data matrix of 3498 genes was yielded. These 3498 genes were aggregated in meta-genes (average 10 genes each), resulting in a matrix of 18×18 meta-genes. Consensus unsupervised clustering was applied on the meta-gene data, revealing three clusters of samples.

The cluster had well-defined boundaries, as shown by the consensus heatmap (Figure 1a). To exclude the existence of under-represented clusters, the consistency of sample assignment was evaluated by silhouette plot analysis. The resulting clustering configuration was appropriate (Figure 1b), since most samples in each cluster had a positive value (average < s >: Cluster 1, Cl1 = 0.68; Cluster 2, Cl2 = 0.53; Cluster 3, Cl3 = 0.48). Only seven samples (two belonging to Cl2 and five belonging to Cl3), corresponding to 2% of the entire case material, had negative values but were in the range between −0.01 and −0.04. These seven samples were assigned by silhouette analysis, as follows: two Cl2 samples to Cl1, three Cl3 samples to Cl2, and three Cl3 samples to Cl1. We assessed the sample size adequacy by estimating the power for the detection of the three clusters; the robustness of the classification was ensured since at least 87% of genes had a power level of 0.9 (Figure S1, Supplementary Materials). By training the SOM algorithm, each sample was portrayed by displaying its molecular fingerprint. The generated subtype SOM images revealed a series of adjacent mosaic tiles coherently over- or under-expressed, and the resulting gallery of SOM portraits was used to intuitively visualize the coherent cluster patterns. In this way, we highlighted cluster-specific tiles in the SOM portraits, independent of the patient's individuality (Figure 1c).

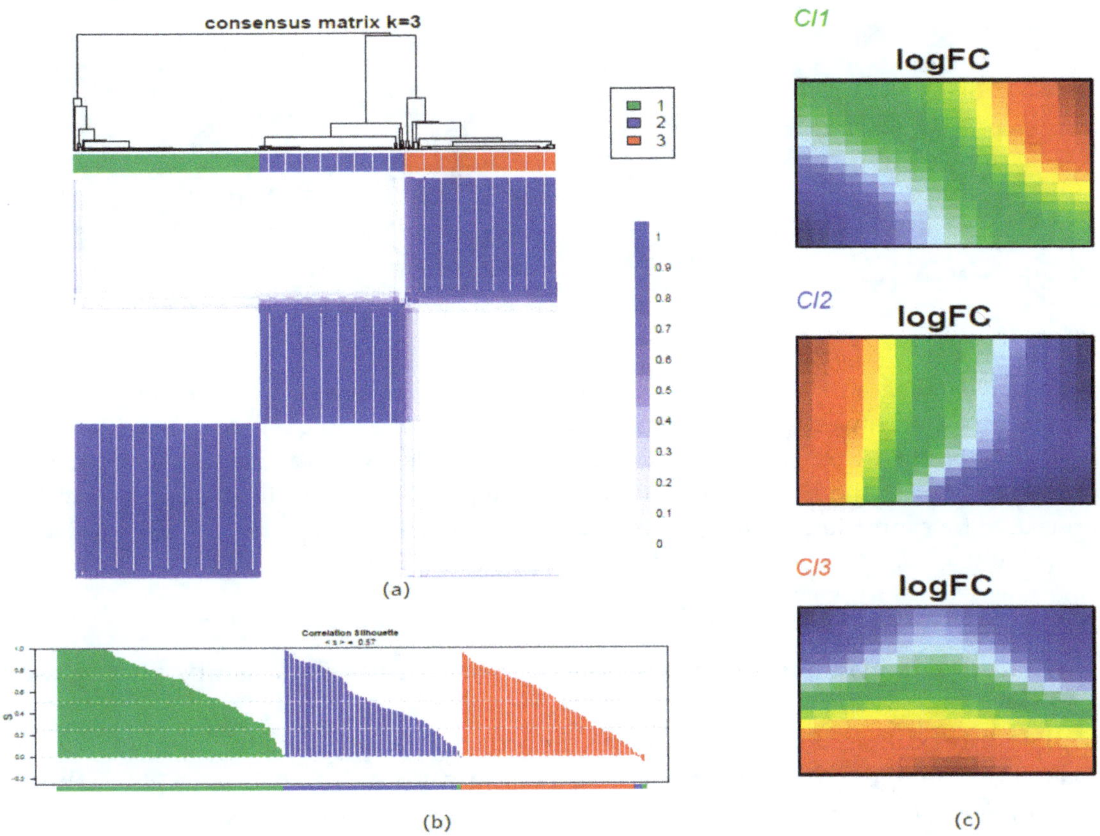

Figure 1. Human papillomavirus (HPV)-positive head and neck squamous cell carcinoma (HNSCC) tumor clusters: first-level self-organizing map (SOM) and unsupervised clustering analysis. (**a**) Consensus matrix heatmap imposing three clusters: Cl1 (n = 134; 39%), Cl2 (n = 104; 30%), and Cl3 (n = 108; 31%). The consensus values are reported in a range from 0 (white, samples that never cluster together) to 1 (blue, samples showing the highest clustering affinity). (**b**) Silhouette plot analysis. The samples are ranked based on silhouette values (S) in each cluster. The heights indicate a strong similarity of the samples within their clusters compared with the samples belonging to other clusters. The colors in the lower bar show the predicted membership by silhouette analysis; the colors correspond to the consensus clustering assignment for all samples with the exception of the seven samples with a negative number but close to 0. (**c**) First level of the SOM gallery of the three clusters with cluster-specific tiles highlighted. The expression patterns are translated into a color code indicating over- and under-expression in a range from red to blue spots, respectively.

We also investigated the influence related to technical sources of variability on our findings. An alluvial diagram was used to show the three-cluster membership, based on the study of origin and the platform used for the expression profiling (Figure 2). The percentage of variation, explained by these variables, was investigated compared with the variation associated with the present cluster stratification, and this is summarized in the violin plots (Figure S2, Supplementary Materials). Our findings supported the biological value behind our three-subtype stratification, with a negligible influence of technical covariates.

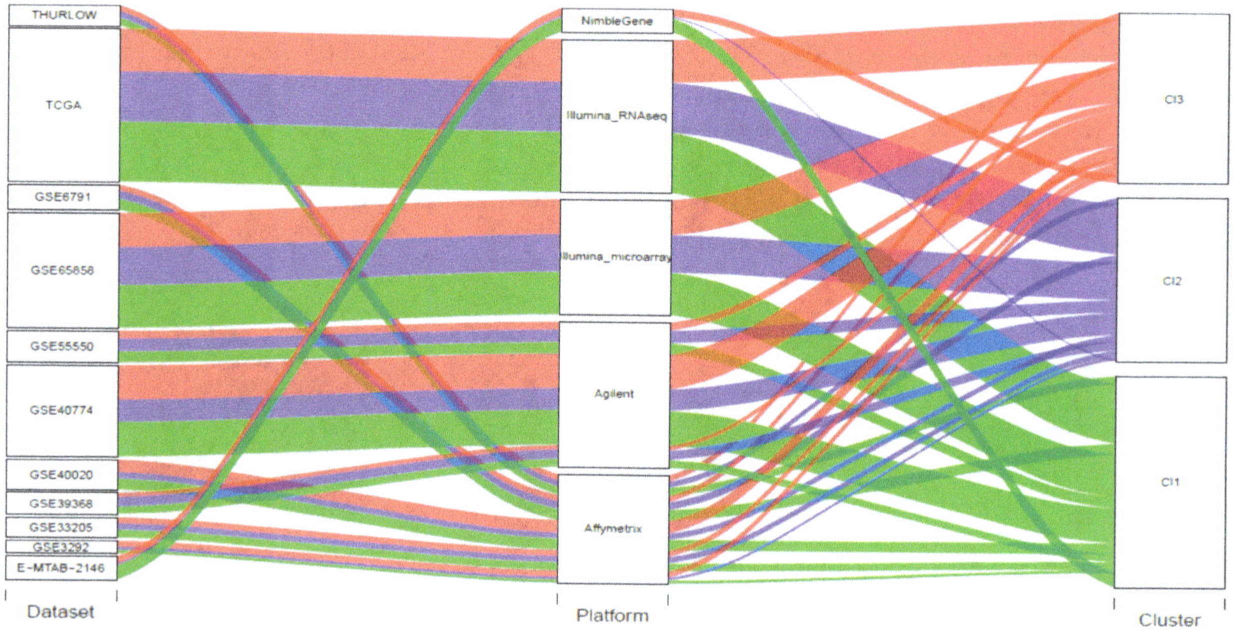

Figure 2. Alluvial diagram. In the diagram, each of the blocks corresponds to the number of features, and the stream fields between the blocks represent changes in the composition of the different blocks. The sizes of the blocks are proportional to the number of samples. We explored the cluster membership taking into account (i) the study of origin of each sample (11 strata); (ii) the different technology platforms used for expression profiling (five strata). Study of the origin: χ^2 test = 12.08, p-value = 0.913; Platform χ^2 test = 5.93, p-value = 0.655.

2.3. HPV-Positive HNSCC Cluster Similarity Relationships: Second-Level SOM

The second-level SOM analysis investigated the similarity relationships among the first-level sample SOM portraits.

We applied three different sample similarity approaches to estimate the mutual distances among samples, based on metagene expression data and using different metrics and algorithms. The first approach, independent component analysis (ICA), displayed three clusters supporting the identified stratification, although the boundaries between them were not strictly defined (Figure 3a, left panel). Additional information could be retrieved from the three independent components (component 1, component 2, and component 3): the projections onto the component 1/component two axes (Figure 3a, right lower panel) segregated Cluster 1 (Cl1, green spots) from Cl2 and Cl3 (blue and red spots, respectively); however, regions of high density Cl2 and Cl3 showed distinct behavior without clear separation. On the contrary, when the component 1/component three axes were considered, Cl2 and Cl3 were more clearly divided (Figure 3a, right upper panel).

As a second alternative metric, we investigated a correlation network approach: the resulting structure was visualized into a graph to highlight the correlation network (Figure 3b), and it confirmed the presence of a main cluster including Cl1 with few connections to Cl2 and Cl3.

The third approach exploited a Euclidean distance-based approach through the resolution of neighbor-joining (NJ) clustering, which projects the relationships among samples in phylogenetic trees

(Figure 3c). The NJ dendrogram was able to disclose finer details than the previous approaches, and it revealed inherent substructures and their connections in each cluster. By visual inspection, most Cl1 samples were segregated into clearly different branches from Cl2 and Cl3 branches, which, in contrast, appeared tightly correlated.

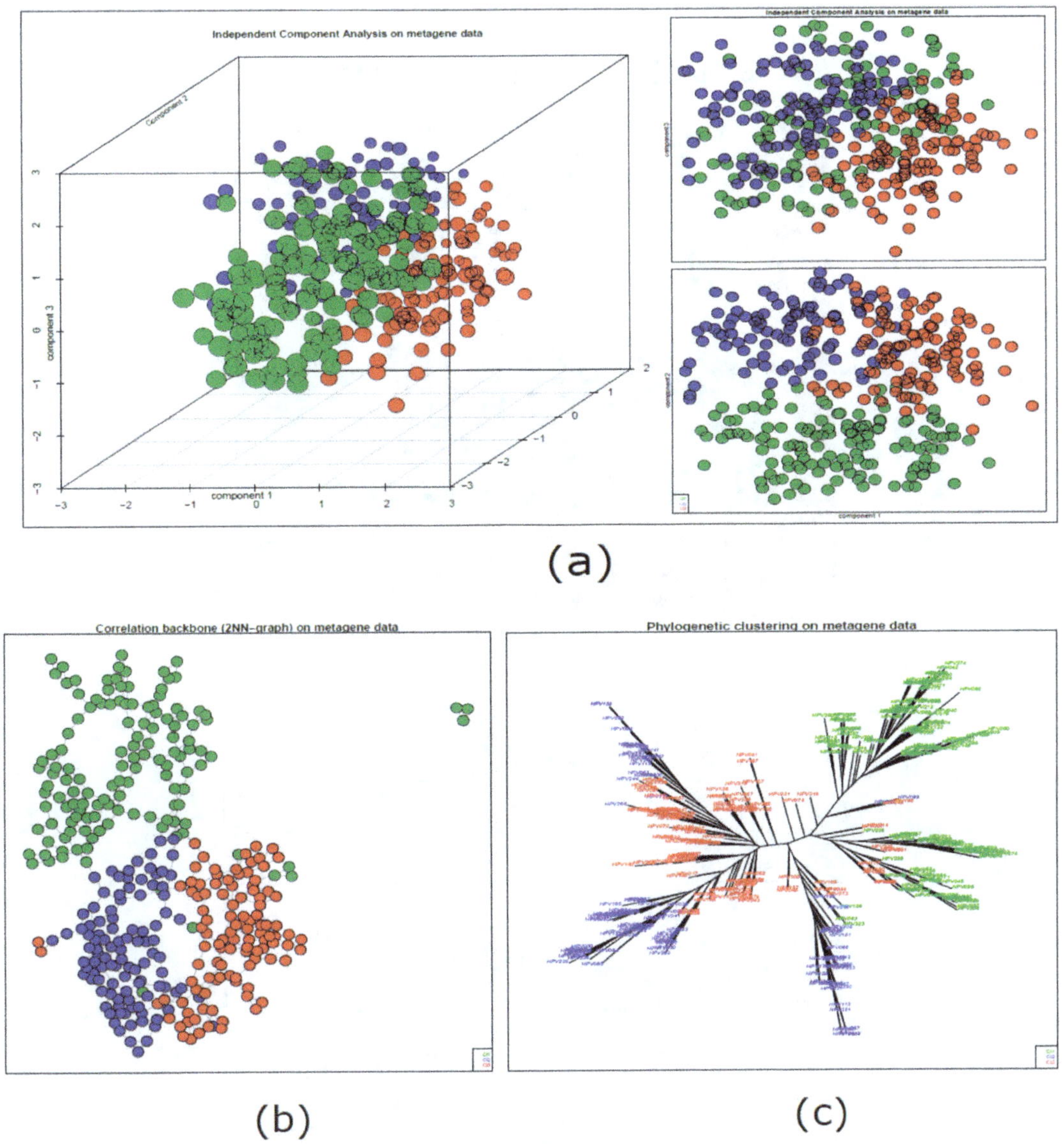

Figure 3. HPV-positive HNSCC cluster similarity relationships: second-level SOM. (**a**) Independent component analysis of meta-gene data. Samples were distributed along the three leading independent components; the plots show the three-dimensional distribution and the projections into the component 1/component 2 (lower panel) and component 1/component 3 (upper panel) dimensions. (**b**) Sample correlation network. The samples are visualized by nodes connected by edges with a backbone structure linking samples with the highest correlation. The similarity between samples is represented by their reciprocal distance; closer nodes have higher similarity and distant nodes have lower similarity. (**c**) Neighbor-joining analysis. The sample similarities are summarized in a phylogenetic tree structure computed using Euclidean distance. The neighbor-joining (NJ) analysis visualizes "bush-like" groups of similar samples by assessing their mutual dissimilarity.

Finally, we investigated the relationship among meta-genes characterizing the three identified subtypes. The process of detection of coherent expression of meta-genes in SOM portraits highlighted specific molecular features for each subtype. Indeed, the resulting map defined three over-expression regions, each of them located in distinct corners of the map. These regions corresponded to SOM clusters of co-regulated meta-genes (Figure 4a). The association of meta-genes to each cluster in precise map locations (left panels) and to a bar plot of expression intensity (right panels) better confirmed and defined the differences between subtypes: 54, 93, and 57 meta-genes had positive correlations with Clusters 1, 2, and 3, respectively ($r = 0.77$, $r = 0.53$, $r = 0.67$) (Figure 4b).

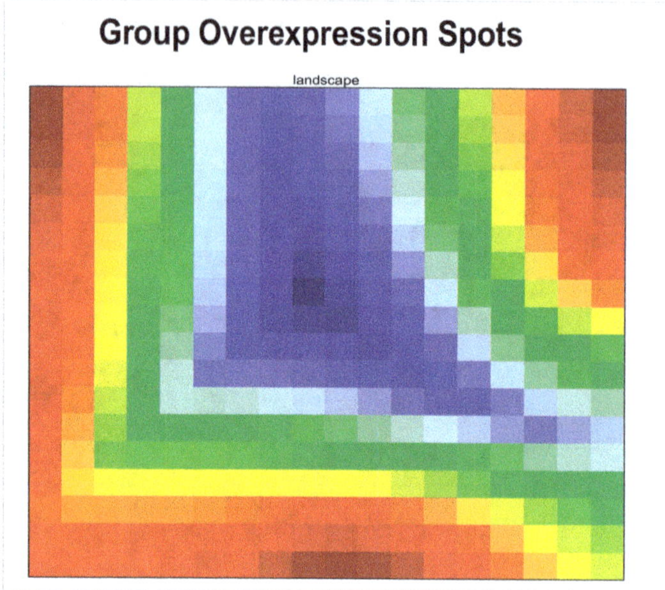

(a)

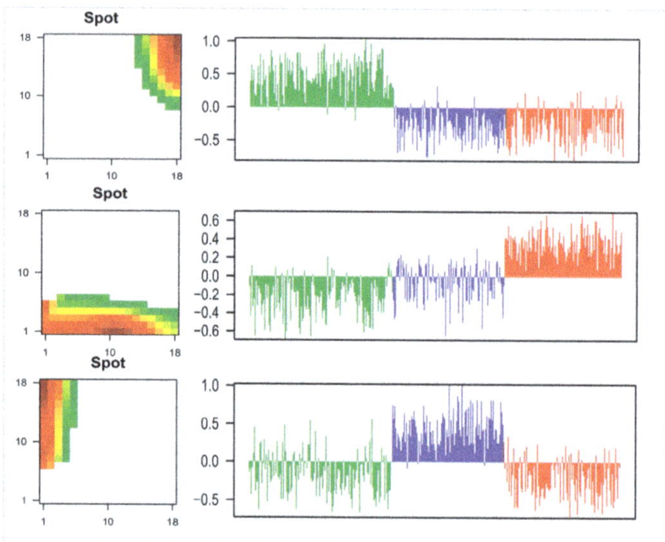

(b)

Figure 4. Subtype characterization by group overexpression maps. (**a**) The 18 × 18 map of meta-genes summarizes the expression landscapes over the three subtypes; according to this analysis, co-regulated meta-genes are located in the opposite corners of the map. (**b**) Detailed analysis of metagenes overexpressed in each subtype: map location (left panels) and bar plot of expression intensity (right panels). The bar plot represents the average meta-gene expression of each sample for the selected tiles.

2.4. *Tumor Microenvironment Landscape*

The xCell tool was applied for the detection and evaluation, if present, of any differences in the three clusters, regarding microenvironment components. According to a dimensionality reduction technique (t-distributed stochastic neighbor embedding, t-SNE), we obtained two-dimensional coordinates that clearly segregated the three molecular clusters. It provided evidence about the existence of unique and defined biological subtypes (Figure 5a). To better disclose the properties of each subtype, the composite scores of immune cells (ImmuneScore), stromal cells (StromaScore), and the score of keratinocytes were calculated. Cl1, compared to Cl2 and Cl3, was characterized by enrichment of immune components (p-value = 9.9×10^{-29}) (Figure 5b) and under-expression of keratinocytes (p-value = 2.03×10^{-32}) (Figure 5c). On the contrary, Cl2 and Cl3 showed similar enrichment in keratinocytes, but a lower immunoscore. Cl2 and Cl3 were clearly separated when compared in terms of stromal components, with Cl3 significantly decreased (p-value = 6.3×10^{-18}) compared with the two other two subtypes (Figure 5d).

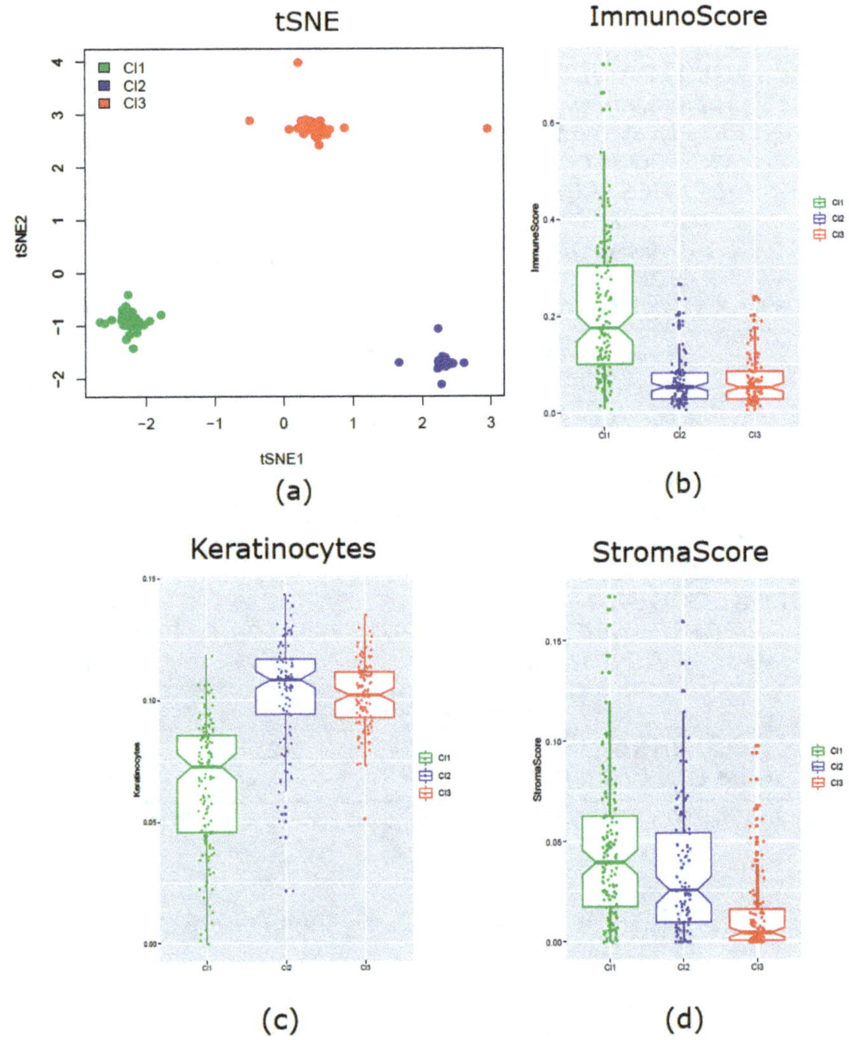

Figure 5. Tumor microenvironment landscape. (**a**) Visualization of the immune and "other cell" infiltrates assessed by xCell. Individual patients are summarized based on two-dimensional coordinates from the t-distributed stochastic neighbor embedding (t-SNE) method. The notched boxplots show the ImmuneScores (p-value = 9.9×10^{-29}) (**b**), keratinocytes scores (p-value = 2.03×10^{-32}) (**c**), and stromal cell infiltrates (p-value = 6.3×10^{-18}) (**d**) split into the three different subtypes.

2.5. Functional Analyses of Subtypes

To disclose the biological properties associated with each of the three resulting clusters, further functional characterization was performed using Gene Set Enrichment Analysis (GSEA). GSEA is a method used to test the overrepresentation of genes in gene sets, which are characterized by independent studies. We investigated the "Hallmark" gene set collection representing specific well-defined biological processes. In particular, our analysis provided evidence of a specific enrichment for each cluster. Cl1 showed enrichment in immune-related hallmarks, such as "allograft rejection", "IFN, interferon gamma", and "IL6 JAK STAT3 signaling"; Cl2 overexpressed genes related to the hallmarks "epithelial–mesenchymal transition" (EMT), "myogenesis", and "hypoxia"; Cl3 displayed enrichment in proliferation-related hallmarks, e.g., "E2F targets" and "G2M checkpoint" (Table 2 and Figure 6).

Table 2. Gene-sets significantly up-regulated in each cluster.

Gene-set ID	HALLMARK Gene-Set Name	Genes [a]	NES [b]	Nom *p*-Value	FDR q-val
	Cl1 vs. Cl2 and Cl3				
GS-1	*ALLOGRAFT REJECTION (immune resp)*	130	2.89	<0.00001	<0.00001
GS-2	*INTERFERON GAMMA RESPONSE*	151	2.18	<0.00001	<0.00001
GS-3	*IL6 JAK STAT3 SIGNALING*	60	1.94	<0.00001	<0.00001
GS-4	*INFLAMMATORY RESPONSE*	132	1.76	<0.00001	0.0018
GS-5	*KRAS SIGNALING UP*	114	1.75	<0.00001	0.0019
	Cl2 vs. Cl1 and Cl3				
GS-1	*EPITHELIAL MESENCHYMAL TRANSITION*	140	3.01	<0.00001	<0.00001
GS-2	*MYOGENESIS*	119	2.42	<0.00001	<0.00001
GS-3	*COAGULATION*	77	2.23	<0.00001	<0.00001
GS-4	*ANGIOGENESIS*	19	2.02	<0.00001	<0.00001
GS-5	*HYPOXIA*	133	1.90	<0.00001	<0.00001
GS-6	*HEDGEHOG SIGNALING*	17	1.89	0.0020	<0.00001
GS-7	*UV RESPONSE DN*	97	1.78	<0.00001	0.0020
GS-8	*APICAL JUNCTION*	137	1.78	<0.00001	0.0020
	Cl3 vs. Cl1 and Cl2				
GS-1	*E2F TARGETS*	143	2.56	<0.00001	<0.00001
GS-2	*G2M CHECKPOINT*	150	2.24	<0.00001	0.0020

GS: geneset; thresholds: FDR ≤ 0.005; NES≥1.75, [a] Number of total genes present in the geneset, [b] NES = normalized enrichment score.

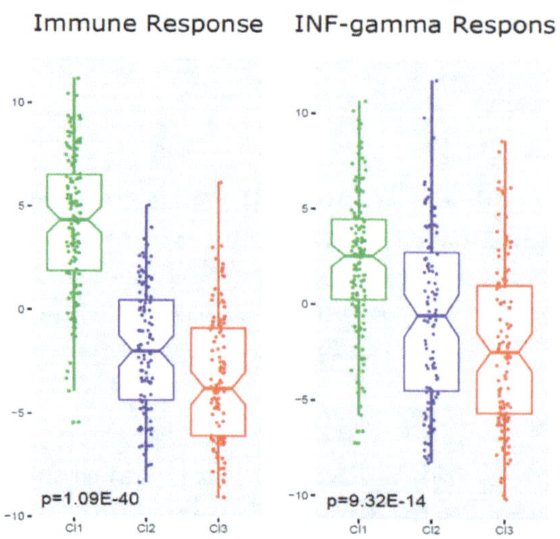

Figure 6. *Cont.*

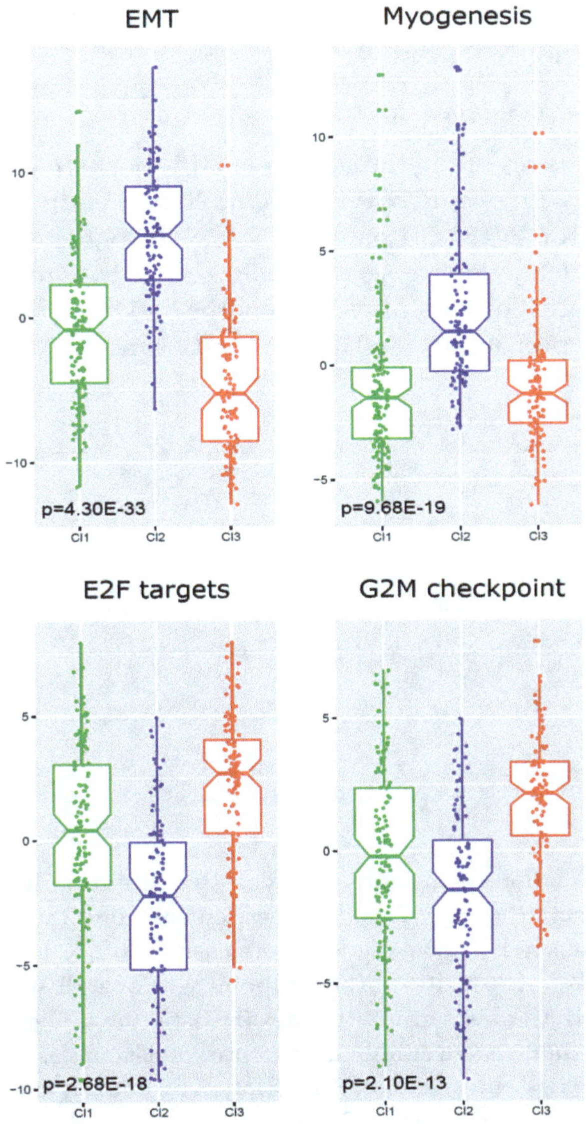

Figure 6. Visualization of the Gene Set Enrichment Analysis (GSEA) functional analysis for each of the three clusters. The boxplots show how the gene set Z score (GSZ) values (depicted in y-axis) are distributed within each of the three clusters (Cl1, green; Cl2, blue; Cl3 red). In each row, comparisons of the GSZ score values for the two most enriched hallmark gene sets are shown: for Cl1, over-expression is shown for the "immune response" hallmark (p-value 1.09×10^{-40}) and "interferon (IFN)-gamma response" hallmark (p-value = 9.32×10^{-14}); for Cl2, enrichment is shown in the "epithelial–mesenchymal transition (EMT)" hallmark (p-value = 4.30×10^{-33}) and "myogenesis" hallmark (p-value = 9.68×10^{-19}); for Cl3, over-expression is shown in the "E2F targets" hallmark (p-value = 2.68×10^{-18}) and "G2M checkpoint" (p-value 2.10×10^{-13}). The p-values were obtained by means of Kruskal–Wallis tests.

2.6. HPV Presence/Integration and Its Association with Clusters

We investigated the association between HPV viral integration and our three clusters, using the data provided by Koneva et al. [20]. Table S2 (Supplementary Materials) shows the contingency table for the TCGA cases analyzed in Koneva et al., reaching a significant association of χ^2 =12.32 and a p-value = 0.00212; the relative presence of HPV integrated cases in each subtype increased in the order Cl1 < Cl3 < Cl2, with relative frequencies of 0.45, 0.77, and 1, respectively. Moreover, we explored the expression of viral genes (E2, E4, and E5). The expression patterns in Cluster 2 are consistent with viral integration. When integrated, the expression of the E2 gene is reduced, since it is truncated along with downstream genes such as E4 and E5 (Figure S3).

2.7. Prognostic Values of the Three-Subtype Classification

Due to the robust analysis revealing three distinct HPV-positive HNSCC subtypes, we aimed to investigate their associations with overall survival as the clinical endpoint. Outcome data (i.e., overall survival; OS) were available for 75/134 Cl1 patients, 56/108 Cl2 patients, and 66/104 Cl3 patients, for a total of 197 patients. As depicted in Figure 7a, the results showed a significantly better outcome for Cl1 subtype patients, with a survival probability at 60 months of 0.809, and a worst outcome for Cl3 and Cl2 subtypes, with a survival probability at 60 months of 0.47 and 0.197, respectively (log-rank p-value $= 4.76 \times 10^{-9}$).

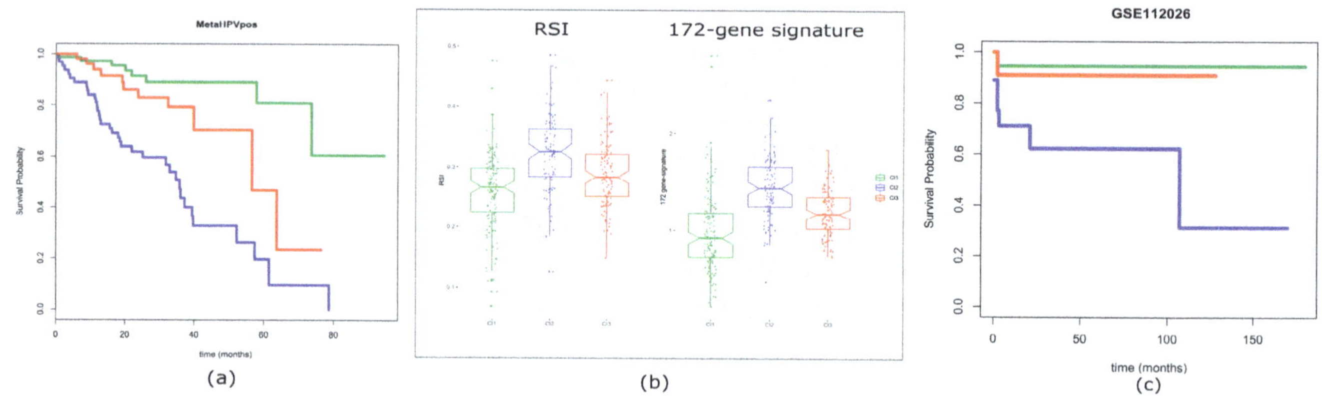

Figure 7. Prognostic evaluation of the three-subtype stratification. (**a**) Survival analysis on the meta-analysis dataset (MetaHPVpos). The 197 cases, entered into the three subtypes (75/134 Cl1 patients; 56/108 Cl2 patients; 66/104 Cl3 patients), were used for the Kaplan–Meier analysis, yielding a log-rank score of p-value $= 4.76 \times 10^{-9}$. The endpoint was overall survival. (**b**) Gene-signature. Two models were evaluated: (i) radiosensitivity index (RSI), (ii) the 172-gene prognostic model. RSI is directly proportional to radioresistance (high index = radioresistance), while the 172-gene model is directly proportional to the risk of recurrence. Stratification by both signatures reached p-value $= 8.76 \times 10^{-13}$ and p-value $= 7.98 \times 10^{-22}$ for the RSI and 172-gene model, respectively. (**c**) Validation on GSE112026. The 47 cases belonging to GSE112026 were stratified based on our three subtypes: 18, 18, and 11 cases were predicted as belonging to Cl1, Cl2, and Cl3, respectively. The cases, entered into the three identified subtypes, were used for the Kaplan–Meier analysis, yielding a p-value $= 0.0152$ (log-rank test).

Furthermore, we applied two different gene expression published signatures to the 197 HPV-positive HNSCC patients with available follow-up information: (i) the 172-gene model, a prognostic model for HNSCC [21]; (ii) the radiosensitivity index (RSI) [22], a gene signature developed as a pan-marker of cellular radiosensitivity. In order to assess whether and to what extent the signatures were associated with HPV-related subtypes, we applied the algorithms developed [21,22] to our cohort. The resulting scores were compared to the three-subtype stratification. A significant relationship was found between our stratification and these molecular signatures (Figure 7b). In detail, the Cl1 subtype showed the lowest 172-gene signature related score, meaning that Cl1 has the minimum predicted risk, as confirmed by OS. Furthermore, Cl1 displayed the lowest RSI value, which predicted its radiosensitivity. On the contrary, Cl2 subtype exhibited the highest score in the 172-gene signature, and the maximum RSI score, compared with the other two subtypes, predicting its high risk and intrinsic radioresistance, respectively. The Cl3 subtype showed an "intermediate" behavior, with all three analyses (OS, 172-gene signature score, and RSI).

The clinical relevance of our classification was additionally investigated and associated with the outcome in an external validation dataset. For our analysis, we retrieved the RNA-sequencing (RNA-seq) data of Ando et al. [23], which included 47 HPV-positive oropharyngeal squamous cell carcinomas. With this external validation, we confirmed that the three-subtype stratification provides useful prognostic information. As a matter of fact, better outcomes were associated with patients belonging to Cl1/Cl3 subtypes, and worse outcomes were associated with patients belonging to Cl2 subtype (Figure 7c) (log-rank p-value = 0.0152). Finally, we investigated the association between clinal features and our molecular stratification. Table S3 (Supplementary Materials) reports the data related to gender, age, smoking habit, site, and TNM v7 stage. We found a significant association with site having Cl2 a higher percentage of cases other than oropharynx. In addition, due to its potential prognostic role, smoking habit was associated with the three subtypes. There was a trend in the different distribution of the smoking habit with higher percentage of smokers in Cl2. Table S4 (Supplementary Materials) reports the association for Ando's dataset including gender, age, smoking, Ang et al. (2010) classification system, smoked packs per year, alcohol use, t-stage, and n-stage. We found a significant association with t-stage, having Cl2 cases a higher percentage of T3–4.

3. Discussion

Among HNSCCs, the HPV-positive tumors are an independent entity with specific clinical and molecular characteristics. Moreover, inside the HPV-positive subgroup, it is additionally possible to observe an intrinsic heterogeneity, in terms of patients' outcomes. This assumption questions whether treatment de-intensification could be applied to all HPV-positive HNSCCs. Clinical factors, such as large tumor burden and smoking history, correlate with a worse prognosis, but the biological mechanisms elucidating the complexity of the HPV-positive subgroup are still not fully understood. In the present meta-analysis of transcriptomic data, we applied a rigorous and up-to-date bioinformatics analysis to 346 HPV-positive HNSCCs with published sample data. To the best of our knowledge, this is the largest cohort of HPV-positive HNSCCs analyzed up until now. Specifically, our study identified three tumor subtypes, and it further dissected a population, which was previously divided into only two subgroups by published studies [12,13,24]. In agreement with these findings, we clearly identified an immune-associated cluster (named Cl1 in our analysis). In addition, we stratified the remaining patients (previously described as one "keratinocyte subtype" cluster [13,24]) into two well distinct subtypes with clearly defined biological and prognostic characteristics. The stratification refinement could be attributed not only to the dimension of the analyzed cohort (from two to three times larger than in previous studies), but also to the application of the NJ analysis, which revealed a degree of heterogeneity moving from Cl2 to Cl3 samples with disjointed branches.

In general, HPV-related HNSCCs are known to have better outcomes when compared with HPV-negative HNSCCs [25]. The observed overall survival of our cohort of patients is aligned with the reported prognostic data. However, our analysis displayed a specific prognosis for each cluster, identifying those HPV-positive cases with the best, intermediate, and poorest prognoses. Interestingly, the subtype stratification did not provide evidence of a significant association with smoking habit, but highlighted some specific biological traits for each cluster that could help in interpreting their different outcomes.

Cluster 1 patients exhibited the best outcome at five years and it showed similar behavior to those patients identified as having low-risk HPV-related HNSCC [25]. Additionally, Cl1 was clearly separated from the other two clusters by its high immune score in the xCell analysis, and by upregulation of the hallmarks "IFN, interferon gamma signaling" and "IL6 JAK STAT3 signaling". The high immune score, associated with a good outcome, could be in agreement with the hypothesis that, in these patients, the immune system plays an important role in the clearance of viral proteins expressed in HPV-positive cancers [26]. Indeed, tumors enriched by the IFN-gamma signature may benefit from immunotherapy [27]. On the contrary, the IL6/JAK/STAT3 pathway hyper-activation is more difficult to interpret in the context of a better prognosis. In fact, IL6/JAK/STAT3 signaling is expected to drive proliferation, survival, and invasiveness of tumor cells, and to suppress the anti-tumor immune response. Overall, we could assume that, in Cl1, the immune infiltrate, as determined by the ImmuneScore, and the high "IFN, interferon gamma signaling" could counterbalance the pro-tumoral action of IL6 JAK STAT3 signaling; however, specific functional assays are necessary to confirm this assumption. Considering the better prognosis and the biological profile, we could hypothesize that Cl1 patients would be the best candidate for de-escalating treatment strategies, even including checkpoint inhibitors.

Cluster 2 exhibited the worst outcomes, and it strongly differed from the other two subtypes by its high stromal score. Essentially, this score reflects fibroblast infiltration, and it frequently leads to deregulation of EMT-inducing factors, EMT upregulation, and hallmark "hypoxia" overexpression. The EMT changes in tumor cells were reported to be linked to the acquisition of aggressive behaviors including (i) increased invasive properties, (ii) resistance to DNA damage, (iii) chemotherapy-induced apoptosis, (iv) immunosuppression, and (v) acquisition of stem-like features [28]. In addition, the increase in the hallmark "hypoxia" is in agreement with the radioresistance detected by RSI [29]. We hypothesize that treatment intensification could be beneficial for these patients. As an example, an accelerated fractionation schedule of radiotherapy should be considered as a strategy to overcome radioresistance.

Cluster 3, characterized by an intermediate outcome compared with the other two clusters, was clearly defined by upregulation of the hallmarks "E2F targets" and "G2M checkpoint", both associated with increased proliferation. A possible explanation for these data may be the interpretation of boosted proliferation as a result of the integration of the viral genome in the host cell. Moreover, upregulation of the hallmarks "E2F targets" and "G2M checkpoints" is in agreement with the observation that the HPV genome does not encode enzymes necessary for viral replication [26]. Instead, the virus utilizes host cell proteins to replicate its DNA. Therefore, basal cells containing HPV genomes remain active in the pathway related to the cell cycle, also due to Rb degradation. The E2F transcription factor, without Rb function, is free to drive the expression of S-phase genes [26,30]. A first explorative investigation, between the viral integration and our three clusters using data provided by Koneva et al. [20], revealed a significant association between the integration of HPV in the host genome and each of our subtypes in the following order: Cl1 < Cl3 < Cl2 (Figure S2, Supplementary Materials). Despite the analysis being performed on a limited number of samples, Cl2 seemed to be in accordance with cases already described in literature, in which HPV was integrated and viral integration was associated with a poor prognosis [31]. Nevertheless, in this regard, Cl3 shows an intermediate behavior, which may possibly be explained through Nulton discovery [32]. Indeed, HPV infection is described not only as its usual integrated and episomal state but, additionally, as a third state where the viral genome exists as both episomal and integrated states. Anyway, the proposed associations require further evaluation, for not only exploring the HPV state, in terms of integration, episomal, and intermediate states, but also to examine possible target amplification.

Some limitations of this study and some differences with more recent data should be mentioned. Based on the clinical characteristics of the analyzed patients, we observed a relatively high number of missing clinical data (near to 30% in age and stage). The possible explanation for the unavailability of these data could reside in the nature of the studies included in our meta-analysis, which had the biological description of the HPV tumors as a primary endpoint and, accordingly, an inconsistent collection of clinical data was performed.

It is noteworthy that HPV-related tumors in subsites, other than the oropharynx, reached a higher percentage than expected (10%). We hypothesize that this difference could be attributed to the sample collection in the years before the clear prognostic role of HPV infection in oropharynx cancers. In fact, the new TNM staging system (American Joint Committee on Cancer, 8th edition) distinguishes, for the first time, HPV-related from HPV-unrelated oropharynx cancers by stratifying according to p16 expression. The prognostic value for other subsites (i.e., oral cavity, hypopharynx, larynx) other than the oropharynx is still debatable, although a recent review demonstrated a prognostic role for HPV infection in all HNSCC subsites [33].

Considering the prognostic role of our stratification, three subtypes, with different outcomes, were described for the first time. An identified limitation could be the fact that treatment was not systematically recorded, and the overall survival of our case series was poorer than the expected outcome [25]. Moreover, another limitation was identified: the association of subtypes and prognoses should be underscored, although we should highlight that the follow-up was only available for 197 out of 346 (57%) cases. A further bias is related to the differences in treatment techniques used in the last 15 years (e.g., three-dimensional (3D) vs. intensity-modulated radiotherapy; trans-oral robotic surgery, TORS, robotics vs. traditional open surgery).

In conclusion, ongoing trials on de-escalation treatment approaches in HPV-positive HNSCC are based only on HPV status and do not take the contributions of genomics and molecular profiles into consideration [34]. It is conceivable that, upon rigorous validation, our stratification could help develop a "precision treatment approach" based on the genomic profile of HPV-related HNSCC to select patients.

4. Materials and Methods

4.1. Case Material: Gene Expression and Clinical Data

A survey of gene-expression data on HNSCC (available at 31 August 2018) was accomplished. The cases entered into our study were selected based on the following eligibility criteria: (i) primary lesions of squamous cell carcinoma; (ii) reported HPV status, according to the clinical practice in the reference center; (iii) MIAME (Minimum Information about a Microarray Experiment) [35] complaint data with the availability of raw data deposited on publicly accessible repositories and full gene annotation (Gene Bank accession or EntrezID). After literature revision, there were 11 datasets [12,36–45]. See Table S1 (Supplementary Materials) for details regarding the datasets including the accession numbers and methods of HPV detection. Raw microarray data were retrieved from the NCBI (National Center for Biotechnology Information) Gene Expression Omnibus (GEO) database [46], ArrayExpress (the EMBL European Bioinformatics Institute, UK) [47], MIAME-Vice [48], and TCGA repositories [49] and were integrated into a unique dataset through a meta-analysis approach, as previously described [50].

In addition, we collected available clinical data related to this case material, comprising age at diagnosis, gender, smoking habits, tumor subsite, stage, and overall survival.

For validation purposes, we retrieved the data from Ando et al. [23], which are publicly available on the GEO repository (identifier (ID): GSE112026). A cohort of 47 primary tumor tissues with HPV-related oropharyngeal squamous cell carcinoma was collected for RNA-seq analysis and microdissected to yield at least 80% tumor purity. HPV tumor status was confirmed by in situ hybridization for high-risk HPV subtypes or p16 immunohistochemistry. According to the TCGA RSEM (RNA-Seq by Expectation Maximization) pipeline, RNA-seq data were processed using RSEM version 1.2.9 and upper quartile normalization. For class prediction purposes, analyses were performed through R-based BRB-ArrayTools software (version 3.5.0) developed by Richard Simon and the BRB-ArrayTools development team [51]. A class prediction method based on a supervised learning method was applied for classifying GSE112026 cases. Prediction was based on the support vector machine (SVM) method by incorporating genes at the univariate significance level ($\alpha = 0.001$) in a binary tree classification framework, which was chosen due to its ability to classify more than two classes. SVM is specifically designed to address binary classification; however, it can be adapted to handle multi-class classification by building a sequence of binary classifiers. The prediction error of the binary tree classifier was estimated by the leave-one-out cross-validation method.

4.2. *Data Preprocessing for Meta-Analysis Dataset Generation*

The selected studies were analyzed with four platforms, including three microarray platforms (Affymetrix, Agilent, and Nimblegene) and one RNA-seq (Illumina). For Affymetrix data, signal intensities were normalized within each individual dataset using a robust multi-array average (RMA) tool. For Agilent data, the normexp background correction and loess normalization were used for two-channel arrays, while quantile normalization procedures were applied to the probe-level data. For Illumina microarray data, quantile normalization was applied. For RNA-seq data, TCGA level 3 files were downloaded along with the clinical annotations and used for the analysis. The redundancy of probes mapping the same EntrezID was removed by selecting the probe with the highest variance among multiple probe-sets by identifying the same gene; collapse was performed using WGCNA package 1.63 (function: *collapseRows*) and the "*maxRowVariance*" method [52]. To reduce the likelihood of systemic non-biological technical experimental biases among data from different platforms, after log2 transformation, the ComBat algorithm was applied [53]. Then, the expression value of each gene was averaged over all samples of our data matrix, converting the expression data into the change in log-expression ($\Delta e_{i,m}$) of gene i in sample m; $\Delta e_{i,m} = 0$ implies an expression level according to its mean value, while a relative positive or negative value refers to over- or under-expression, respectively, according to the mean gene expression.

4.3. *Tumor Clusters: First-Level SOM*

The $\Delta e_{i,m}$ data matrix was used to train a SOM, an unsupervised machine learning method based on the artificial neural network, enabling the dimensionality reduction of complex data structures of size N × M (N: number of genes; M: number of samples) to K × M (K: number of meta-genes), where K << N, promoting the discovery of qualitative relationships among samples [54]. Each meta-gene represents a cluster of genes sharing similar expression profiles and was selected by an interactive machine learning process by SOM; the process was trained until the meta-genes captured the entire range of expression patterns present in the data matrix. SOM algorithm data analysis and landscape visualization were performed using the "*oposSOM*" R package (version 1.18.0) [55], which uses the "som" R package [56]. A statistical significance criterion based on expression variance was applied to discard the non-informative features in our data matrix through the BRB-ArrayTools developed by Dr. Richard Simon and the BRB-ArrayTools Development Team [57]. The procedure assigns each input gene measured in M samples into a meta-gene of the same length, and each gene is included in a meta-gene, $\Delta e_{i,m}{}^{meta}$, of closest similarity established by the Euclidian distance. The meta-genes are organized in a two-dimensional grid of K = x × y tiles with the most similar expression profiles of meta-genes adjacent each to another, while the dissimilar ones are more distant. In the present study, we adopted a tile size with an average of $n_k \approx 10$ genes per meta-gene, corresponding to a two-dimensional grid of size K = 18 × 18 meta-genes with square topology and the Gaussian neighborhood function [14]. The meta-genes were normalized to fit into the range $-1 \leq e_{i,m}{}^{meta} \leq 1$ and coded by a color scale from blue (low expression) to red (high expression).

4.4. *Tumor Clusters: Unsupervised Clustering Analysis*

The R-package "*ConsensusClusterPlus*" [58] was applied to portion the samples into molecular coherent subtypes. The meta-data $\Delta e_{i,m}{}^{meta}$ were used as input for unsupervised class identification using partition around medoids (PAM) clustering with 1-Pearson correlation as the distance matrix. The PAM algorithm [59] is similar to the K-means algorithm, with both being partitional algorithms that split the dataset into clusters and try to minimize the error. However, while K-means works with centroids, which are artificially created entities that are representative of each cluster, PAM chooses real data-points as cluster centers. An unsupervised clustering procedure was applied to the data through 1000 re-sampling interactions by randomly selecting a fraction of the samples. Cluster numbers ranging from 2 to 10 were tested, and the empirical cumulative distribution function (CDF) and delta area plots displaying consensus distributions were assessed to identify the number of clusters giving maximum stability with a negligible increase in the CDF area [60]. To estimate the accuracy of the classification, the silhouette correlation width values were calculated for all samples (R-package: *"oposSOM"*), providing a graphical representation of how well the samples lay within their assigned cluster. The silhouette values ranged from +1 to −1, indicating the degree of similarity of a sample to the assigned cluster (cohesion) or to other clusters (separation). The evaluation of sample size adequacy of the identified clusters was assessed according to Warnes and Liu (R-package: *"ssize"*) [61] and computed by imposing the type I error rate (false discovery rate, FDR), $\alpha = 0.05$, and a minimum effect size (log fold-change) of $\Delta = 1$. Cluster-specific portraits represent the mean value of each meta-gene of the samples belonging to the cluster in detail. The portraits are depicted in a log (fold-change) scale where the fold-change is the expression difference compared with the mean expression in all samples. To ascertain to what degree technical variability (i.e., study of origin and platform) affects our subtype clustering analysis, we used the "alluvial diagram", a variant of the parallel coordinates plot that is helpful for exploring categorical data by grouping them into flows that can easily be traced in the diagram [62]. The plots were generated using the R-package *"alluvial"*. In addition, we used a linear mixed model to quantify the extent of technical variability in each sample through the *"variancePartition"* R package [63]. To visualize the contribution of each variable, violin plots were depicted to show the trend and rank the distribution of variance explained by each variable across all genes. The plots summarize the results in terms of the percentage of variance explained.

4.5. Cluster Similarity Relationships: Second-Level SOM Cartography

Second-level SOM analysis aims to address the issue of similarity relationships among groups of samples. It estimates the hierarchy of similarities and mutual distances based on the expression of meta-genes, and it provides improved visualization and representativeness of the results. To infer the main structures present in our data, we applied three approaches for computing the distance metrics.

Independent component analysis (ICA) [64] was applied to the SOM meta-genes using the *"fastICA"* R package [65], a method based on the covariance matrix assessed by Pearson's correlation to decompose the input meta-genes into independent and non-Gaussian components in order to ensure that each one is statistically as independent from the others as possible.

The correlation backbone through a two-nearest-neighbor graph is a correlation network approach where Pearson correlations are computed between all pairwise combinations of samples, and their structures are visualized in a graph.

The NJ algorithm (*"ape"* R package [66]) is a distance-based method offering phylogenetic tree reconstruction where similarity trees are defined between samples into an Euclidian space, allowing "bush-like clusters" displaying mutual dissimilarity to be revealed [67].

To visualize the main meta-genes related to subtype stratification, we assessed the group over-expression spots. We exploited SOM portraits by detection of the coherent expression of meta-genes. Using group overexpression maps, we linked selected meta-genes (correlation with $r > 0.5$) in different regions of the SOM with groups of samples. The group overexpression portrait was calculated as the mean map profile by averaging the meta-gene expression over the three subtypes. To identify the over-expression tiles, a 98th percentile criterion was applied to the meta-gene expression SOM training aggregate meta-genes with similar profiles in the adjacent neighbored tiles of the map. These tiles' profiles grouped over-expressed (or under-expressed) samples that differed from the others. The samples belonging to each subtype were summarized in an average representative portrait. The mining of biological functions from SOM portraits was performed using *"oposSOM"* R package (version 1.18.0).

4.6. Tumor Microenvironment Landscape

To evaluate the heterogeneity in the tumor microenvironment, the immune, stromal, and other cell components were inferred by an in silico approach using the xCell tool [68,69]. This approach enables the assessment of 64 cell types using the bulk gene expression profiles of the tumors as input and comparing them across samples, as described by the authors of Reference [69]. The tool outputs include the transformed xCell scores for the immune, stromal, and other cell types. The adjusted ImmuneScore included 10 populations (B-cells, CD4+ T-cells, CD8+ T-cells, DC, eosinophils, macrophages, monocytes, mast cells, neutrophils, and NK cells) and StromaScore 3 populations (adipocytes, endothelial cells, fibroblasts). In addition, to identify potential keratinocyte differentiation, the xCell score for keratynocytes was computed. To visualize the cellular heterogeneity of the clusters, we applied a dimension reduction method by t-distributed stochastic neighbor embedding (t-SNE) using the "*Rtsne*" package [70], which projected the cell type enrichment scores onto two-dimensional axes [71]. We presented the scores of each subtype in notched boxplots using the "*ggplot2*" R package. Notch boxplots display a confidence interval around the median based on the median $\pm 1.58 \times$ IQR (interquartile range) /sqrt(n). They are useful graphs for comparing groups of samples, because an absence in notch overlapping provides strong visual evidence that the medians differ. The p-values were calculated by the Kruskal–Wallis test, a nonparametric test that compares the means among three or more groups, as in our subtype classification.

4.7. Functional Analyses

To disclose the biological functional properties associated with the proposed molecular subtypes, gene set analysis was applied. This approach estimates gene set over-representation (probability of finding genes in a list compared to their random appearance) and over-expression (difference in expression compared to the mean expression over the samples). The gene sets were defined from a priori knowledge from independent studies and they were summarized in a list of genes specifically related to molecular pattern/biological function. A large collection of gene sets was retrieved from the Gene Set Enrichment Analysis (GSEA Broad Institute; software.broadinstitute.org/gsea/) and the Molecular Signatures Database (MSigDB) repository, including 50 hallmark gene sets. We used the gene set Z-score (GSZ) to summarize the profile of a gene set across all samples [72]. GSZ is a Z-score function that merges both over-representation and over-expression features from a gene set to give a defined gene set and provides a representative score of the gene set for each sample. Boxplots were generated using the "*ggplot2*" R package with the notched boxplot function (see Section 4.6).

4.8. Analysis of Viral Presence/Integration and Its Association with Clusters

The association between viral integration and our subtype stratification was investigated using the results provided by Koneva et al. [20]. Based on TCGA RNA-seq data and exploiting VirusSeq software [73], they detected known virus strains and identified the integration sites. Thus, the authors disclosed the HPV integration status of 65 TCGA cases present in our meta-analysis and assessed viral gene expression (E2, E4, and E5). We investigated the relative presence of integrated HPV cases defined as integrated cases/(integrated + non-integrated cases) in each subtype, and significance was calculated by the χ^2 test. Counts per million (CPM) were retrieved from Koneva et al. and transformed into the log scale by $\log_2(\text{CPM} + 1)$ [74]. Associations with viral gene expression were visualized by a heatmap. The samples were ranked by the Gene Set Variation Analysis (GSVA [75]) based on the three viral genes. GSVA was used to estimate the variation of a gene set over the samples in an unsupervised manner. The p-values were calculated by the Kruskal–Wallis test.

4.9. Evaluation of Prognostic Signatures

Statistical analysis was performed using R (version 3.5.1) [76] and Bioconductor (release 3.7) [77]. Survival curves were assessed according to the Kaplan–Meier method, and overall survival was used as the endpoint. Differences between the subtypes were assessed using the log-rank test and R package "*survival*". Two signatures were evaluated: (i) the 172-gene prognostic model [21]; (ii) the radiosensitivity index (RSI) [22]. The list of genes and the algorithm used for model assessment were retrieved from the original papers.

Supplementary Materials
Figure S1: Estimation of sample size adequacy. The relationship between the genes in our data matrix and power to detect a sample size defined by our three-subtype stratification (Cl1 = 134; Cl2 = 104; Cl3 = 108) is shown in the plots. The percentage of genes achieving a power level of at least 0.9 is displayed by the red bars and was calculated by performing a pairwise comparison between subtypes; Figure S2: Violin and boxplot of the percent variation in gene expression explained by the study of origin, platform, and our three-cluster stratification. Median percentage variation explained: cluster = 50.4%; study <1%; platform <1%; Figure S3: Expression heatmap of viral genes. The expression values for HPV E2, E4, and E5 in the TCGA cases were retrieved from Koneva et al. For visualization purposes, samples were ranked based on Gene Set Variation Analysis (GSVA) from low to high viral gene enrichment. The membership of each TCGA sample is depicted in the bar below the heatmap. Low E2, E4, and E5 expression was found in Cl2 cases compared with Cl1 and Cl3 (p-value = 0.00156, p-value = 0.00204, and p-value = 0.00147 determined by Kruskal–Wallis Tests, respectively); Table S1: List of used datasets. Dataset name, platform used, provider, technology, repository (included websource), number of samples, assignment to the three clusters, and methods of HPV detection are detailed in the table for each of the 11 sources utilized; Table S2: Contingency table for TCGA HPV cases annotated for HPV integration status by Koneva et al; Table S3: Association to clinical parameters in the meta-analysis dataset. The table includes the evaluation of the following clinical parameters: (i) gender; (ii) age; (iii) smoking habit (current or former smokers vs. never smoke); (iv) site (oropharynx vs. other sites); (v) stage. p-values by χ^2 test, with the exception for age determined by Kruskal–Wallis Tests; Table S4: Association to clinical parameters in the validation dataset (GSE112026). The table includes the evaluation of the following clinical parameters: (i) gender; (ii) age; (iii) smoking, (iv) Ang et al. (2010) classification system; (v) smoked packs per year; (vi) alcohol use; (vii) t-stage; (viii) n-stage. p-values by χ^2 test, with the exception for age determined by Kruskal–Wallis Tests.

Author Contributions: Conceptualization, L.D.L. and L.D.C.; Data curation, L.D.C., E.O., S.C., P.B., S.C. and L.D.C.; Formal analysis, M.S.S., M.F.I. and A.C.; Funding acquisition, L.L. and L.D.C.; Investigation, C.R.; Methodology, M.S.S., A.C. and L.D.C.; Writing—original draft, L.D.C., M.S.S. and S.C.; Writing—review & editing, L.D.L., M.S.S. and L.D.C.

References

1. Fitzmaurice, C.; Allen, C.; Barber, R.M.; Barregard, L.; Bhutta, Z.A.; Brenner, H.; Dicker, D.J.; Chimed-Orchir, O.; Dandona, R.; Dandona, L.; et al. Global, regional, and national cancer incidence, mortality, years of life lost, years lived with disability, and disability-adjusted life-years for 32 cancer groups, 1990 to 2015: A systematic analysis for the global burden of disease study. *JAMA Oncol.* **2017**, *3*, 524–548. [PubMed]
2. Chaturvedi, A.K.; Engels, E.A.; Anderson, W.F.; Gillison, M.L. Incidence trends for human papillomavirus-related and -unrelated oral squamous cell carcinomas in the United States. *J. Clin. Oncol.* **2008**, *26*, 612–619. [CrossRef] [PubMed]
3. Rettig, E.M.; D'Souza, G. Epidemiology of head and neck cancer. *Surg. Oncol. Clin. N. Am.* **2015**, *24*, 379–396. [CrossRef] [PubMed]
4. Gillison, M.L.; Castellsagué, X.; Chaturvedi, A.; Goodman, M.T.; Snijders, P.; Tommasino, M.; Arbyn, M.; Franceschi, S. Eurogin Roadmap: Comparative epidemiology of HPV infection and associated cancers of the head and neck and cervix. *Int. J. Cancer* **2014**, *134*, 497–507. [CrossRef] [PubMed]
5. Marur, S.; Forastiere, A.A. Head and neck cancer: Changing epidemiology, diagnosis, and treatment. *Mayo Clin. Proc.* **2008**, *83*, 489–501. [CrossRef]
6. Fakhry, C.; Westra, W.H.; Li, S.; Cmelak, A.; Ridge, J.A.; Pinto, H.; Forastiere, A.; Gillison, M.L. Improved survival of patients with human papillomavirus-positive head and neck squamous cell carcinoma in a prospective clinical trial. *J. Natl. Cancer Inst.* **2008**, *100*, 261–269. [CrossRef] [PubMed]
7. Martín-Hernán, F.; Sánchez-Hernández, J.G.; Cano, J.; Campo, J.; del Romero, J. Oral cancer, HPV infection and evidence of sexual transmission. *Med. Oral Patol. Oral Cir. Bucal* **2013**, *18*, e439–e444. [CrossRef]
8. Lechner, M.; Fenton, T.; West, J.; Wilson, G.; Feber, A.; Henderson, S.; Thirlwell, C.; Dibra, H.K.; Jay, A.; Butcher, L.; et al. Identification and functional validation of HPV-mediated hypermethylation in head and neck squamous cell carcinoma. *Genome Med.* **2013**, *5*, 15. [CrossRef]
9. Sepiashvili, L.; Bruce, J.P.; Huang, S.H.; O'Sullivan, B.; Liu, F.F.; Kislinger, T. Novel insights into head and neck cancer using next-generation "omic" technologies. *Cancer Res.* **2015**, *75*, 480–486. [CrossRef]
10. Leemans, C.R.; Snijders, P.J.F.; Brakenhoff, R.H. The molecular landscape of head and neck cancer. *Nat. Rev. Cancer* **2018**, *18*, 269–282. [CrossRef]
11. Mirghani, H.; Blanchard, P. Treatment de-escalation for HPV-driven oropharyngeal cancer: Where do we stand? *Clin. Transl. Radiat. Oncol.* **2017**, *8*, 4–11. [CrossRef] [PubMed]

12. Keck, M.K.; Zuo, Z.; Khattri, A.; Stricker, T.P.; Brown, C.D.; Imanguli, M.; Rieke, D.; Endhardt, K.; Fang, P.; Brägelmann, J.; et al. Integrative analysis of head and neck cancer identifies two biologically distinct HPV and three non-HPV subtypes. *Clin. Cancer Res.* **2015**, *21*, 870–881. [CrossRef] [PubMed]
13. Zhang, Y.; Koneva, L.A.; Virani, S.; Arthur, A.E.; Virani, A.; Hall, P.B.; Warden, C.D.; Carey, T.E.; Chepeha, D.B.; Prince, M.E.; et al. Subtypes of HPV-Positive Head and Neck Cancers Are Associated with HPV Characteristics, Copy Number Alterations, PIK3CA Mutation, and Pathway Signatures. *Clin. Cancer Res.* **2016**, *22*, 4735–4745. [CrossRef] [PubMed]
14. Wirth, H.; Loffler, M.; von Bergen, M.; Binder, H. Expression cartography of human tissues using self organizing maps. *BMC Bioinform.* **2011**, *12*, 306. [CrossRef] [PubMed]
15. Tamayo, P.; Slonim, D.; Mesirov, J.; Zhu, Q.; Kitareewan, S.; Dmitrovsky, E.; Lander, E.S.; Golub, T.R. Interpreting patterns of gene expression with self-organizing maps: Methods and application to hematopoietic differentiation. *Proc. Natl. Acad. Sci. USA* **1999**, *96*, 2907–2912. [CrossRef] [PubMed]
16. Törönen, P.; Kolehmainen, M.; Wong, G.; Castrén, E. Analysis of gene expression data using self-organizing maps. *FEBS Lett.* **1999**, *451*, 142–146. [CrossRef]
17. Loeffler-Wirth, H.; Kreuz, M.; Hopp, L.; Arakelyan, A.; Haake, A.; Cogliatti, S.B.; Feller, A.C.; Hansmann, M.L.; Lenze, D.; Möller, P.; et al. A modular transcriptome map of mature B cell lymphomas. *Genome Med.* **2019**, *11*, 27. [CrossRef]
18. Kunz, M.; Löffler-Wirth, H.; Dannemann, M.; Willscher, E.; Doose, G.; Kelso, J.; Kottek, T.; Nickel, B.; Hopp, L.; Landsberg, J.; et al. RNA-seq analysis identifies different transcriptomic types and developmental trajectories of primary melanomas. *Oncogene* **2018**, *37*, 6136–6151. [CrossRef]
19. Venuti, A.; Paolini, F. HPV detection methods in head and neck cancer. *Head Neck Pathol.* **2012**, *6* (Suppl. 1), S63–S74. [CrossRef]
20. Koneva, L.A.; Zhang, Y.; Virani, S.; Hall, P.B.; McHugh, J.B.; Chepeha, D.B.; Wolf, G.; Carey, T.E.; Rozek, L.S.; Sartor, M.A. HPV Integration in HNSCC Correlates with Survival Outcomes, Immune Response Signatures, and Candidate Drivers. *Mol. Cancer Res.* **2017**. [CrossRef]
21. De Cecco, L.; Bossi, P.; Locati, L.; Canevari, S.; Licitra, L. Comprehensive gene expression meta-analysis of head and neck squamous cell carcinoma microarray data defines a robust survival predictor. *Ann. Oncol.* **2014**, *25*, 1628–1635. [CrossRef] [PubMed]
22. Eschrich, S.A.; Pramana, J.; Zhang, H.; Zhao, H.; Boulware, D.; Lee, J.H.; Bloom, G.; Rocha-Lima, C.; Kelley, S.; Calvin, D.P.; et al. A gene expression model of intrinsic tumor radiosensitivity: Prediction of response and prognosis after chemoradiation. *Int. J. Radiat. Oncol. Biol. Phys.* **2009**, *75*, 489–496. [CrossRef]
23. Ando, M.; Saito, Y.; Xu, G.; Bui, N.Q.; Medetgul-Ernar, K.; Pu, M.; Fisch, K.; Ren, S.; Sakai, A.; Fukusumi, T.; et al. Chromatin dysregulation and DNA methylation at transcription start sites associated with transcriptional repression in cancers. *Nat. Commun.* **2019**, *10*, 2188. [CrossRef]
24. Gleber-Netto, F.O.; Rao, X.; Guo, T.; Xi, Y.; Gao, M.; Shen, L.; Erikson, K.; Kalu, N.N.; Ren, S.; Xu, G.; et al. Variations in HPV function are associated with survival in squamous cell carcinoma. *JCI Insight* **2019**. [CrossRef] [PubMed]
25. Ang, K.K.; Harris, J.; Wheeler, R.; Weber, R.; Rosenthal, D.I.; Nguyen-Tân, P.F.; Westra, W.H.; Chung, C.H.; Jordan, R.C.; Lu, C.; et al. Human papillomavirus and survival of patients with oropharyngeal cancer. *N. Engl. J. Med.* **2010**, *363*, 24–35. [CrossRef] [PubMed]
26. Blitzer, G.C.; Smith, M.A.; Harris, S.L.; Kimple, R.J. Review of the clinical and biologic aspects of human papillomavirus-positive squamous cell carcinomas of the head and neck. *Int. J. Radiat. Oncol. Biol. Phys.* **2014**, *88*, 761–770. [CrossRef]
27. Chen, Y.P.; Wang, Y.Q.; Lv, J.W.; Li, Y.Q.; Chua, M.L.K.; Le, Q.T.; Lee, N.; Colevas, A.D.; Seiwert, T.; Hayes, D.N.; et al. Identification and validation of novel microenvironment-based immune molecular subgroups of head and neck squamous cell carcinoma: Implications for immunotherapy. *Ann. Oncol.* **2019**. [CrossRef]
28. Suarez-Carmona, M.; Lesage, J.; Cataldo, D.; Gilles, C. EMT and inflammation: Inseparable actors of cancer progression. *Mol. Oncol.* **2017**, *11*, 805–823. [CrossRef]
29. Nordsmark, M.; Bentzen, S.M.; Rudat, V.; Brizel, D.; Lartigau, E.; Stadler, P.; Becker, A.; Adam, M.; Molls, M.; Dunst, J.; et al. Prognostic value of tumor oxygenation in 397 head and neck tumors after primary radiation therapy. An international multi-center study. *Radiother. Oncol.* **2005**, *77*, 18–24. [CrossRef]

30. Speel, E.J. HPV Integration in Head and Neck Squamous Cell Carcinomas: Cause and Consequence. *Recent Results Cancer Res.* **2017**, *206*, 57–72.
31. Nulton, T.J.; Nak-Kyeong, K.; DiNardo, L.J.; Morgan, I.M.; Windle, B. Patients with integrated HPV16 in head and neck cancer show poor survival. *Oral Oncol.* **2018**, *80*, 52–55. [CrossRef] [PubMed]
32. Nulton, T.J.; Olex, A.L.; Dozmorov, M.; Morgan, I.M.; Windle, B. Analysis of The Cancer Genome Atlas sequencing data reveals novel properties of the human papillomavirus 16 genome in head and neck squamous cell carcinoma. *Oncotarget* **2017**, 17684–17699. [CrossRef]
33. Li, H.; Torabi, S.J.; Yarbrough, W.G.; Mehra, S.; Osborn, H.A.; Judson, B. Association of Human Papillomavirus Status at Head and Neck Carcinoma Subsites With Overall Survival. *JAMA Otolaryngol. Head Neck Surg.* **2018**, *144*, 519–525. [CrossRef] [PubMed]
34. Orlandi, E.; Alfieri, S.; Simon, C.; Trama, A.; Licitra, L.; RARECAREnet Working Group. Treatment challenges in and outside a network setting: Head and neck cancers. *Eur. J. Surg. Oncol.* **2019**, *45*, 40–45. [CrossRef] [PubMed]
35. Brazma, A.; Hingamp, P.; Quackenbush, J.; Sherlock, G.; Spellman, P.; Stoeckert, C.; Aach, J.; Ansorge, W.; Ball, C.A.; Causton, H.C.; et al. Minimum information about a microarray experiment (MIAME)-toward standards for microarray data. *Nat. Genet.* **2001**, *29*, 365–371. [CrossRef]
36. Slebos, R.J.; Yi, Y.; Ely, K.; Carter, J.; Evjen, A.; Zhang, X.; Shyr, Y.; Murphy, B.M.; Cmelak, A.J.; Burkey, B.B.; et al. Gene expression differences associated with human papillomavirus status in head and neck squamous cell carcinoma. *Clin. Cancer Res.* **2006**, *12 Pt 1*, 701–709. [CrossRef]
37. Pyeon, D.; Newton, M.A.; Lambert, P.F.; den Boon, J.A.; Sengupta, S.; Marsit, C.J.; Woodworth, C.D.; Connor, J.P.; Haugen, T.H.; Smith, E.M.; et al. Fundamental differences in cell cycle deregulation in human papillomavirus-positive and human papillomavirus-negative head/neck and cervical cancers. *Cancer Res.* **2007**, *67*, 4605–4619. [CrossRef]
38. Walter, V.; Yin, X.; Wilkerson, M.D.; Cabanski, C.R.; Zhao, N.; Du, Y.; Ang, M.K.; Hayward, M.C.; Salazar, A.H.; Hoadley, K.A.; et al. Molecular subtypes in head and neck cancer exhibit distinct patterns of chromosomal gain and loss of canonical cancer genes. *PLoS ONE* **2013**, *8*, e56823. [CrossRef]
39. Sun, W.; Gaykalova, D.A.; Ochs, M.F.; Mambo, E.; Arnaoutakis, D.; Liu, Y.; Loyo, M.; Agrawal, N.; Howard, J.; Li, R.; et al. Activation of the NOTCH pathway in head and neck cancer. *Cancer Res.* **2014**, *74*, 1091–1104. [CrossRef]
40. Thibodeau, B.J.; Geddes, T.J.; Fortier, L.E.; Ahmed, S.; Pruetz, B.L.; Wobb, J.; Chen, P.; Wilson, G.D.; Akervall, J.A. Gene Expression Characterization of HPV Positive Head and Neck Cancer to Predict Response to Chemoradiation. *Head Neck Pathol.* **2015**, *9*, 345–353. [CrossRef]
41. Tomar, S.; Graves, C.A.; Altomare, D.; Kowli, S.; Kassler, S.; Sutkowski, N.; Gillespie, M.B.; Creek, K.E.; Pirisi, L. Human papillomavirus status and gene expression profiles of oropharyngeal and oral cancers from European American and African American patients. *Head Neck* **2016**, *38* (Suppl. 1), E694–E704. [CrossRef]
42. Wichmann, G.; Rosolowski, M.; Krohn, K.; Kreuz, M.; Boehm, A.; Reiche, A.; Scharrer, U.; Halama, D.; Bertolini, J.; Bauer, U.; et al. The role of HPV RNA transcription, immune response-related gene expression and disruptive TP53 mutations in diagnostic and prognostic profiling of head and neck cancer. *Int. J. Cancer* **2015**, *137*, 2846–2857. [CrossRef]
43. Mirghani, H.; Ugolin, N.; Ory, C.; Lefèvre, M.; Baulande, S.; Hofman, P.; St Guily, J.L.; Chevillard, S.; Lacave, R. A predictive transcriptomic signature of oropharyngeal cancer according to HPV16 status exclusively. *Oral Oncol.* **2014**, *50*, 1025–1034. [CrossRef]
44. Thurlow, J.K.; Peña Murillo, C.L.; Hunter, K.D.; Buffa, F.M.; Patiar, S.; Betts, G.; West, C.M.; Harris, A.L.; Parkinson, E.K.; Harrison, P.R.; et al. Spectral clustering of microarray data elucidates the roles of microenvironment remodeling and immune responses in survival of head and neck squamous cell carcinoma. *J. Clin. Oncol.* **2010**, *28*, 2881–2888. [CrossRef]
45. Cancer Genome Atlas Network. Comprehensive genomic characterization of head and neck squamous cell carcinomas. *Nature* **2015**, *517*, 576–582. [CrossRef]
46. Edgar, R.; Domrachev, M.; Lash, A.E. Gene Expression Omnibus: NCBI gene expression and hybridization array data repository. *Nucleic Acids Res.* **2002**, *30*, 207–210. [CrossRef]
47. Kolesnikov, N.; Hastings, E.; Keays, M.; Melnichuk, O.; Tang, Y.A.; Williams, E.; Dylag, M.; Kurbatova, N.; Brandizi, M.; Burdett, T.; et al. ArrayExpress update—Simplifying data submissions. *Nucleic Acids Res.* **2015**, *43*, D1113–D1116. [CrossRef]

48. BIOINFORMATICS @ MANCHESTER. Available online: http://bioinformatics.picr.man.ac.uk/vice/Welcome.vice (accessed on 31 March 2016).
49. National Cancer Institute GDC Data Portal. Available online: https://portal.gdc.cancer.gov/repository (accessed on 30 April 2018).
50. De Cecco, L.; Nicolau, M.; Giannoccaro, M.; Daidone, M.G.; Bossi, P.; Locati, L.; Licitra, L.; Canevari, S. Head and neck cancer subtypes with biological and clinical relevance: Meta-analysis of gene-expression data. *Oncotarget* **2015**, *6*, 9627–9642. [CrossRef]
51. Simon, R.; Lam, A.; Li, M.C.; Ngan, M.; Menenzes, S.; Zhao, Y. Analysis of gene expression data using BRB-ArrayTools. *Cancer Inform.* **2007**, *3*, 11–17. [CrossRef]
52. Langfelder, P.; Horvath, S. WGCNA: An R package for weighted correlation network analysis. *BMC Bioinform.* **2008**, *9*, 559. [CrossRef]
53. Johnson, W.E.; Li, C.; Rabinovic, A. Adjusting batch effects in microarray expression data using empirical Bayes methods. *Biostatistics* **2007**, *8*, 118–127. [CrossRef]
54. Kohonen, T. Self-organized formation of topologically correct feature maps. *Biol. Cybern.* **1982**, *43*, 59–69. [CrossRef]
55. Löffler-Wirth, H.; Kalcher, M.; Binder, H. oposSOM: R-package for high-dimensional portraying of genome-wide expression landscapes on bioconductor. *Bioinformatics* **2015**, *31*, 3225–3227. [CrossRef]
56. Yan, J. Som: Self-Organizing Map. 2010 R Package. Available online: Cran.r-project.org/web/packages/som (accessed on 30 November 2018).
57. National Cancer Institute. Available online: https://brb.nci.nih.gov/BRB-ArrayTools/index.html (accessed on 30 November 2018).
58. Wilkerson, M.D.; Hayes, D.N. ConsensusClusterPlus: A class discovery tool with confidence assessments and item tracking. *Bioinformatics* **2010**, *26*, 1572–1573. [CrossRef]
59. Kaufman, L.; Rousseeuw, P. Clustering by Means of Medoids. In Proceedings of the Statistical Data Analysis Based on the L1 Norm and Related Methods, Neuchâtel, Switzerland, 31 August–4 September 1987; Dodge, Y., Ed.; Elsevier Science Pub. Co.: Amsterdam, The Netherlands, 1987; pp. 405–416.
60. Monti, S.; Tamayo, P.; Mesirov, J.; Todd, G. Consensus Clustering: A Resampling-Based Method for Class Discovery and Visualization of Gene Expression Microarray Data. *Mach. Learn.* **2003**, *52*, 91–118. [CrossRef]
61. Warnes, G.; Liu, P.; Li, F. Ssize: Estimate Microarray Sample Size. R Package Version 1.54.0. Available online: http://bioconductor.org/packages/release/bioc/html/ssize.html (accessed on 31 May 2017).
62. Rosvall, M.; Bergstrom, C.T. Mapping Change in Large Networks. *PLoS ONE* **2010**, *5*, e8694. [CrossRef]
63. Hoffman, G.E.; Schadt, E.E. variancePartition: Interpreting drivers of variation in complex gene expression studies. *BMC Bioinform.* **2016**, *17*. [CrossRef]
64. Hyvärinen, A.; Oja, E. Independent component analysis: Algorithms and applications. *Neural Netw.* **2000**, *13*, 411–430. [CrossRef]
65. FastICA. Available online: https://CRAN.R-project.org/package=fastICA (accessed on 30 November 2018).
66. Paradis, E.; Claude, J.; Strimmer, K. APE: Analyses of Phylogenetics and Evolution in R language. *Bioinformatics* **2004**, *20*, 289–290. [CrossRef]
67. Saitou, N.; Nei, M. The neighbor-joining method: A new method for reconstructing phylogenetic trees. *Mol. Biol. Evol.* **1987**, *4*, 406–425.
68. xCell. Available online: http://xcell.ucsf.edu/ (accessed on 28 February 2019).
69. Aran, D.; Hu, Z.; Butte, A.J. xCell: Digitally portraying the tissue cellular heterogeneity landscape. *Genome Biol.* **2017**, *18*, 220. [CrossRef]
70. Krijthe, J.H. Rtsne: T-Distributed Stochastic Neighbor Embedding Using a Barnes-Hut Implementation. Available online: https://github.com/jkrijthe/Rtsne (accessed on 28 February 2019).
71. van der Maaten, L.; Hinton, G. Visualizing data using t-SNE. *J. Mach. Learn. Res.* **2008**, *9*, 2579–2605.
72. Törönen, P.; Ojala, P.J.; Marttinen, P.; Holm, L. Robust extraction of functional signals from gene set analysis using a generalized threshold free scoring function. *BMC Bioinform.* **2009**, *10*, 307. [CrossRef]
73. Chen, Y.; Yao, H.; Thompson, E.J.; Tannir, N.M.; Weinstein, J.N.; Su, X. VirusSeq: Software to identify viruses and their integration sites using next-generation sequencing of human cancer tissue. *Bioinformatics* **2013**, *29*, 266–267. [CrossRef]
74. Law, C.W.; Chen, Y.; Shi, W.; Smyth, G.K. voom: Precision weights unlock linear model analysis tools for RNA-seq read counts. *Genome Biol.* **2014**, *15*, R29. [CrossRef]

75. Hänzelmann, S.; Castelo, R.; Guinney, J. GSVA: Gene set variation analysis for microarray and RNA-Seq data. *BMC Bioinform.* **2013**, *14*, 7. [CrossRef]
76. R Development Core Team. R: A Language and Environment for Statistical Computing. Vienna, Austria: R Foundation for Statistical Computing 2007. Available online: http://www.R-project.org (accessed on 30 September 2018).
77. Gentleman, R.C.; Carey, V.J.; Bates, D.M.; Bolstad, B.; Dettling, M.; Dudoit, S.; Ellis, B.; Gautier, L.; Ge, Y.; Gentry, J.; et al. Bioconductor: Open software development for computational biology and bioinformatics. *Genome Biol.* **2004**, *5*, R80. [CrossRef]

13

Association Analysis of Deep Genomic Features Extracted by Denoising Autoencoders in Breast Cancer

Qian Liu [1] and Pingzhao Hu [1,2,3,*]

1 Department of Biochemistry and Medical Genetics, College of Medicine, Faculty of Health Sciences, University of Manitoba, Winnipeg, MB R3E 0J9, Canada; qianl@myumanitoba.ca
2 Research Institute in Oncology and Hematology, CancerCare Manitoba, Winnipeg, MB R3E 0V9, Canada
3 Department of Computer Science, University of Manitoba, Winnipeg, MB R3T 2N2, Canada
* Correspondence: pingzhao.hu@umanitoba.ca;

Abstract: Artificial intelligence-based unsupervised deep learning (DL) is widely used to mine multimodal big data. However, there are few applications of this technology to cancer genomics. We aim to develop DL models to extract deep features from the breast cancer gene expression data and copy number alteration (CNA) data separately and jointly. We hypothesize that the deep features are associated with patients' clinical characteristics and outcomes. Two unsupervised denoising autoencoders (DAs) were developed to extract deep features from TCGA (The Cancer Genome Atlas) breast cancer gene expression and CNA data separately and jointly. A heat map was used to view and cluster patients into subgroups based on these DL features. Fisher's exact test and Pearson' Chi-square test were applied to test the associations of patients' groups and clinical information. Survival differences between the groups were evaluated by Kaplan–Meier (KM) curves. Associations between each of the features and patient's overall survival were assessed using Cox's proportional hazards (COX-PH) model and a risk score for each feature set from the different omics data sets was generated from the survival regression coefficients. The risk scores for each feature set were binarized into high- and low-risk patient groups to evaluate survival differences using KM curves. Furthermore, the risk scores were traced back to their gene level DAs weights so that the three gene lists for each of the genomic data points were generated to perform gene set enrichment analysis. Patients were clustered into two groups based on concatenated features from the gene expression and CNA data and these two groups showed different overall survival rates (p-value = 0.049) and different ER (Estrogen receptor) statuses (p-value = 0.002, OR (odds ratio) = 0.626). All the risk scores from the gene expression and CNA data and their concatenated one were significantly associated with breast cancer survival. The patients with the high-risk group were significantly associated with patients' worse outcomes (p-values ≤ 0.0023). The concatenated risk score was enriched by the AMP-activated protein kinase (AMPK) signaling pathway, the regulation of DNA-templated transcription, the regulation of nucleic acid-templated transcription, the regulation of apoptotic process, the positive regulation of gene expression, the positive regulation of cell proliferation, heart morphogenesis, the regulation of cellular macromolecule biosynthetic process, with FDR (false discovery rate) less than 0.05. We confirmed DAs can effectively extract meaningful genomic features from genomic data and concatenating multiple data sources can improve the significance of the features associated with breast cancer patients' clinical characteristics and outcomes.

Keywords: denoising autoencoders; breast cancer; feature extraction and interpretation; concatenated deep feature

1. Introduction

Advanced hardware technologies have highly increased computational power, which makes the implementation of computation-consuming algorithms possible. At the same time, the development of biological technologies has greatly reduced the cost of genomic sequencing, which produced a huge amount of high-dimensional genomic data. Under these circumstances, bioinformatics becomes an exciting research field for researchers to explore the possibility to interpret genomic data using advanced computational technologies [1].

Different types of high-dimensional genomic data have been associated with cancer clinical characteristics and outcomes. The most commonly used ones are gene expression data and copy number alteration (CNA) data [2]. The activity of gene expression in tumor tissues is quite different from that in normal tissues [3] and has been established to have the ability to distinguish the characteristics of cancers [4]. There are some repeated segments in normal DNA, and during the process of cancer development, the repeated number of the segments may be changed due to abnormal DNA replication in tumor cells. This phenomenon is called copy number alteration [5]. CNA may result in chromosome structure changes in the forms of duplication or deletion in DNA segments. It has been shown that CNA plays an important role in the development of many types of cancers including breast cancer [6]. Therefore, it is highly necessary to mine the prognostic and diagnostic significance of the genome-wide cancer genomic data. From a clinical point of view, the prognosis of the genomic factors is always a necessary consideration because of its importance in making treatment plans [7]. In previous studies, prognosis significance was evaluated mainly based on clinical features, such as tumor grades and tumor subtypes [7] and molecular features, such as expression related gene signatures (e.g., PAM50 subtypes) [8,9]. Results from these studies showed that the gene signatures tend to have better prognosis significance than traditional pathological assessment [7]. This might be due to the integration ability of these gene signatures. For instance, PAM50 can combine the information from the tumor stage, tumor grade and tumor subtype together [9]. However, the known gene signatures are only based on single genomic data source such as gene expression. This might be not adequate since other types of genomic data such as copy number alterations should also include important cancer prognosis information [9]. Advanced algorithms now give us new tools to explore the possibility of integrating different data sources together. For example, Chi, et al. identified several genes and pathways with a high prognostic significance for young breast cancer patients based on their gene expression and copy number alteration data using a graph-based machine learning (ML) method [9].

Traditional ML methods such as artificial neural networks (ANN) and support vector machines (SVM) may suffer some problems in dealing with the high-dimensional, noisy and massive genomic data [10]. Recently, a special case of ANN with more nodes and layers has emerged as an efficient method to handle these high-dimensional and noisy data. The idea of ANN was originated from the information processing and communication patterns in a human nervous system [11]. As the new development of the traditional ANN, deep learning (DL) presents a large group of interconnected artificial neurons with many more layers. Like other learning methods, DL could be implemented in a supervised or unsupervised way, which depends on whether the input data is labeled or not. Although both supervised and unsupervised DL algorithms have been successfully applied to the analysis of genomic data, they could be used to solve different biology problems. Supervised learning algorithms are often used to predict gene functions and gene-gene interactions or to identify new driver genes [12], while unsupervised learning algorithms are often used to cluster the strong signals in the data [13,14]. Among the unsupervised learning algorithms, autoencoder is a new technology that uses the data itself as the learning objective or label. Therefore, it is also known as self-labeled or self-supervised deep learning. Traditional autoencoders may face the invalid learning problem when the number of hidden nodes is larger than the input size. To avoid this potential risk, denoising autoencoders (DAs) came up with the solution of adding some noise into the input data on purpose.

Vincent, et al. brought the concept of DAs into DL and built a specialized feature extraction DL architecture [15]. The key idea of DAs as mentioned above is to add random noise into the raw data before it is input into the network. After the encode and decode processes, the raw data would be reconstructed from the noisy data, while the compact and efficient representations from the raw data could be learned as well [15]. These representations are the DAs-based genomic features.

DL as a special case of ML and ANN has been applied to mine deep information from complex genomic data and has generated interesting results [16]. Its high integration and reconstruction abilities give us large flexibility to combine different types of genomic data to extract valuable information from them. It has been expected that deep features extracted by DL models would perform better in clinical association and prognosis prediction than standard gene or pathway signatures [17]. For example, Tan, et al. reported a deep feature representing ER status and a deep feature with high prognosis significance based on breast cancer gene expression data [13]. These deep features were constructed by a DAs and performed better in the downstream analyses [13]. However, these studies were based on only a single genomic source.

This study aims to extract the integrated features from both the gene expression and CNA data by a concatenated DAs model. As a comparison, we also built a standard DAs model to extract deep features from gene expression and CNA data separately. The comparisons were made in terms of the performance in association analysis as well as prognosis analysis. The study design and analysis procedures are shown in Figure 1.

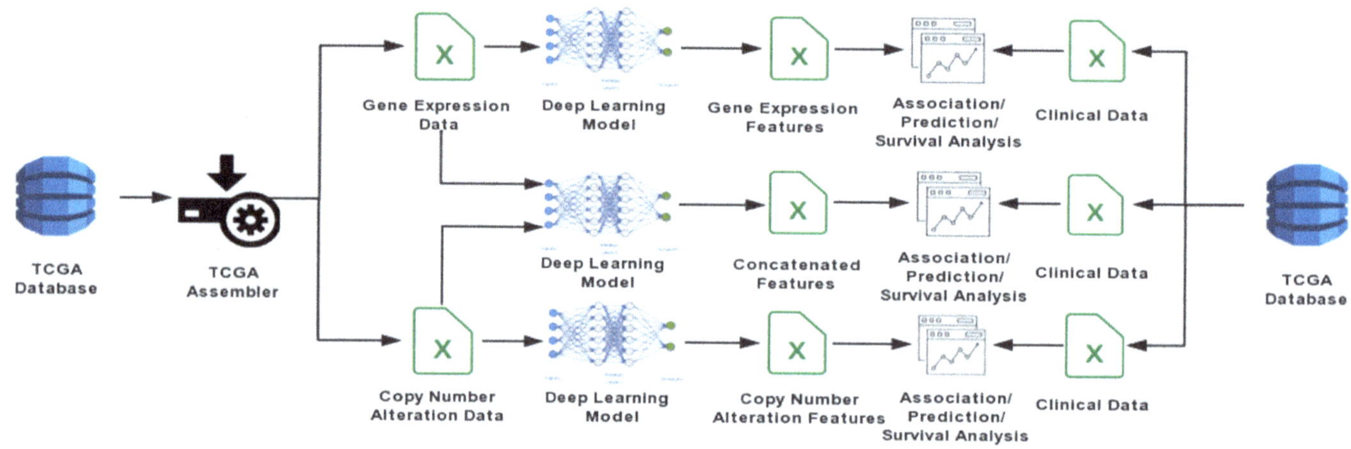

Figure 1. A flowchart illustrating the analysis procedures in this study.

2. Materials and Methods

2.1. Data Sources

Datasets used in this study came from The Cancer Genome Atlas (TCGA) [18], which is one of the most comprehensive genomic databases. TCGA provides 1098 breast cancer patients' clinical data along with their genomic data. These genomic data include gene expressions, CNA, protein expressions, micro RNA (miRNA) expressions, and somatic mutations.

For gene expression data, the sequencing, alignment, quality control and quantification were performed previously [18]. Using the TCGA-Assembler tool [19], we downloaded the gene expression raw count, then filtered out unexpressed genes and those genes with a count per million (CPM) less than 1 in 3 patients. We performed normalization of the data using Upper Quartile Fragments per Kilobase of transcript per Million mapped reads (FPKM-UQ) [20]. FPKM-UQ is a modified FPKM algorithm in which the total read count is replaced by the 75th percentile read count for a given sample.

Similar to the gene expression data, upstream processes of CNA data were done previously as well [18]. Using the downloaded chromosome-region specific log2 copy number data, we calculated the gene-level CNA values using the TCGA-Assembler tool. Several data cleaning procedures such as removing all-NAs were also performed to avoid potential format issues in the follow-up analysis.

After normalization and preprocessing, there were 18,163 genes from each of the 1095 patients left for gene expression data and 23,563 genes from the 1098 patients left for CNA data. To keep the gene dimension and scale matched in the two data sources, both of them were linearly transformed into a range between 0 and 1, resulting in the decreasing of the data dimension to 16,197 (genes) × 1085 (patients) for both data sources.

2.2. DA Models

Two DAs models were developed using Keras [21] with Tensorflow [22] as the backend to extract deep genomic features. One model was for feature extraction from a single genomic source, named as one-input DAs model (Figure 2). The other, named as the two-input DAs model (Figure 3), was for concatenated feature extraction from the integrated genomic sources.

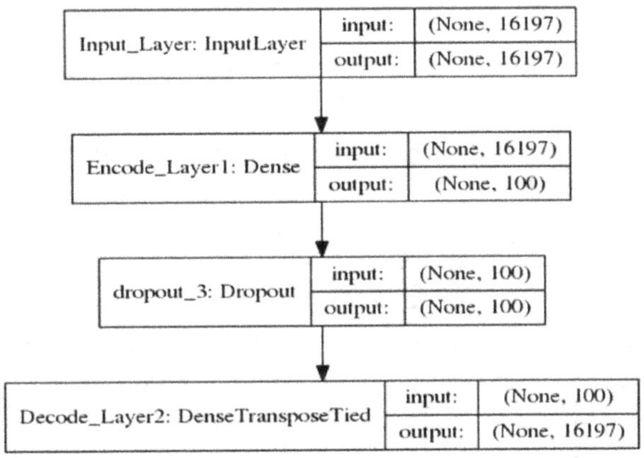

Figure 2. The one-input denoising autoencoders model. There are two hidden layers in the encode phase and two decode layers. The input can be either gene expression data or copy number alteration data.

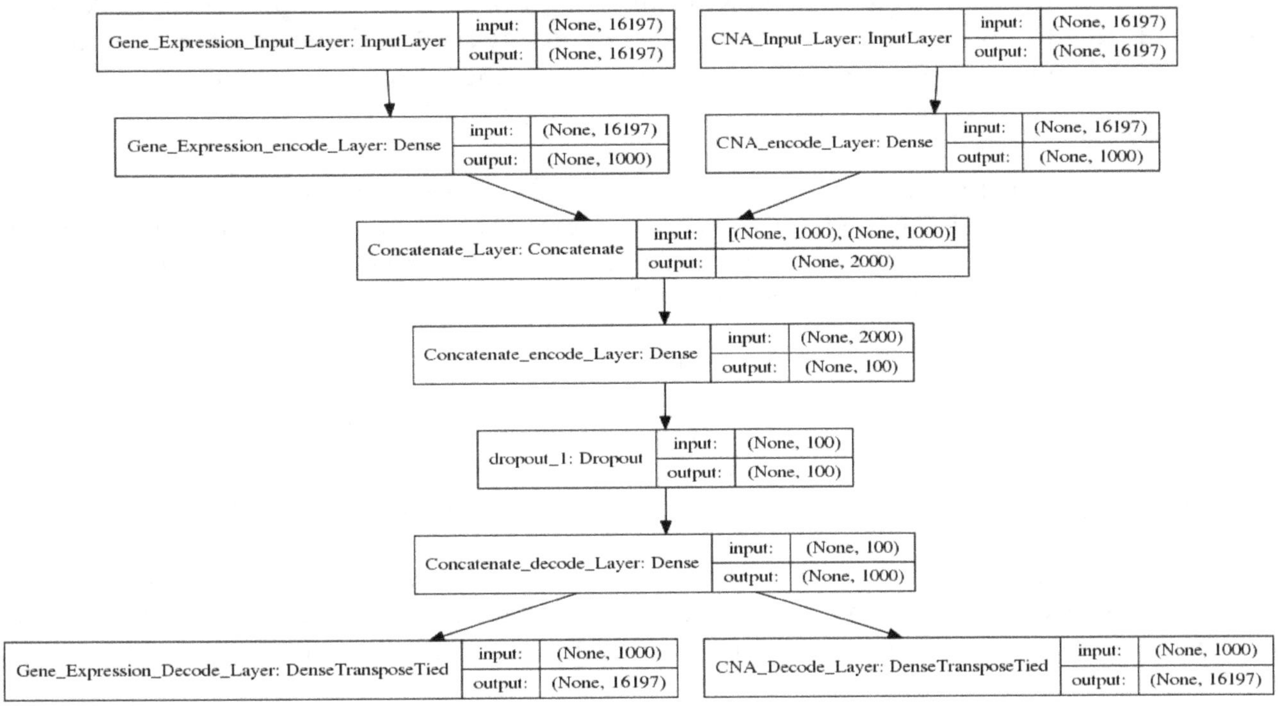

Figure 3. The two-input DAs model. There are two hidden layers in the encode phase and one decode layer. Concatenation was performed between the two encode layers.

2.2.1. One-Input DAs Model

This architecture was composed of one input layer, one fully connected encode hidden layer with 100 nodes which were chosen to be the deep features used in this study and one decode layer which uses the transpose of encoding layer′ weights. This procedure can be formulated as below:

$$\begin{aligned} \text{encode} &= \text{sigmoid}\ (W \times \text{input} + b) \\ \text{decode} &= \text{sigmoid}\ (W' \times \text{encode} + b') \end{aligned} \tag{1}$$

where W is the weight metrics between the layers with the size of 16,197 × 100, b is the bias for each node, and the sigmoid function is sigmoid $(x) = 1 / (1 + e^{-x})$. The counterparts with the superscript refer to the transpose metrics. A dropout layer was added after the encode layer, which randomly set 50% of the output of encode layer to 0 to prevent overfitting. The encode item was chosen to be the activity values of the deep features in this model.

2.2.2. Two-Input DAs Model

Literally, the two-input DAs model contained two input layers, followed by one encode layer with 1000 nodes for each input layer, then followed by a concatenated layer, and another encode layer with 100 nodes which were chosen to be the deep concatenated features. Finally, there were two decode layers. The procedure can be formulated as follow:

$$\begin{aligned} \text{input}_1\text{\_encode}_1 &= \text{sigmoid}\ (input_1\_W_1 \times \text{input}_1 + input_1\_b_1) \\ \text{input}_2\text{\_encode}_1 &= \text{sigmoid}\ (input_2\_W_1 \times \text{input}_2 + input_2\_b_1) \\ \text{concate\_encode}_1 &= \text{concatenate}\ (\text{input}_1\text{\_encode}_1, \text{input}_2\text{\_encode}_1) \\ \text{concate\_encode}_2 &= \text{sigmoid}\ (concate\_W_2 \times \text{concate\_encode}_1 + concate\_b_2) \\ \text{output}_1 &= \text{sigmoid}\ (input_1\_W_1{}' \times \text{concate\_encode}_2 + input_1\_b_1{}') \\ \text{output}_2 &= \text{sigmoid}\ (input_2\_W_1{}' \times \text{concate\_encode}_2 + input_2\_b_1{}') \end{aligned} \tag{2}$$

where $input_1\_W_1$, $input_2\_W_1$, and $concate\_W_2$ are the weight metrics between the layers with the size of 16,197 × 1000, 16,197 × 1000, 2000 × 100 respectively. The $input_1\_b_1$, $input_2\_b_1$, and $concate\_b_2$ are the biases for each node. The counterparts with superscript refer to the transpose metrics. A dropout layer was added after concate_encode$_2$ layer, which randomly set 50% of the output of that layer to 0. The concate_encode$_2$ was chosen to be the activity values of the deep features in this model.

2.3. Train the Models

Before the training process, the input data sets were disrupted by a noise factor of 0.25, which is the proportion of the number of genes in the data sources. These genes were selected randomly and their values were set to 0. The binary cross-entropy function shown below was used to measure the difference between the input layer and the output layer:

$$L\ (input, output) = -(1/N)\ \Sigma\ (input_k \times log(output_k) + (1 - input_k) \times log(1 - output_k)) \tag{3}$$

where $L\ (input, output)$ is the binary cross-entropy, K is the index of batches, N is the total number of batches. Thus, the training task is to minimize the $L\ (input, output)$.

For the optimizer, e.g., the strategy to update the weights and bias so that the minima could be found, we selected stochastic gradient descent (SGD), which has several arguments to be set freely. After having different trials, the learning rate was finally set to 0.1; the batch size and epoch were set to 64 and 100 respectively. The models were finally trained under the parameters mentioned above. The activity values and weight metrics related to deep features were read out.

2.4. Visualization and Clustering

Heatmap3 [23] was used to visualize the activity values of these deep feature sets. We used the complete linkage function in the hierarchical clustering process and visual-guided criteria by analysis of the dendrogram to decide the number of clusters. First, the clinical data downloaded from TCGA were carefully scanned and the most clinical-relevant characteristics such as pathological status (T, N, M), tumor stage, estrogen receptor (ER) status, progesterone receptor (PR) status, human epidermal growth factor receptor 2 (HER2) status, triple negative status, and PAM50 subtypes (i.e., Luminal A, Luminal B, Basal-like, HER2-enriched, and Normal-like) were extracted. These clinical characteristics were shown as the sidebar of the heat map.

2.5. Association Analysis

To test whether the identified patient clusters are associated with known clinical and molecular characteristics, we applied both Fisher's exact test and Pearson' Chi-square test.

Survival differences between the identified patients groups were evaluated by Kaplan–Meier (KM) curves. Furthermore, associations between each deep feature in the three feature sets (gene expression, CNA, the concatenated one) and patient's overall survival was assessed using Cox's proportional hazards (COX-PH) model [24]. The hazard function is

$$h(t) = h_0\ (t) \times exp\ (bx) \tag{4}$$

where t represents the survival time. b is the coefficient which measures the impact of the covariate x. Later, a risk score for each feature set was generated from the COX-PH coefficients:

$$r = \Sigma\ (b_i \times a_i) \tag{5}$$

where r is the risk score, b_i is the coefficient from the COX-PH model and a_i is the related activity value of the given feature. Afterward, the risk scores were binarized into high-risk and low-risk groups using R package xtile function with a *prob* parameter set to 0.55, which means we use the 55% quantile as the cutoff to bin the patients into the high-risk and low-risk groups. Finally, the survival differences between these two groups were evaluated by the KM curve.

2.6. Gene Sets Enrichment Analysis

For each of the three DAs models for gene expression, CNA and their concatenated one, we traced back their gene-level weights based on

$$W_g = W \times B \tag{6}$$

where W is the 16,197 $\times$ 100 dimensional weights that were extracted from a given DAs model previously. B is the vector of COX-PH coefficients. The gene-specific weights W_g were filtered by a cutoff 0.01, which resulted in the three selected gene lists with 6954, 5381 and 6297 genes, respectively. Finally, the three gene lists were used to perform gene set enrichment analysis (GSEA) by the Enricr tool [25] to identify the up-regulated and down-regulated pathways. Kyoto Encyclopedia of Genes and Genomes (KEGG) [26] and Gene Ontology (GO) [27] Biological Process 2018 version were chosen to be the reference gene sets.

3. Results

Based on the normalized and processed breast cancer genomic data, our models were trained and the activity values of the 100 deep features for each of the three data sets as well as the weights matrices were extracted (Table 1). Then we clustered these activity values for each of the three data sets. Overall, there were no clear patterns shown in the deep features from a single genomic source (gene expression or CNA data). However, patients were roughly clustered into 2 groups according to the activity values of the concatenated deep features (Figure 4).

Table 1. The size and organization of deep features obtained from the models. The size and structure of the deep features extracted from gene expression data and copy number alteration data by the two denoising autoencoders (DAs) models.

Model	Data Source	Deep Features (Noise Factors = 0.25)	
One-input DAs	Gene expressions	Activity values	1085 × 100
		weights	16,197 × 100
	Copy number alterations	Activity values	1085 × 100
		weights	16,197 × 100
Two-input DAs	Gene expressions Copy number alterations	Activity values	1085 × 100
		weights	16,197 × 100

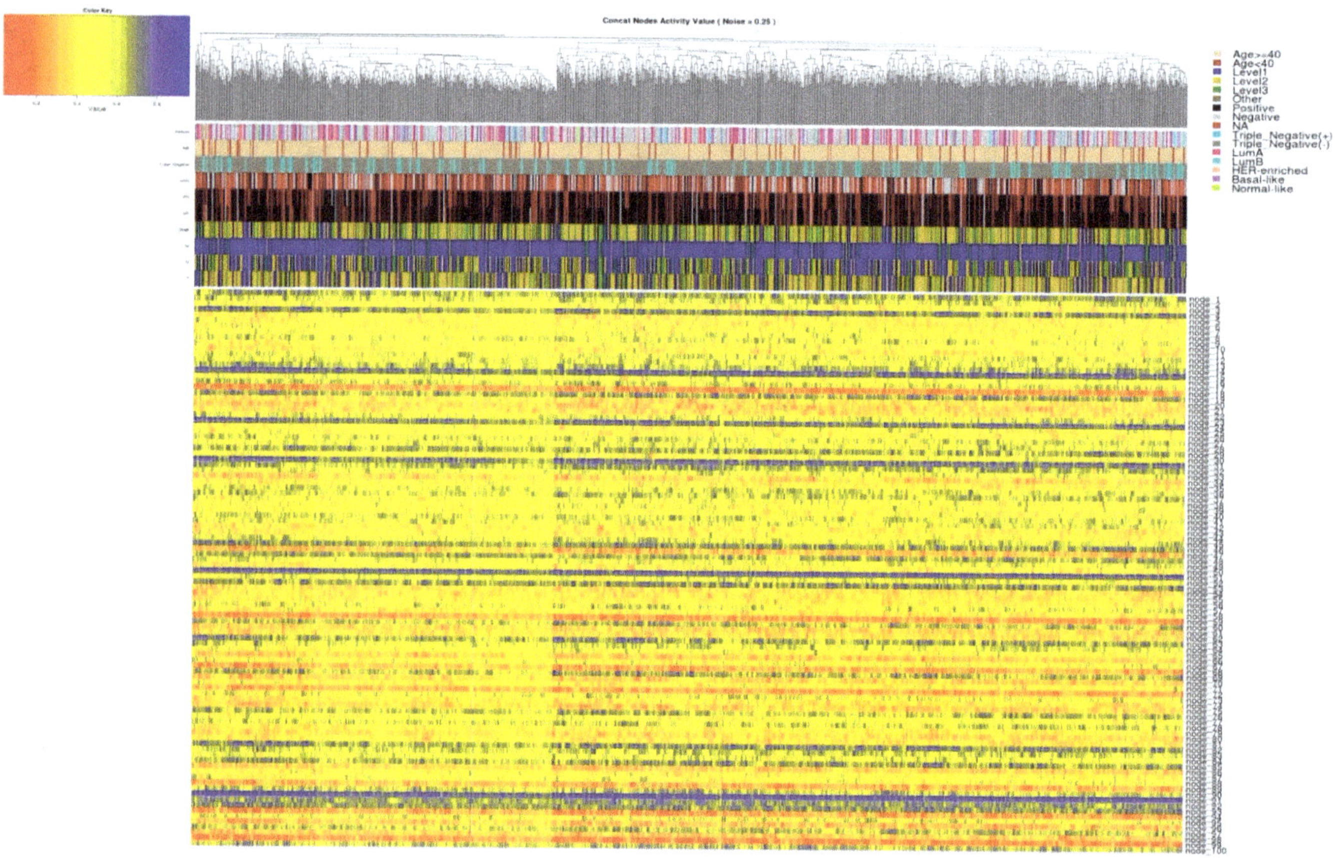

Figure 4. The clustering of activity values of concatenated deep features extracted under the noise factor of 0.25. The columns are the 1085 patients and the rows are the 100 deep features. The sidebar contains the corresponding clinical information of the patients. Values are clustered by both columns and rows.

Results from the association tests between the two patient groups and their clinical characteristics are shown in Table 2. The two patient groups showed significant survival (Figure 5) and ER status difference (Table 2) with p-values 0.049 and 0.002, respectively, which mean that the concatenated features have learned the ER information and performed well in predicting patient's prognosis. The odds ratio of ER status is 0.626, indicating that the second group tends to be associated with ER-negative patients. From the KM plot (Figure 5), we can see that the patients in Group 2 suffered from a poor prognosis, which happens to be associated with ER-negative status. It has been shown that ER-negative breast cancer patients usually have a poor prognosis.

Table 2. The results of clinical association analysis. * patients were classified as young (age < 40) and old (age $\geq$ 40) groups.

Clinical Characteristics	Fisher's Exact p-Value	Chi-Square Test p-Value
Pathological T	0.69	0.69
Pathological N	0.95	0.96
Pathological M	0.95	0.94
Tumor Stage	0.93	0.93
ER Status	0.002	0.002
PR Status	1.00	0.99
HER Status	0.43	0.44
Age *	0.58	0.67
Triple Negative Status	0.15	0.17
Tumor Subtype	0.35	0.36

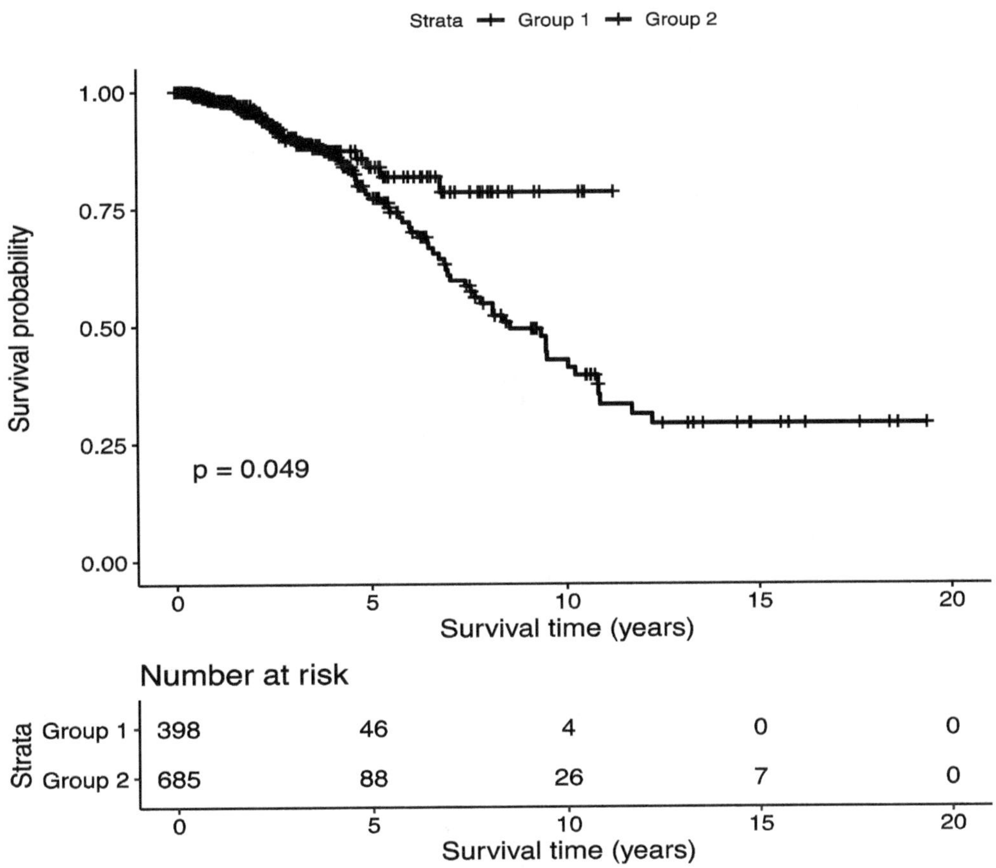

Figure 5. The Kaplan–Meier (KM) plot of the two patient groups clustered by the concatenated features.

According to the results of COX-PH models, the high-risk scores generated from each of the three deep feature sets are all significantly associated with a poor overall survival with p-values less than 1×10^{-5} (Table 3). The concatenated features showed a higher hazard ratio (HR) with 95% confidence interval (CI) (1.27, 1.16–1.40) than gene expression features (1.009, 1.005–1.013) and CNA features (1.23, 1.15–1.32). These results indicated that the risk scores from the deep features, especially the concatenated risk score, predict patient's poor prognosis. The similar patterns were observed in KM plots (Figure 6), where the patient group with high-risk scores always suffered from a poor prognosis.

Table 3. Cox's proportional hazards (COX-PH) results for risk scores.

Risk Score	HR	Lower.95_HR	Upper.95_HR	*p*-Value
Gene expression	1.009	1.005	1.013	1.06×10^{-5}
CNA	1.23	1.15	1.32	7.86×10^{-9}
Concatenated	1.27	1.16	1.40	5.62×10^{-7}

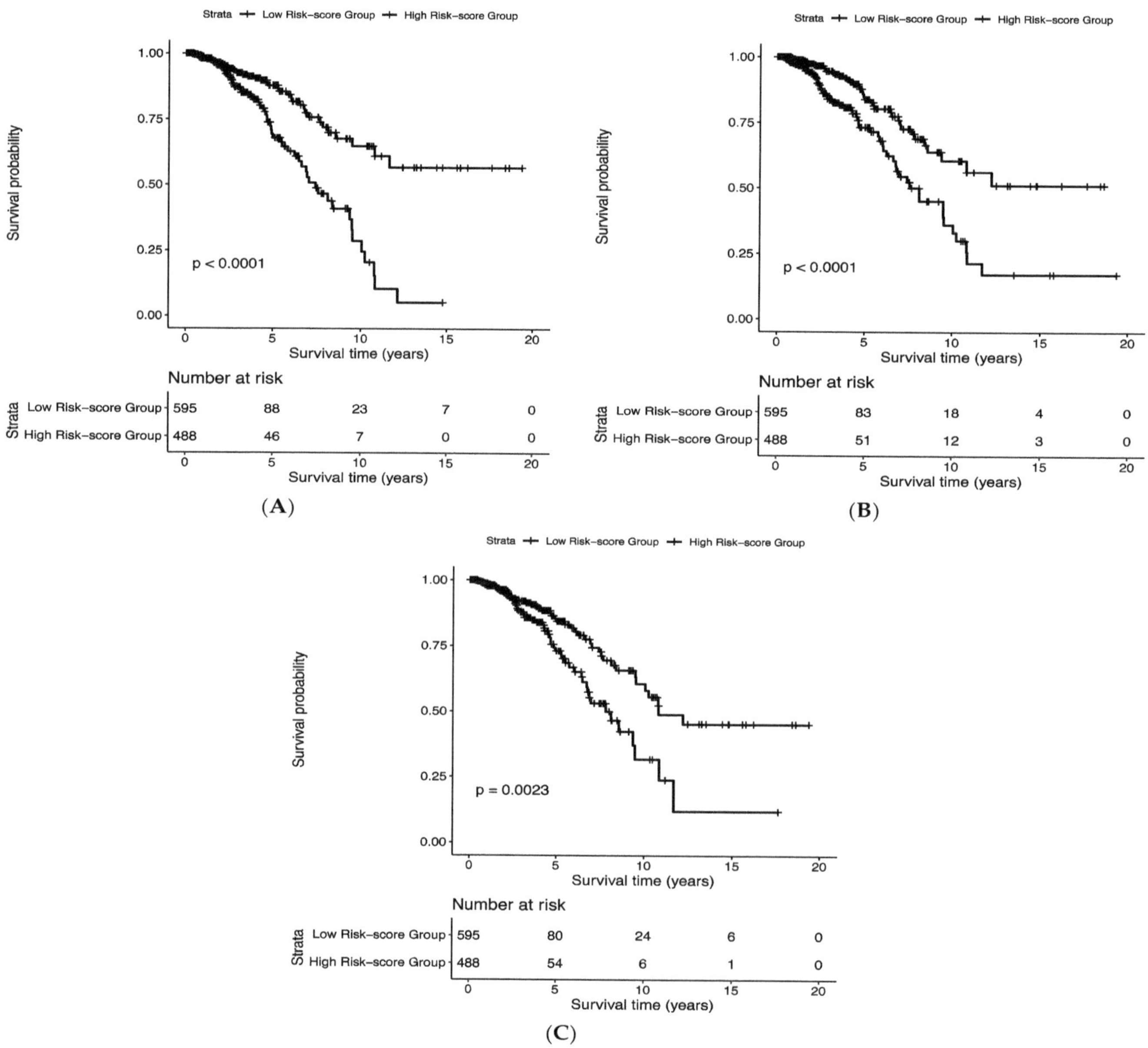

Figure 6. The KM-plots for risk scores based on the deep feature sets. (**A**) Gene expression data; (**B**) copy number alteration data; (**C**) the concatenated data.

GSEA using the 6,297 genes selected based on the concatenated deep feature set showed that the AMP-activated protein kinase (AMPK) signaling pathway in the KEGG family was significantly down-regulated with a false discovery rate (FDR) less than 0.05, and several GO-based regulation processes, such as the regulation of DNA-templated transcription, the regulation of nucleic acid-templated transcription, the regulation of apoptotic process, the positive regulation of gene expression, the positive regulation of cell proliferation, and the regulation of cellular macromolecule biosynthetic process were significantly enriched as well, with an FDR less than 0.05 (Table 4).

Table 4. The gene set enrichment analysis using Enricr.

Gene Sets	p-Value	Adjusted p-Value
regulation of transcription, DNA-templated	2.25×10^{-7}	0.001
regulation of nucleic acid-templated transcription	6.03×10^{-5}	0.04
regulation of apoptotic process	6.19×10^{-5}	0.04
positive regulation of gene expression	5.89×10^{-5}	0.04
positive regulation of cell proliferation	4.78×10^{-5}	0.04
AMPK signaling pathway_Homo sapiens_hsa04152	6.08×10^{-5}	0.018

AMPK is an important cellular metabolism and energy homeostasis regulator in mammalian tissues. It is situated in the center of a signaling network which contains tumor suppressors such as LKB1, TSC2 and p53 [25]. Some evidence has been reported that AMPK plays an anti-tumorigenic role and a lot of work are ongoing to involve agonists of AMPK for cancer treatment [28]. Furthermore, all those enriched GO regulation processes are critical as hallmarks in cancer occurrence and progression [29].

4. Discussion

In building the DA model, one of the key parameters we need to set up is the noise level used to partially destroy the inputs. We tried to add different levels of noise (e.g., 0%, 10%, 25% and 50%) into the DA model. Similar to the observations made by Vincent et al. [15], we also found that the more noise was added the better the network learns dependencies between the features. With low noise levels, the learned features do not stand out. As we set the noise level at 0.25, denoising training can capture more distinctive deep features.

Comparing with conventional breast cancer biomarkers, such as CA15-3 for measuring how breast cancer treatment is working and looking for cancer that has come back or recurred, after treatment [30], and NCC-ST-439 for measuring breast cancer progression [31], the explanation of the deep genomic features or biomarkers from the DA model for breast cancers is more complicated. Each of the extracted deep features is a high-level summary of the raw features or conventional biomarkers. These high-level features or biomarkers can be more robust against noise in the conventional biomarkers. Furthermore, these high-level features can potentially significantly improve the breast cancer outcome prediction by integrating information from both breast cancer histology images and genomic biomarkers [32]. The extracted features based on the proposed deep learning model can be also used to predict the statuses of malignancy, relapse, and reactivity for anticancer if the related data sources are available. We will explore the method in other large data sets and cancer types in the future. This can further validate the usefulness of the method for risk stratification of cancer patients.

In order to extract robust deep features using the proposed DA model, we took a strategy to add noise into the input genomic data by the partial corruption of the input pattern. It is expected that the learned deep features from the partially destroyed inputs can yield almost the same representation of the raw genomic data. In order to further boost the performance of using the learned deep features to predict breast cancer outcome or traits, another interesting strategy is to incorporate the prior knowledge about breast cancer hallmarks, which can be represented by a few molecular or signaling networks [33], into the deep learning procedure. This can be potentially implemented in different ways. For example, the interaction information among different genes or mutations collected in the molecular or signaling network databases can be used to assign the weights in different layers of the network among different neurons. We will explore the interesting strategy in future studies.

5. Conclusions

In this study, we showed that unsupervised DAs as an effective model to extract meaningful deep genomic features from either single- or multi- genomic sources from breast cancer patients. These features were significantly associated with the breast cancer ER status and had the prognosis significance. We also showed that the concatenated deep features were enriched by breast cancer relevant pathways.

This study can be improved in two potential ways. The first one is to develop new DAs model structures such as stacking more layers into DAs or adding a regression layer to make it supervised [34]. The second one is to combine all types of possible data sources together, such as somatic mutation data, protein expressions, miRNA expressions, etc. We will explore these ideas in future analyses.

Author Contributions: Q.L. and P.H. were involved in the conceptualization, development of methodologies and manuscript writing; P.H. was involved in supervision, project administration and funding acquisition.

Abbreviations

DL	Deep learning
CNA	Copy number alteration
DAs	Denoising autoencoders
TCGA	The Cancer Genome Atlas
KM	Kaplan-Meier
COX-PH	Cox's proportion hazard
OR	Odds ratio
AMPK	AMP-activated protein kinase
FDR	False discovery rate
GSEA	Gene sets enrichment analysis
ML	Machine learning
ANN	Artificial neural network
SVM	Support vector machine
ER	Estrogen receptor
miRNA	Micro RNA
CPM	Count per million
FPKM-UQ	Upper quartile fragments per kilobase of transcript per Million mapped reads
SGD	Stochastic gradient descent
KEGG	Kyoto Encyclopedia of Genes and Genomes
GO	Gene Ontology

References

1. Lesk, A.M. *Introduction to Bioinformatics*, 3rd ed.; Oxford University Press: Oxford, UK, 2008.
2. Bergamaschi, A.; Kim, Y.H.; Wang, P.; Sørlie, T.; Hernandez-Boussard, T.; Lonning, P.E.; Tibshirani, R.; Borresen-Dale, A.L.; Pollack, J.R. Distinct patterns of DNA copy number alteration are associated with different clinicopathological features and gene-expression subtypes of breast cancer. *Genes Chromosomes Cancer* **2006**, *45*, 1033–1040. [CrossRef]
3. Ramaswamy, S.; Tamayo, P.; Rifkin, R.; Mukherjee, S.; Yeang, C.H.; Angelo, M.; Ladd, C.; Reich, M.; Latulippe, E.; Mesirov, J.P.; et al. Multiclass cancer diagnosis using tumor gene expression signatures. *Proc. Natl. Acad. Sci. USA* **2001**, *98*, 15149–15154. [CrossRef]
4. Sorlie, T.; Tibshirani, R.; Parker, J.; Hastie, T.; Marron, J.S.; Nobel, A.; Deng, S.; Johnsen, H.; Pesich, R.; Geisler, S.; et al. Repeated observation of breast tumor subtypes in independent gene expression data sets. *Proc. Natl. Acad. Sci. USA* **2003**, *100*, 8418–8423. [CrossRef] [PubMed]

5. Wu, H.T.; Hajirasouliha, I.; Raphael, B.J. Detecting independent and recurrent copy number aberrations using interval graphs. *Bioinformatics* **2014**, *30*, i195–i203. [CrossRef]
6. Beroukhim, R.; Mermel, C.H.; Porter, D.; Wei, G.; Raychaudhuri, S.; Donovan, J.; Barretina, J.; Boehm, J.S.; Dobson, J.; Urashima, M.; et al. The landscape of somatic copy-number alteration across human cancers. *Nature* **2010**, *463*, 899–905. [CrossRef]
7. Boughorbel, S.; Al-Ali, R.; Elkum, N. Model Comparison for Breast Cancer Prognosis Based on Clinical Data. *PLoS ONE* **2016**, *11*, e0146413. [CrossRef] [PubMed]
8. Nielsen, T.O.; Parker, J.S.; Leung, S.; Voduc, D.; Ebbert, M.; Vickery, T.; Davies, S.R.; Snider, J.; Stijleman, I.J.; Reed, J.; et al. A comparison of PAM50 intrinsic subtyping with immunohistochemistry and clinical prognostic factors in tamoxifen-treated estrogen receptor-positive breast cancer. *Clin. Cancer Res.* **2010**, *16*, 5222–5232. [CrossRef] [PubMed]
9. Chi, C.; Murphy, L.C.; Hu, P. Recurrent copy number alterations in young women with breast cancer. *Oncotarget* **2018**, *9*, 11541–11558. [CrossRef] [PubMed]
10. Auria, L.; Moro, R.A. *Support Vector Machines (SVM) as a Technique for Solvency Analysis*; DIW Discussion Papers 811; DIW Berlin, German Institute for Economic Research: Berlin, Germany, 2008.
11. Olshen, A.B.; Venkatraman, E.S.; Lucito, R.; Wigler, M. Circular binary segmentation for the analysis of array-based DNA copy number data. *Biostatistics* **2004**, *5*, 557–572. [CrossRef]
12. Schadt, E.E.; Lamb, J.; Yang, X.; Zhu, J.; Edwards, S.; Guhathakurta, D.; Sieberts, S.K.; Monks, S.; Reitman, M.; Zhang, C.; et al. An integrative genomics approach to infer causal associations between gene expression and disease. *Nat. Genet.* **2005**, *37*, 710–717. [CrossRef]
13. Tan, J.; Ung, M.; Cheng, C.; Greene, C.S. Unsupervised feature construction and knowledge extraction from genome-wide assays of breast cancer with denoising autoencoders. *Pac. Symp. Biocomput.* **2014**, *20*, 132–143.
14. Guyon, I.; Elisseeff, A. Feature Extraction, Foundations and Applications: An introduction to feature extraction. *Stud. Fuzziness Soft Comput.* **2006**, *207*, 1–25.
15. Vincent, P.; Larochelle, H.; Bengio, Y.; Manzagol, P.A. Extracting and composing robust features with denoising autoencoders. In Proceedings of the 25th International Conference on Machine Learning, Helsinki, Finland, 5–9 July 2008; ACM: New York, NY, USA, 2008; pp. 1096–1103.
16. Khan, J.; Wei, J.S.; Ringnér, M.; Saal, L.H.; Ladanyi, M.; Westermann, F.; Berthold, F.; Schwab, M.; Antonescu, C.R.; Peterson, C.; et al. Classification and diagnostic prediction of cancers using gene expression profiling and artificial neural networks. *Nat. Med.* **2001**, *7*, 673–679. [CrossRef] [PubMed]
17. Angermueller, C.; Pärnamaa, T.; Parts, L.; Oliver, S. Deep Learning for Computational Biology. *Mol. Syst. Biol.* **2016**, *12*, 878. [CrossRef] [PubMed]
18. Tomczak, K.; Czerwińska, P.; Wiznerowicz, M. The Cancer Genome Atlas (TCGA): An immeasurable source of knowledge. *Wspolczesna Onkol.* **2015**, *19*, A68–A77. [CrossRef] [PubMed]
19. Zhu, Y.; Qiu, P.; Ji, Y. TCGA-assembler: Open-source software for retrieving and processing TCGA data. *Nat. Methods* **2014**, *11*, 599–600. [CrossRef]
20. Bullard, J.H.; Purdom, E.; Hansen, K.D.; Dudoit, S. Evaluation of statistical methods for normalization and differential expression in mRNA-Seq experiments. *BMC Bioinform.* **2010**, *11*, 94. [CrossRef] [PubMed]
21. Chollet, F. Building Autoencoders in Keras. *The Keras Blog*, 2016. Available online: https://blog.keras.io/building-autoencoders-in-keras.html (accessed on 20 January 2019).
22. Abadi, M.; Barham, P.; Chen, J.; Chen, Z.; Davis, A.; Dean, J.; Devin, M.; Ghemawat, S.; Irving, G.; Isard, M.; et al. TensorFlow: A System for Large-Scale Machine Learning. In Proceedings of the 12th USENIX Symposium on Operating Systems Design and Implementation (OSDI'16), Savannah, GA, USA, 2–4 November 2016; pp. 265–284.
23. Wu, G.; Xing, M.; Mambo, E.; Huang, X.; Liu, J.; Guo, Z.; Chatterjee, A.; Goldenberg, D.; Gollin, S.M.; Sukumar, S.; et al. Somatic mutation and gain of copy number of PIK3CA in human breast cancer. *Breast Cancer Res.* **2005**, *7*, R609–R616. [CrossRef]
24. Ching, T.; Zhu, X.; Garmire, L.X. Cox—Nnet: An artificial neural network method for prognosis prediction on high—Throughput omics data. *PLoS Comput. Biol.* **2016**, *14*, e1006076. [CrossRef]
25. Chen, E.Y.; Tan, C.M.; Kou, Y.; Duan, Q.; Wang, Z.; Meirelles, G.V.; Clark, N.R.; Ma'ayan, A. Enrichr: Interactive and collaborative HTML5 gene list enrichment analysis tool. *BMC Bioinform.* **2013**, *14*, 128. [CrossRef]

26. Ogata, H.; Goto, S.; Sato, K.; Fujibuchi, W.; Bono, H.; Kanehisa, M. KEGG: Kyoto encyclopedia of genes and genomes. *Nucleic Acids Res.* **1999**, *27*, 29–34. [CrossRef]
27. Ashburner, M.; Ball, C.A.; Blake, J.A.; Botstein, D.; Butler, H.; Cherry, J.M.; Davis, A.P.; Dolinski, K.; Dwight, S.S.; Eppig, J.T.; et al. Gene ontology: Tool for the unification of biology. *Nat. Genet.* **2000**, *25*, 25–29. [CrossRef]
28. Giordanetto, F.; Karis, D. Direct AMP-activated protein kinase activators: A review of evidence from the patent literature. *Expert Opin. Ther. Pat.* **2012**, *22*, 1467–1477. [CrossRef]
29. Hanahan, D.; Weinberg, R.A. Hallmarks of cancer: The next generation. *Cell* **2011**, *144*, 646–674. [CrossRef]
30. Harris, L.; Fritsche, H.; Mennel, R.; Norton, L.; Ravdin, P.; Taube, S.; Somerfield, M.R.; Hayes, D.F.; Bast, R.C., Jr. American Society of Clinical Oncology 2007 update of recommendations for the use of tumor markers in breast cancer. *J. Clin. Oncol.* **2007**, *25*, 5287–5312. [CrossRef]
31. Miyahara, E.; Toi, M.; Wada, T.; Yamada, H.; Osaki, A.; Yanagawa, E.; Toge, T. The expression of NCC-ST-439, a tumor marker, in human breast cancer patients. *Gan No Rinsho* **1990**, *36*, 2023–2026.
32. Mobadersany, P.; Yousefi, S.; Amgad, M.; Gutman, D.A.; Barnholtz-Sloan, J.S.; Vega, J.E.V.; Brat, D.J.; Cooper, L.A.D. Predicting cancer outcomes from histology and genomics using convolutional networks. *Proc. Natl. Acad. Sci. USA* **2018**, *115*, E2970–E2979. [CrossRef]
33. Wang, E.; Zaman, N.; Mcgee, S.; Milanese, J.S.; Masoudi-Nejad, A.; O'Connor-McCourt, M. Predictive genomics: A cancer hallmark network framework for predicting tumor clinical phenotypes using genome sequencing data. *Semin. Cancer Biol.* **2015**, *30*, 4–12. [CrossRef]
34. Vincent, P.; Larochelle, H.; Lajoie, I.; Bengio, Y.; Manzagol, P.A. Stacked denoising autoencoders: Learning useful representations in a deep network with a local denoising criterion. *J. Mach. Learn. Res.* **2010**, *11*, 3371–3408.

Permissions

All chapters in this book were first published by MDPI; hereby published with permission under the Creative Commons Attribution License or equivalent. Every chapter published in this book has been scrutinized by our experts. Their significance has been extensively debated. The topics covered herein carry significant findings which will fuel the growth of the discipline. They may even be implemented as practical applications or may be referred to as a beginning point for another development.

The contributors of this book come from diverse backgrounds, making this book a truly international effort. This book will bring forth new frontiers with its revolutionizing research information and detailed analysis of the nascent developments around the world.

We would like to thank all the contributing authors for lending their expertise to make the book truly unique. They have played a crucial role in the development of this book. Without their invaluable contributions this book wouldn't have been possible. They have made vital efforts to compile up to date information on the varied aspects of this subject to make this book a valuable addition to the collection of many professionals and students.

This book was conceptualized with the vision of imparting up-to-date information and advanced data in this field. To ensure the same, a matchless editorial board was set up. Every individual on the board went through rigorous rounds of assessment to prove their worth. After which they invested a large part of their time researching and compiling the most relevant data for our readers.

The editorial board has been involved in producing this book since its inception. They have spent rigorous hours researching and exploring the diverse topics which have resulted in the successful publishing of this book. They have passed on their knowledge of decades through this book. To expedite this challenging task, the publisher supported the team at every step. A small team of assistant editors was also appointed to further simplify the editing procedure and attain best results for the readers.

Apart from the editorial board, the designing team has also invested a significant amount of their time in understanding the subject and creating the most relevant covers. They scrutinized every image to scout for the most suitable representation of the subject and create an appropriate cover for the book.

The publishing team has been an ardent support to the editorial, designing and production team. Their endless efforts to recruit the best for this project, has resulted in the accomplishment of this book. They are a veteran in the field of academics and their pool of knowledge is as vast as their experience in printing. Their expertise and guidance has proved useful at every step. Their uncompromising quality standards have made this book an exceptional effort. Their encouragement from time to time has been an inspiration for everyone.

The publisher and the editorial board hope that this book will prove to be a valuable piece of knowledge for researchers, students, practitioners and scholars across the globe.

List of Contributors

Ryuji Hamamoto, Kazuma Kobayashi and Norio Shinkai
Division of Molecular Modification and Cancer Biology, National Cancer Center Research Institute, 5-1-1 Tsukiji, Chuo-ku, Tokyo 104-0045, Japan
Cancer Translational Research Team, RIKEN Center for Advanced Intelligence Project, 1-4-1 Nihonbashi, Chuo-ku, Tokyo 103-0027, Japan
Department of NCC Cancer Science, Graduate School of Medical and Dental Sciences, Tokyo Medical and Dental University, 1-5-45 Yushima, Bunkyo-ku, Tokyo 113-8510, Japan

Kruthi Suvarna
Indian Institute of Technology Bombay, Powai, Mumbai 400 076, India

Masayoshi Yamada
Division of Molecular Modification and Cancer Biology, National Cancer Center Research Institute, 5-1-1 Tsukiji, Chuo-ku, Tokyo 104-0045, Japan
Department of Endoscopy, National Cancer Center Hospital, 5-1-1 Tsukiji, Chuo-ku Tokyo 104-0045, Japan

Mototaka Miyake
Department of Diagnostic Radiology, National Cancer Center Hospital, 5-1-1 Tsukiji, Chuo-ku, Tokyo 104-0045, Japan

Masamichi Takahashi
Division of Molecular Modification and Cancer Biology, National Cancer Center Research Institute, 5-1-1 Tsukiji, Chuo-ku, Tokyo 104-0045, Japan
Department of Neurosurgery and Neuro-Oncology, National Cancer Center Hospital, 5-1-1 Tsukiji, Chuoku, Tokyo 104-0045, Japan

Shunichi Jinnai
Department of Dermatologic Oncology, National Cancer Center Hospital, 5-1-1 Tsukiji, Chuo-ku, Tokyo 104-0045, Japan

Ryo Shimoyama, Kanto Shozu and Ai Dozen
Division of Molecular Modification and Cancer Biology, National Cancer Center Research Institute, 5-1-1 Tsukiji, Chuo-ku, Tokyo 104-0045, Japan

Akira Sakai
Division of Molecular Modification and Cancer Biology, National Cancer Center Research Institute, 5-1-1 Tsukiji, Chuo-ku, Tokyo 104-0045, Japan
Department of NCC Cancer Science, Graduate School of Medical and Dental Sciences, Tokyo Medical and Dental University, 1-5-45 Yushima, Bunkyo-ku, Tokyo 113-8510, Japan

Ken Takasawa, Amina Bolatkan, Hidenori Machino, Satoshi Takahashi, Ken Asada, Masaaki Komatsu and Syuzo Kaneko
Division of Molecular Modification and Cancer Biology, National Cancer Center Research Institute, 5-1-1 Tsukiji, Chuo-ku, Tokyo 104-0045, Japan
Cancer Translational Research Team, RIKEN Center for Advanced Intelligence Project, 1-4-1 Nihonbashi, Chuo-ku, Tokyo 103-0027, Japan

Jun Sese
Division of Molecular Modification and Cancer Biology, National Cancer Center Research Institute, 5-1-1 Tsukiji, Chuo-ku, Tokyo 104-0045, Japan
Humanome Lab, 2-4-10 Tsukiji, Chuo-ku, Tokyo 104-0045, Japan

Lei Qin
School of Statistics, University of International Business and Economics, Beijing 100029, China

Tsung-Ming Chen
Department of Otorhinolaryngology, Shuang-Ho Hospital, Taipei Medical University, New Taipei City 23561, Taiwan

Yi-Wei Kao
Graduate Institute of Business Administration, Fu Jen Catholic University, Taipei 116, Taiwan

Kuan-Chou Lin
Department of Oral and Maxillofacial Surgery, Wanfang Hospital, Taipei Medical University, Taipei 116, Taiwan

Kevin Sheng-Po Yuan
Department of Otorhinolaryngology, Wanfang Hospital, Taipei Medical University, Taipei 116, Taiwan

Alexander T. H. Wu
Ph.D. Program for Translational Medicine, Taipei Medical University, Taipei 116, Taiwan

Ben-Chang Shia
College of Management, Taipei Medical University, Taipei 106, Taiwan

Szu-Yuan Wu
Department of Radiation Oncology, Wanfang Hospital, Taipei Medical University, Taipei 116, Taiwan
Department of Internal Medicine, School of Medicine, College of Medicine, Taipei Medical University, Taipei 110, Taiwan

Davide Angeli
Department of Paediatric Haematology, IRCCS Ospedale Pediatrico Bambino Gesù, 00146 Rome, Italy

Maurizio Fanciulli and Matteo Pallocca
SAFU Unit, IRCCS Regina Elena National Cancer Institute, 00144 Rome, Italy

Johannes Vey
Functional Genomics and Systems Biology Group, Department of Bioinformatics, University of Würzburg, 97074 Würzburg, Germany
Institute of Medical Biometry and Informatics, University of Heidelberg, Im Neuenheimer Feld 130.3, 69120 Heidelberg, Germany

Lorenz A. Kapsner
Center of Medical Information and Communication Technology, Erlangen University Hospital, 91054 Erlangen, Germany

Maximilian Fuchs
Functional Genomics and Systems Biology Group, Department of Bioinformatics, University of Würzburg, 97074 Würzburg, Germany
Chair of Medical Informatics, Friedrich-Alexander University of Erlangen-Nürnberg, 91058 Erlangen, Germany

Philipp Unberath and Meik Kunz
Chair of Medical Informatics, Friedrich-Alexander University of Erlangen-Nürnberg, 91058 Erlangen, Germany

Giulia Veronesi
Unit of Thoracic Surgery, Humanitas Research Hospital, Via Manzoni 56, 20089 Rozzano (Milan), Italy

Xueli Zhang
School of Medicine, Institute of Medical Sciences, Örebro University, SE-70182 Örebro, Sweden
Centre for Systems Biology, Soochow University, Suzhou 215006, China

Xiao-Feng Sun
Department of Oncology and Clinical and Experimental Medicine, Linköping University, SE-58183 Linköping, Sweden

Bairong Shen
Centre for Systems Biology, Soochow University, Suzhou 215006, China

Hong Zhang
School of Medicine, Institute of Medical Sciences, Örebro University, SE-70182 Örebro, Sweden

Mafalda Ramos de Matos, Ioana Posa, Filipa Sofia Carvalho, Vanessa Alexandra Morais and Sérgio Fernandes de Almeida
Instituto de Medicina Molecular João Lobo Antunes, Faculdade de Medicina da Universidade de Lisboa, 1649-028 Lisboa, Portugal

Ana Rita Grosso
Instituto de Medicina Molecular João Lobo Antunes, Faculdade de Medicina da Universidade de Lisboa, 1649-028 Lisboa, Portugal
UCIBIO, Departamento de Ciências da Vida, Faculdade de Ciências e Tecnologia, Universidade NOVA de Lisboa, 2829-516 Caparica, Portugal

Luca Falzone and Rossella Salemi
Department of Biomedical and Biotechnological Sciences, Oncologic, Clinic and General Pathology Section, University of Catania, 95123 Catania, Italy

Gabriella Lupo, Carmelina Daniela Anfuso, Massimo Libra and Saverio Candido
Department of Biomedical and Biotechnological Sciences, Oncologic, Clinic and General Pathology Section, University of Catania, 95123 Catania, Italy
Research Center for Prevention, Diagnosis and Treatment of Cancer, University of Catania, 95123 Catania, Italy

Giusy Rita Maria La Rosa and Ernesto Rapisarda
Department of General Surgery and Surgical-Medical Specialties, University of Catania, 95125 Catania, Italy

Salvatore Crimi
Department of Surgical and Biomedical Sciences, University of Catania, 95123 Catania, Italy

Patrizia Ferroni and Fiorella Guadagni
BioBIM (InterInstitutional Multidisciplinary Biobank), IRCCS San Raffaele Pisana, Via di Val Cannuta 247, 00166 Rome, Italy
Department of Human Sciences & Quality of Life Promotion, San Raffaele Roma Open University, Via di Val Cannuta 247, 00166 Rome, Italy

Fabio M. Zanzotto
Department of Enterprise Engineering, University of Rome "Tor Vergata", Viale Oxford 81, 00133 Rome, Italy

Silvia Riondino
BioBIM (InterInstitutional Multidisciplinary Biobank), IRCCS San Raffaele Pisana, Via di Val Cannuta 247, 00166 Rome, Italy
Department of Systems Medicine, Medical Oncology, Tor Vergata Clinical Center, University of Rome "Tor Vergata", Viale Oxford 81, 00133 Rome, Italy

Noemi Scarpato
Department of Human Sciences & Quality of Life Promotion, San Raffaele Roma Open University, Via di Val Cannuta 247, 00166 Rome, Italy

Mario Roselli
Department of Systems Medicine, Medical Oncology, Tor Vergata Clinical Center, University of Rome "Tor Vergata", Viale Oxford 81, 00133 Rome, Italy

Igor B. Rogozin and Frida Belinky
National Center for Biotechnology Information, National Library of Medicine, National Institutes of Health, Bethesda, MD 20894-6075, USA

Abiel Roche-Lima
Center for Collaborative Research in Health Disparities-RCMI Program, Medical Sciences Campus, University of Puerto Rico, San Juan, PR 00936, USA

Artem G. Lada
Department Microbiology and Molecular Genetics, University of California, Davis, CA 95616, USA

Ivan A. Sidorenko and Vladimir N. Babenko
Institute of Cytology and Genetics, Novosibirsk 630090, Russia

Galina V. Glazko
Department of Biomedical Informatics, University of Arkansas for Medical Sciences, Little Rock, AR 72205, USA

David N. Cooper
Institute of Medical Genetics, Cardiff University, Cardiff CF14 4AY, UK

Youri I. Pavlov
Departments of Microbiology and Pathology; Biochemistry and Molecular Biology; Genetics, Cell Biology and Anatomy, University of Nebraska Medical Center, Omaha, NE 68198, USA
Eppley Institute for Research in Cancer and Allied Diseases, Omaha, NE 68198, USA

Pulak R. Manna, Ahsen U. Ahmed and Kevin Pruitt
Departments of Immunology and Molecular Microbiology, School of Medicine, Texas Tech University Health Sciences Center, Lubbock, TX 79430, USA

Shengping Yang
Internal Medicine, School of Medicine, Texas Tech University Health Sciences Center, Lubbock, TX 79430, USA

Madhusudhanan Narasimhan
Pharmacology and Neuroscience, School of Medicine, Texas Tech University Health Sciences Center, Lubbock, TX 79430, USA

Joëlle Cohen-Tannoudji
Physiologie de l'axe gonadotrope U1133, Institut National de la Santé et de la Recherche Médicale, CNRS, Biologie Fonctionnelle et Adaptative UMR 8251, Université Paris Diderot, 75205 Paris, France

Andrzej T. Slominski
Department of Dermatology and Laboratory Medicine, Comprehensive Cancer Center, Cancer Chemoprevention Program, University of Alabama at Birmingham, Birmingham, AL 35294, USA
Veterans Administration Medical Center, Birmingham, AL 35294, USA

Arlina Shen
The Blake School, 511 Kenwood Pkwy, Minneapolis, MN 55403, USA

Han Fu, Kevin He and Hui Jiang
Department of Biostatistics, University of Michigan, 1415 Washington Heights, Ann Arbor, MI 48109, USA

Laura D. Locati, Carlo Resteghini, Stefano Cavalieri and Paolo Bossi
Head and Neck Medical Oncology Department, Fondazione IRCCS Istituto Nazionale dei Tumori di Milano, 20133 Milan, Italy

Mara S. Serafini, Maria F. Iannò, Andrea Carenzo, Silvana Canevari and Loris De Cecco
Integrated Biology Platform, Department of Applied Research and Technology Development, Fondazione IRCCS Istituto Nazionale dei Tumori di Milano, 20133 Milan, Italy

Ester Orlandi
Radiation Oncology Department, Fondazione IRCCS Istituto Nazionale dei Tumori di Milano, 20133 Milan, Italy

Lisa Licitra
Head and Neck Medical Oncology Department, Fondazione IRCCS Istituto Nazionale dei Tumori di Milano, 20133 Milan, Italy
Department of Oncology, University of Milan, 20122 Milan, Italy

Qian Liu
Department of Biochemistry and Medical Genetics, College of Medicine, Faculty of Health Sciences, University of Manitoba, Winnipeg, MB R3E 0J9, Canada

Pingzhao Hu
Department of Biochemistry and Medical Genetics, College of Medicine, Faculty of Health Sciences, University of Manitoba, Winnipeg, MB R3E 0J9, Canada
Research Institute in Oncology and Hematology, Cancer Care Manitoba, Winnipeg, MB R3E 0V9, Canada
Department of Computer Science, University of Manitoba, Winnipeg, MB R3T 2N2, Canada

Index

www.ingramcontent.com/pod-product-compliance
Lightning Source LLC
LaVergne TN
LVHW060941220926
848485LV00015B/1233
9781639276134